Kundalini Yoga Meditation for Complex Psychiatric Disorders

Techniques Specific for Treating the Psychoses, Personality, and Pervasive Developmental Disorders

Other titles by David Shannahoff-Khalsa

Kundalini Yoga Meditation: Techniques Specific for Psychiatric Disorders, Couples Therapy, and Personal Growth

Psychophysiological States: The Ultradian Dynamics of Mind-Body Interactions

A Norton Professional Book

Kundalini Yoga Meditation for Complex Psychiatric Disorders

Techniques Specific for Treating the Psychoses, Personality, and Pervasive Developmental Disorders

David S. Shannahoff-Khalsa

W. W. Norton & Company
New York • London

The techniques and protocols taught in this book are not meant to be a substitute for medical care and advice. You are advised to consult with your health care professional with regard to matters relating to your health, including matters that may require diagnosis or medical attention. In particular, if you have been diagnosed with schizophrenia or any form of psychosis, a personality disorder in any form including paranoid, schizoid, schizotypal, antisocial, borderline, histrionic, narcissistic, avoidant, dependent, or obsessive-compulsive personality disorder, autism, Asperger's Disorder, or any other pervasive developmental disorder, or any other psychiatric or related disorder, or if you are taking or have been advised to take any medication, you should consult regularly with your physician regarding any changes in medication use.

Unless otherwise noted, all illustrations and meditation protocols are the property of the author.

Photos by Beatrice Ring

For reader comments or to order a video mentioned in the book, please visit the author's web site at www.theinternetyogi.com (to order videos), or email him at dsk@ucsd.edu

For information about permission to reproduce selections from this book, write to Permissions, W. W. Norton & Company, Inc., 500 Fifth Avenue, New York, NY 10110

For information about special discounts for bulk purchases, please contact W. W. Norton Special Sales at specialsales@wwnorton.com or 800-233-4830

Manufacturing by World Color Fairfield Graphics
Book design by Martha Meyer
Production manager: Leeann Graham

Library of Congress Cataloging-in-Publication Data

Shannahoff-Khalsa, David.
    Kundalini yoga meditation for complex psychiatric disorders : techniques specific for treating the psychoses, personality, and pervasive developmental disorders / David S. Shannahoff-Khalsa. — 1st ed.
    p. cm. — (A Norton professional book)
    Includes bibliographical references and index.
    ISBN 978-0-393-70568-3 (hardcover)
1. Meditation—Therapeutic use. 2. Kundalini—Therapeutic use. I. Title.
RC489.M43S528 2010
616.89´1653—dc22   2009044749

ISBN: 978-0-393-70568-3

W. W. Norton & Company, Inc., 500 Fifth Avenue, New York, N.Y. 10110
        www.wwnorton.com
W. W. Norton & Company Ltd., Castle House, 75/76 Wells Street, London W1T 3QT

1 2 3 4 5 6 7 8 9 0

To Raj Yog Guru Ram Das, my Guru in the Divine;

Raj Yog Yogi Bhajan, Master of Kundalini Yoga,
my Spiritual Teacher in the Divine;

David (deceased) and Sarah Shannahoff, my parents for their
life-long loving support;

Bubba, JJ, and Patrick, my three Golden Sons,
for their eternal love and devotion.

Contents

CONTENTS

Acknowledgments

It would not have been possible to write this book without all of the efforts of my many colleagues over the past 36 years that helped to establish a scientific foundation that led to my first book with W. W. Norton & Co., which surely set the stage for this companion book. However, without the teachings of Yogi Bhajan on Kundalini yoga, this book would have been impossible. Therefore, I first want to thank Yogi Bhajan for the teachings that have made my scientific studies possible and for his tireless efforts to share the individual meditation techniques that are now included in this book. He spent 35 years devoting his life to publicly sharing the sacred and ancient knowledge of Kundalini yoga that previously had only been passed secretly from master to disciple over the past 3,000 years. Second, I want to thank Floyd E. Bloom, MD, for his efforts as my first scientific collaborator on yogic research when we were both at the Salk Institute, and for helping to launch this work and making it a respectable and important scientific endeavor. His active participation inspired many others to collaborate. I am truly grateful for the many years of his support, guidance, and wisdom. He gave me the idea for establishing a nonprofit foundation to help facilitate the funding of this work and he committed to be the first vice president on the board of directors and first scientific advisor in the early years. I am also grateful to Drs. David

Schubert, Tony Hunter, and Walter Eckhart, who gave me many years of institutional support at the Salk Institute for Biological Studies to help establish my scientific career. I am indebted to Sheldon S. Hendler, MD, PhD, for his role as my first scientific mentor, for facilitating my initial research engagement at the Salk, for his role as a vice president at the Khalsa Foundation for Medical Science, and for his sage advice for the last 41 years. I am grateful to Michael G. Ziegler, MD, for nearly 20 years of collaboration on pioneering psychophysiological studies during waking and sleep in his laboratory and at the General Clinical Research Center at the University of California, San Diego (UCSD). I am immensely grateful to F. Eugene Yates, MD, University of California, Los Angeles, for his many years of collaboration, which helped to ensure the success of the multivariate physiological and psychophysiological studies that are briefly discussed in my first book (Shannahoff-Khalsa, 2006) and are now described in complete detail in my second book (Shannahoff-Khalsa, 2008). These studies have led to defining psychophysiological states in a completely new way, and they have led to the discovery of the lateralized ultradian rhythms of the autonomic and central nervous systems, which play a key regulatory role in mind-body states. Today, it is also clear that these "neural rhythms are a unique step in the evolution of the nervous system that have mostly been ignored or missed in our understanding of physiology, mental activities, brain rhythms, and in the treatment of psychiatric disorders" (Shannahoff-Khalsa, 2008). The basic science on how to alter these mind-body states using yogic techniques has now led to new discoveries and a new direction and successful application in psychiatry. All of these scientific studies would not have been possible without my many colleagues that directly and indirectly have set the stage for this book.

I am grateful to J. Christian Gillin, MD (deceased), Department of Psychiatry, UCSD, for his collaboration in sleep research and his generous collegial tutoring on the nature of the academic world. I am grateful to Liana Beckett, MA, MFCC, who was in the Department of Psychiatry, UCSD, for the first invitation to collaborate using Kundalini yoga meditation techniques for treating ob-sessive-compulsive disorder (OCD). I am grateful to Saul Levine, MD, Departments of Psychiatry, UCSD and Children's Hospital, San Diego, for his interest and collaboration to help further the OCD clinical trial work and making the National Institutes of Health (NIH)–funded randomized controlled trial a success. I want to express my gratitude to Christopher C. Gallen, MD, PhD, for his collaboration on the second OCD trial. If not for Chris, we proba-bly would not have had the study design that gave the trial so much credibility and recognition. I am also grateful to Chris for initiating the research opportunities employing magnetoencephalography (MEG) for studying OCD patients, healthy controls, and the study of the OCD breath technique when he was the director of the MEG lab at the Scripps Research Institute. I am grateful to Leslie Ellen Ray, MA, MFCC, for running the control group in the OCD clinical trial, and to Barry J. Schwartz, PhD, when he was at the Scripps Research Institute, and John Sidorowich, PhD, UCSD, for their collaborative efforts on the randomized and controlled OCD trial. In addition, I am grateful to Henry D. I. Abarbanel, PhD, who was the director of the Institute for Nonlinear Science (INLS), UCSD, for providing the institutional support for conducting many of these studies in a wonderfully open, rigorous, creative, and pro-ductive atmosphere. I want to thank my other colleagues at the former INLS (now the BioCircuits Institute), Drs. Jon A. Wright, Roy Schult, Evgeny Novikov, and Barry J. Schwartz for collabora-tion on pioneering MEG studies. I also want to thank Drs. Luigi Fortuna, Maide Bucolo, Manuela La Rosa, Mattia Fresca, Francesca Sapuppo, and Federica Di Grazia at the University of Catania, Di-partimento di Ingegneria Elettrica Elettronica e dei Sistemi, for their creative and productive collaborative efforts on the MEG studies on the yogic meditation techniques, normals, and OCD pa-tients. I am grateful to Stuart W. Jamieson, MB, head of the Divi-sion of Cardiothoracic Surgery, UCSD, Matthew B. Kennel, UCSD, and B. Bo Sramek, PhD, Czech Technical University Prague, De-partment of Mechanical Engineering, for collaboration on yogic techniques for altering cardiovascular function and for novel work on defining hemodynamic states. I want to thank Brian Fallon, MD, Columbia University, Department of Psychiatry, and New York State Psychiatric Institute, for inviting me to present at a 2003 symposium on OCD at the Annual American Psychiatric Association (APA) Conference, which helped to lead to a 90-minute APA workshop and four 6-hour APA courses where I have taught many of these Kundalini yoga meditation techniques for treating psychiatric disorders. The 2004 APA workshop led to the invitation by my editor, Deborah Malmud, to write the first book for W. W. Norton & Co. I want to thank Sidney Zisook, MD, Director of Residency Training, Department of Psychiatry, UCSD, for his special interest in this work and the opportunity to lecture on these techniques to the second-year UCSD psychiatry residents.

I also want to thank T. M. Srinivasan, PhD, for his successful efforts to fund some of the studies on multivariate physiology when he was the Director of Research at the Fetzer Institute. In addition, I gladly acknowledge the Daunting One for her help. There are many other scientific collaborators and support staff that have helped to make this work and these books possible over the last 33 years, and I am grateful to all of them for their key roles.

I want to especially acknowledge with my deepest gratitude Mr. John DeBeer and Dr. Mona Baumgartel for financial support to the Khalsa Foundation for Medical Science every year since its inception in 1984, which has helped to give this work continuity. In addition, I want to thank Jeremy Waletsky, MD, for his financial contributions in the early years of this work, and finally the NIH for funding the OCD randomized controlled clinical trial (Shannahoff-Khalsa et al., 1999), which helped to set a precedent for much of the patient care that is described in this book.

And last but not least, I am very grateful and indebted to my dear editor, Deborah Malmud, Director of Professional Books at W. W. Norton & Co. Her wisdom, courage, patience, and tireless creative support have made this book and the first book possible. I

Acknowledgments

am also deeply grateful to my associate editors, Andrea Costella, Kristen Holt-Browning, and Vani Kannan, for helping to ensure the quality and success of this book, and for their patience with me. In addition, I am grateful to my assistant editor, Libby Burton, for helping to bring this book to fruition.

Preface

This book was written as an extension and companion to my first book, *Kundalini Yoga Meditation: Techniques Specific for Psychiatric Disorders, Couples Therapy, and Personal Growth*, published by W. W. Norton & Co. While writing the first book, which covered most of the Axis I disorders, I realized that there was still a need to specifically address the treatment of the psychoses, the personality, and the pervasive developmental disorders. Even though many of the patient case histories in the first book were complex and multimorbid, I thought that much more information on multimorbidity is essential. The people that come to me for treatment usually do so because their previous therapeutic efforts have not led to satisfactory results. Most do not come because they have an interest in yoga per se. Consequently, over the years I have had an opportunity to learn what is required to help make a real difference in their lives using Kundalini yoga meditation techniques. Now six additional multipart disorder-specific protocols and a variety of individual disorder-related techniques that can be used as substitutes are included in this book. Because of the poor overall success rate and complications with the antipsychotic medications, we have a need for new approaches for treating and reducing the symptomatology of the schizophrenic patient, including ways to help minimize the duration of their hallucinations. A multipart protocol is now included that I have tested over the years for the variants of the psychoses. I have also included a new short miniprotocol that is being used to help minimize the severity and duration of the hallucinations for these patients. Many of my clients have had personality disorders. But, as is par for the course, they only request help for their Axis I symptoms. Therefore, I have devised three multipart cluster-specific protocols that I now use for the three American Psychiatric Association–defined personality disorder cluster groups, called Clusters A, B, and C, respectively. Included are additional meditation techniques that can be used as substitutions for the three different cluster-specific protocols that can help meet any additional needs for these patients. There is also a new symbol-based classification for each of the 10 different personality disorders with a technique that is unique to each disorder. Therefore, we now have 10 variants of these protocols to help meet the specific needs for each of the 10 different personality disorders. In addition, over the years many people have asked me if I had information on how to treat autism or Asperger's syndrome. That information, which includes a novel approach to treatment, is now also included in this book.

Over the past 35 years I have practiced more than a thousand different Kundalini yoga meditation techniques. When I first started, I realized how important they can be for treating the psychiatric disorders, especially since many of the techniques were taught as being disorder specific. While these individual yogic techniques were devised and discovered many thousands of years ago, these techniques and teachings have their more recent origins from the House of Guru Ram Das and the teachings of Kundalini yoga as taught by Yogi Bhajan. I feel very fortunate to have had the opportunity to learn these techniques and to deliver them in the form of these new multipart disorder-specific protocols that can now more readily serve the needs of those suffering with one or more psychiatric disorders.

Introduction

This book is designed for use by psychiatrists, psychotherapists, psychologists, social workers, physicians, other clinicians, and yoga therapists and yoga teachers who have an interest in working with psychiatric patients, and especially with the nine variants of the psychoses, the 10 variants of the personality disorders, and autism and Asperger's syndrome. This book is also written to more broadly cover the important and common problems of the multimorbidities in psychiatry, and therefore this book is an important complement to my first book, which focuses primarily on how to use Kundalini yoga meditation techniques for treating the other Axis I psychiatric disorders (Shannahoff-Khalsa, 2006). The first book included eight disorder-specific multipart protocols for treating the following disorders: obsessive-compulsive disorder, acute stress disorder, major depressive disorder, bipolar disorders, addictive impulse control and eating disorders, chronic fatigue syndrome, attention-deficit hyperactivity and comorbid disorders, and post-traumatic stress disorder. The first book also had individual meditation techniques, each specific for one of the following disorders or conditions: generalized anxiety disorder, panic attacks, phobias, grief, insomnia, nightmares, fears, anger, to deepen and shorten and induce superefficient sleep, create normal and supernormal states of consciousness; 11 techniques, each specific for treating the abused and battered psyche; and 14 techniques for couples therapy. However, all of the techniques in the first book can also be used to help enhance one's personal growth, performance, and mental health. In addition, it is worth noting that a "7-part protocol for psycho-oncology patients" has also been published for patients suffering from cancer (Shannahoff-Khalsa, 2005).

The presentation of the material in this book, including the detailed definitions of the respective disorders and their prevalence rates, and a review of the most currently published scientific results using conventional treatment modalities, will be especially useful for those who lack formal study of these psychiatric disorders. However, the reviews on treatment may also be useful as a reasonably up-to-date summary for trained clinicians and others in the public health sector.

The reader of this book would be well served by also reading the first book, which introduces a number of landmark scientific discoveries that help give much greater scientific credibility to the Kundalini yogic meditation techniques and protocols that are now included in this book. This is true because all of those scientific studies were also based on concepts from the ancient science of Kundalini yoga as taught by Yogi Bhajan. That work has led to a new perspective for understanding the nature and dynamics of psychophysiological states and mind-body interactions during both waking and sleep, and how the body's major systems are integrated and coregulated by the hypothalamus. Scientific studies are also presented in the first book on several novel endogenous mechanisms for regulating mind-body states, giving further credit to the value of yoga. These mind-body and self-regulation studies are also discussed in another book in complete detail (Shannahoff-Khalsa, 2008). The history and a comprehensive review of the topic of how to self-regulate these states using selective unilateral autonomic activation via unilateral forced nostril breathing is discussed with a review of the studies that show the efficacy of using Kundalini yoga for treating OCD, and how these techniques can have differential effects on heart rate, eye blink rates, glucose levels, intraocular pressures, and hemispheric-dependent cognitive functions (Shannahoff-Khalsa, 2008). The first book also introduces the concept of the chakra system and how yogis define states of consciousness, the *tattvas* or five elements (ether, air, fire, water, and earth) and their role in understanding the disease process, and the basic physical mechanism that helps explain how mantras work (Shannahoff-Khalsa, 2006). Also covered in *Kundalini Yoga Meditation* are the fascinating teachings of Yogi Bhajan on Kundalini yoga called "the 81 facets of the mind," and the "female rhythms of the 11 erogenous centers that influence the psyche." These concepts all help give a much deeper insight into the psyche and they are unique examples of the highly complex understanding of the mind and consciousness that yogis had thousands of years ago. This depth will be apparent when the techniques in this book are explored by the reader.

Chapter 1 in this book presents key studies in the scientific literature on the multimorbidities in the psychiatric disorders in an effort to document the realities and inadequacies of the conventional modalities for treatment in the real world and the greater complexities faced by patients with multimorbidities. A quick snapshot is presented of both the psychiatric problems and general medical multimorbidities that are common for the schizophrenic population. A summary overview is presented for the most expensive trial ever funded by the National Institute of Mental Health, costing $45 million, called the Clinical Antipsychotic Trials of Intervention Effectiveness (CATIE) Study. To date this is the most comprehensive assessment and well-designed multilevel trial that shows us what to expect with the use of the antipsychotic medications in treating the real-world population of schizophrenics. Selected examples are listed for the occurrence rates for the more common psychiatric multimorbidities for schizophrenia, the personality disorders, and the pervasive developmental disorders. In addition, the case is briefly presented for considering the use of Kundalini yoga meditation techniques as an adjunct or alternative approach to help improve treatment for the multimorbid psychiatric disorders.

Chapter 2 gives a brief modern history of the psychoses and the detailed definitions for the nine variants as now described in the American Psychiatric Association's *Diagnostic and Statistical Manual of Mental Disorders*, 4th ed. (text revision) (*DSM-IV-TR*). The prevalence rates and the etiology of the nine variants are presented along with a literature review of the latest studies using conventional modalities for treatment, including an early preliminary study using hatha yoga for treating schizophrenia. The Kundalini yogic view on the etiology is presented. There is a detailed description of the Kundalini yoga protocol called A Protocol for Treating the Variants of Schizophrenia, which is used for treating the nine variants of schizophrenia. Several options are also provided for using different meditation techniques as adjuncts to this protocol. In addition, A Four-Part Miniprotocol for Helping to Terminate Hallucinations is described along with a case history for its treatment efficacy in a complex multimorbid patient. Individual case histories are also presented for schizophrenic patients that have used the primary protocol.

Chapter 3 covers the 10 different personality disorders as defined by the American Psychiatric Association and how they are each included in one of three specific clusters respectively: the Cluster A group (odd-eccentric) includes the paranoid, schizoid, and schizotypal personality disorders; the Cluster B group (dramatic-emotional) includes the histrionic, narcissistic, antisocial, and borderline personality disorders; and the Cluster C group (anxious-fearful) includes the avoidant, dependent, and obsessive-compulsive personality disorders. The history is presented for the personality disorders and the 10 detailed definitions are included as defined by the *DSM-IV-TR*. An up-to-date review of the scientific literature describing the prevalence rates and the efficacy of the conventional treatment modalities is presented. In addition, the yogic view of the etiology of personality disorders is presented. Three complex multipart protocols for treatment are described in detail, one for each cluster group, and where each cluster group also has a meditation that can be substituted that is then even more specific for one of the 10 respective personality disorders. Ten new personality-specific symbols are included called the 10 Symbol-Related Techniques that help make the approach to treatment more understandable, palatable, and effective for this unique population. Suggested substitutions are also presented for some of the key meditations in each of the three clusters. There are also case histories of treatment for patients comorbid for the personality and Axis I disorders.

Chapter 4 covers the five different forms of the pervasive developmental disorders (PDD) as defined by the American Psychiatric Association's *DSM-IV-TR*, autistic disorder, Asperger's disorder (or Asperger's syndrome), Rett's disorder, childhood disintegrative disorder, and pervasive developmental disorder not otherwise specified (PDD-NOS), and each is defined in detail. However, only autistic disorder, Asperger's disorder, and PDD-NOS are discussed in terms of yogic techniques that can be applied in treatment. Some material is presented that covers the controversial etiology and potential mechanisms for the PDD, including some relevant discussion on the related and fascinating topic of savant syndrome. The prevalence rates of the PDD are presented. A brief review of the scientific literature on the clinical results using the major conventional approaches to treatment is presented. There is discussion of the yogic view of the etiology of the PDD. A completely novel approach to treatment using Kundalini yoga meditation is presented, including techniques for the most difficult patients, and four additional elementary brain-balancing techniques for the PDD patient that can be used once the patient is more receptive. Finally, six meditations are included that can be used by more advanced patients, including adults. Case histories of treatment are also included.

Chapter 5 briefly addresses the multimorbidities of the psychiatric disorders in general, and more specifically for schizophrenia, the personality disorders, and pervasive developmental disorders. There is also a presentation on five yogic principles and a hierarchy for treating complex multimorbid psychiatric patients, and how they may be best approached using Kundalini yoga meditation. One additional Kundalini yoga exercise set called Nabhi Kriya is included that can be useful for any and all patients, complex or otherwise, and can further help expedite recovery. A section is included for structuring individual treatment plans for the complex multimorbid psychiatric patient, and two examples are provided. There is also a long case history as self-described by a very complex and difficult multimorbid patient. This patient had bipolar disorder, schizophrenia, and both borderline and narcissistic personality disorders, and has made incredible progress. She has not experienced symptoms of her bipolar condition for a significant time and her hallucinations have been reduced from near daily events lasting 6 to 10 hours to the occasional one-half to one-hour event every 15 to 18 days. She no longer meets the criteria for any personality disorder.

Finally, Chapter 6 is an epilogue, "On the Future of the Prevention and Treatment of Psychiatric Disorders." Included here is a brief but chilling summary of the current status of mental health for children and adolescents in the United States and the United Kingdom. If the status of our youth tells us anything about our future, this summary is worth reading. In addition, I reflect on the potential value of Kundalini yoga and Kundalini yoga meditation techniques in helping to heal the current mental health problems in our country, and how they can be a potent and vital technology for prevention in the future. I also comment on how they can be used to help enhance the dormant human potential and elevate the consciousness of humanity to help make for a much more promising future.

This book is not a review of the scientific literature on yoga, meditation, or other complementary and alternative modalities for treating psychiatric disorders. However, pertinent scientific studies on these select topics are mentioned in the respective chapters. This book also does not review the trade publications on related topics. In this book I also attempt to make the case for a further and rigorous investigation of the concepts and techniques of Kundalini yoga as taught by Yogi Bhajan and the protocols that I have devised for treating psychiatric disorders. Videos are being prepared to assist in the teaching of the techniques and protocols in this book, which will be available through my Website, www.theinternetyogi.com

Kundalini Yoga Meditation for Complex Psychiatric Disorders

Techniques Specific for Treating the Psychoses, Personality, and Pervasive Developmental Disorders

ONE

The Current Need for Advancing Treatment and the Potential for the Therapeutic Application of Yogic Medicine for Complex and Multimorbid Psychiatric Disorders

It is necessity and not pleasure that compels us. [*Necessita c'induce, e non diletto.*]

Dante Alighieri, *Inferno* (XII, 87)

Fear numbs you. Anger aggravates you. Attachment squeezes you to death.

Yogi Bhajan, date unknown

The co-occurrence or "multimorbidity" of the psychiatric disorders is common. "Studies of both clinical and community samples have consistently shown that the frequency of subjects with comorbidity is more common than that of single disorders" (Angst, Sellaro, & Ries Merikangas, 2002). In addition, 46.4% of the U.S. population meet criteria for at least one psychiatric disorder in their lifetime; 27.7% have a lifetime history of two or more disorders; 17.3% have three or more disorders; most had a first onset in childhood or adolescence; later onset disorders are typically temporally secondary comorbid conditions; and disorder severity is strongly associated with high comorbidity (Kessler & Wang, 2008). Most adolescents also exhibit patterns of psychiatric comorbidities (Bird, Gould, & Staghezza, 1993; Kovacs, 1990; Lewinsohn, Rohde, & Seeley, 1995). It is also true that the "most seriously impairing and persistent adult mental disorders are associated with child-adolescent onsets and high comorbidity" (Kessler & Wang, 2008). Adult psychiatric patients also have other medical problems at higher rates than the general population. These multimorbidities and their respective medical complexities deserve much greater attention with increased efforts toward finding new ways to help prevent and resolve this growing health care crisis. The vast majority of clinical research studies are directed toward the treatment of single disorders. There are obvious scientific reasons for this approach to clinical trials; however, this approach does not match the current health status of the average psychiatric patient, nor does it lead to a generalizable clinical result.

First, selected examples are listed for the occurrence rates for the psychiatric multimorbidities for schizophrenia, the personality disorders, and the pervasive developmental disorders. These examples are presented to inform about the complex nature of these psychiatric disorders. For schizophrenics, the "lifetime prevalence rates for any anxiety disorder ranged from 30% to 85% with most studies showing rates higher than in the general population" (Pokos & Castle, 2006). The wide range here for prevalence rates results primarily from the different definitions and scales used for determining the occurrence of anxiety. The anxiety disorder preceded the onset of psychosis in more than 50% of these patients. When it comes to the co-occurrence rates for schizophrenia and panic disorder, two very large surveys with 20,291 individuals from the National Institute of Mental Health Epidemiologic Catchment Area found a range across five study sites of 28% to 63% (Boyd, 1986). "Panic attacks (lifetime) were common among almost half (45%) of those with schizophrenia. Individuals with schizophrenia and panic attacks had significantly elevated rates of co-occurring mental disorders, psychotic symptoms, suicidality, and mental health service utilization compared with individuals with schizophrenia who did not suffer from panic attacks" (Goodwin, Lyons, & McNally, 2002). There is a lifetime odds of >35:1 for having panic disorder in subjects with a diagnosis of schizophrenia, when compared to individuals without schizophrenia (Boyd et al., 1984; Robins & Regier, 1991). Buckley and colleagues reviewed 27 studies looking at the occurrence rates of panic symptoms among patients with schizophrenia and found a prevalence range for panic attacks of 7.1% to 63% and a range for panic disorder of 3.3% to 29.5% with weighted mean estimates of a 25% prevalence rate for panic attacks and a 15% prevalence rate for panic disorder in schizophrenic patients (Buckley, Miller, Lehrer, & Castle, 2009). They also claimed a lifetime prevalence rate of panic disorder in the U.S. general population with a range of 2.0% to 5.1%, which they determined based on three separate publications (Grant et al., 2006; Katerndahl & Realini, 1993; Robins & Regier, 1991).

Post-traumatic stress disorder (PTSD) is another important comorbid and complicating psychiatric disorder for the schizophrenic patient population. Trauma is common in schizophrenic patients and childhood trauma is an important risk factor for psychosis (Morgan & Fisher, 2007). Buckley and colleagues (2009) have reviewed 20 published studies on the association of PTSD in schizophrenics and found a prevalence rate of PTSD among patients with psychosis ranging from 0% to 67% with a weighted average estimating a 29% prevalence rate for PTSD in patients with schizophrenia, compared with a 7.8% estimated lifetime prevalence of PTSD in the U.S. general population. As expected, a schizophrenic patient comorbid for PTSD has a much more severe condition overall and this is known to lead to more cognitive impairment (Fan et al., 2008; Goodman et al., 2007; Kilcommons & Morrison, 2005; Scheller-Gilkey, Moynes, Cooper, Kant, & Miller, 2004), higher rates of suicidal ideation and behavior, and increased outpatient visits and hospitalizations (Strauss et al., 2006).

In a review of 36 studies investigating the co-occurrence of obsessive-compulsive symptoms and obsessive-compulsive disorder (OCD) in schizophrenia patients, Buckley and colleagues (2009) arrived at a prevalence rate for obsessive-compulsive symptoms ranging from 10% to 64% and for OCD a range of 0% to 31.7%, with a crude weighted average for the two conditions, respectively, of 25% and 23% for the schizophrenic patient population. They concluded that these wide ranges are the result "due to difficulties in distinguishing clinically obsessions and delusions, especially when an obsession is held with firm conviction."

Buckley and colleagues (2009) also reviewed the massive literature on schizophrenic patients comorbid for depression, which occurs in an estimated 50% of the schizophrenic patient population. They made the following observations:

1. Depressive symptoms are common in patients with schizophrenia.
2. They add further to the disability of schizophrenia, including being associated with a heightened risk for psychotic relapses.
3. Postpsychotic depression may be a particular *forme fruste* of major depression in schizophrenia.
4. There is some evidence, far from conclusive, that medications might directly impact depressive mood and suicidality to some extent that is not simply less depression because of less psychosis.
5. Although intuitively appealing, there is insufficient evidence in the literature (including a dearth of neurobiological studies) to support the proposition that this represents a distinct subgroup of schizophrenia.

In fact, the relationship of depression to schizophrenia is so complex that there has been a suggestion that depressive symptoms in schizophrenia can be divided into three subgroups: "(1) depressive symptoms secondary to organic factors, (2) nonorganic depression intrinsic to the acute psychotic episode, and (3) depressive symptoms that are not temporally associated with the acute psychotic episode, such as symptoms associated with the prodrome, the postpsychotic interval, as well as those symptoms that resemble depression that may represent negative symptoms of schizophrenia" (Bartels & Drake, 1988).

Buckley and colleagues (2009) also noted one of the more inevitable downsides to the medications used to treat schizophrenia. "Antipsychotic medications themselves produce neurological side effects like Parkinsonism (particularly bradykinesia, diminution of affective expression, masked facies, and verbal delays) and akathitic restlessness that may be confused with the psychomotor retardation or agitation of depression. Antipsychotic drugs may also produce a primary dysphoria, possibly due to dopamine blockade in reward pathways, and it has even been suggested that these drugs are innately depressogenic."

Finally, perhaps the most complicating factor when trying to treat the schizophrenic population is the high rate of abuse of alcohol and illicit drugs, which is remarkably common and "the rule rather than the exception," with an estimated rate of 47% of these patients having a lifetime diagnosis of a substance abuse disorder (Regier et al., 1990).

Buckley and colleagues (2009) listed the seven most pressing problems for schizophrenics that have substance abuse disorders:

1. More positive symptoms
2. Relapse of psychosis
3. Heightened risk of violence
4. Heightened risk of suicide
5. More medical comorbidities
6. Legal complications, including heightened risk of incarceration
7. Greater propensity to antipsychotic-related side effects

In another very recent publication, the authors looked at the types of comorbid disorders from a nationally representative sample of more than 5 million people ages 15 to 64 that were discharged from hospitals from 1979 to 2003. They concluded, "More than 50% of patients with schizophrenia have one or more comorbid psychiatric or general medical conditions" (Weber, Cowan, Millikan, & Niebuhr, 2009). They also found that those diagnosed with schizophrenia and comorbid psychiatric and medical conditions increased significantly over time among both males and females, but the proportion was higher among males, blacks, and those in the Northeast. When they compared the schizophrenic discharges to patients discharged with other primary diagnoses, they found that those discharged with schizophrenia had a higher proportion of all comorbid psychiatric and general medical conditions. The proportional morbidity ratios (PMRs) were "hypothyroidism (PMR = 2.9), contact dermatitis and other eczema (PMR = 2.9), obesity (PMR = 2.0), epilepsy (PMR = 2.0), viral hepatitis (PMR = 1.4), diabetes type II (PMR = 1.2), essential hypertension (PMR = 1.2), and various chronic obstructive pulmonary diseases (PMR range 1.2–1.5)" (Weber et al., 2009). They concluded, "Knowledge of the risks of comorbid psychiatric and general medical conditions is critical both for clinicians and for patients with schizophrenia. Closer attention to prevention, early diagnosis, and treatment of comorbid conditions may decrease associated morbidity and mortality and improve prognosis among patients with schizophrenia."

It is clear that the real world for the majority of schizophrenic patients includes a comorbid psychiatric disorder and often a general medical disorder. However, these complex conditions have not been treated in most clinical drug trials. The typical drug trial preselects for patients that are without psychiatric comorbidities, and there are scientific reasons for excluding other psychiatric disorders. But these drug trials do not yield a generalizable clinical result for the population as a whole. To overcome this major clinical shortcoming, the National Institute of Mental Health conducted a massive, complex clinical trial for schizophrenics, the most important to date, called the Clinical Antipsychotic Trials of Intervention Effectiveness (CATIE) study, which was designed as a multilevel trial to compare the effectiveness and tolerability of antipsychotic drugs. The CATIE study was conducted over a 5-year period at a cost of $42.6 million (Lieberman et al., 2005). The design (Stroup et al., 2003) for CATIE and methods and rationale (Keefe et al., 2003) have been described. CATIE was conducted to compare the effectiveness and tolerability of most of the actively marketed second-generation antipsychotics with those of a typical first-generation antipsychotic, in this case perphenazine. The first level of the trial (Lieberman et al., 2005) included 1,493 schizophrenic patients (mean age 40.6 years; 74% male, 40% nonwhite, and 12% Hispanic; average length of illness of 14.4 years) from 57 U.S. sites comparing olanzapine (7.5–30 mg per day), perphenazine (8–32 mg per day), quetiapine (200–800 mg per day), and risperidone (1.5–6.0 mg per day) for up to 18 months. Ziprasidone (40–160 mg per day) was later included after FDA approval. Overall, 74% of patients discontinued the study medication before 18 months (1,061 of the 1,432 patients who received at least one dose) with the following drug-specific discontinuation results: 64% of those assigned to olanzapine, 75% of those assigned to perphenazine, 82% of those assigned to quetiapine, 74% of those assigned to ris-peridone, and 79% of those assigned to ziprasidone. The time to the discontinuation of treatment for any cause was significantly longer in the olanzapine group than in the quetiapine or risperi-done groups, but not in the perphenazine or ziprasidone groups. The times to discontinuation because of intolerable side effects were similar among the groups, but the rates differed; olanzapine was associated with more discontinuation for weight gain or meta-bolic effects, and perphenazine was associated with more discon-tinuation for extrapyramidal effects. The CATIE Level 1 authors concluded: "The majority of patients in each group discontinued their assigned treatment owing to inefficacy or intolerable side ef-fects or for other reasons. Olanzapine was the most effective in terms of the rates of discontinuation, and the efficacy of the con-ventional antipsychotic agent perphenazine appeared similar to that of quetiapine, risperidone, and ziprasidone. Olanzapine was associated with greater weight gain and increases in measures of glucose and lipid metabolism" (Lieberman et al., 2005). With respect to the Level 1 result, an editor for the *American Journal of Psychiatry* wrote, "That first report thus also showed once again the stark reality of antipsychotic drugs—their therapeutic limitations and their problematic side effects, especially the metabolic effects" (Tamminga, 2006).

Level 2 of the CATIE had two parts: (1) ($N = 444$) comparing the tolerability of olanzapine, quetiapine, risperidone, and ziprasidone with individuals who had stopped their Level 1 medications for intolerable side effects (Stroup et al., 2006); and (2) ($N = 99$) comparison of efficacy of a first-generation antipsychotic (clozapine) with second-generation antipsychotics in individuals who had stopped their Phase 1 medications for poor efficacy (McEvoy et al., 2006). Level 2, Part 1, showed that "the time to treatment discontinuation was longer for patients treated with risperidone (median: 7.0 months) and olanzapine (6.3 months) than with quetiapine (4.0 months) and ziprasidone (2.8 months). Among patients who discontinued their previous antipsychotic because of inefficacy ($N = 184$), olanzapine was more effective than quetiapine and ziprasidone, and risperidone was more effective than quetiapine. There were no significant differences between antipsychotics among those who discontinued their previous treatment because of intolerability ($N = 168$)" (Stroup et al., 2006). The authors concluded that, for Level 2, Part 1, "risperidone and olanzapine were more effective than quetiapine and ziprasidone as reflected by longer time until discontinuation for any reason." For Level 2, Part 2, "median time until treatment discontinuation for any reason was 10.5 months for the clozapine-treated patients, 2.7 months for the olanzapine-treated patients, 3.3 months for the quetiapine-treated patients, and 2.8 months for the risperidone-treated patients" (McEvoy et al., 2006.). Time to discontinuation because of inadequate therapeutic effect was significantly longer for clozapine than for olanzapine, quetiapine, or risperidone. At 3-month assessments, Positive and Negative Syndrome Scale total scores had decreased more in patients treated with clozapine than in patients treated with quetiapine or risperidone but not olanzapine. The authors concluded, "For these patients with schizophrenia who prospectively failed to improve with an atypical antipsychotic, clozapine was more effective than switching to another newer atypical antipsychotic. Safety monitoring is necessary to detect and manage clozapine's serious side effects" (McEvoy et al., 2006).

In sum, for the CATIE, the medications were comparably effective but had very high rates of discontinuation (averaging 74%) because of the inability to control symptoms or intolerable side effects. Tamminga (2006) comments, "the side effect outcomes are staggering in their magnitude and extent and demonstrate the significant medication burden for persons with schizophrenia." In addition, olanzapine was associated with fewer hospitalizations as a result of psychotic relapse, but patients on olanzapine also experienced substantially more weight gain and metabolic changes that are now referred to as "metabolic syndrome" (Lamberti et al., 2006; McEvoy et al., 2005). This new but controversial syndrome includes insulin resistance, abdominal obesity, low levels of high-density lipoprotein cholesterol, high levels of triglycerides, and hypertension. Individuals with metabolic syndrome have a two- to threefold increase in cardiovascular mortality and a twofold increase in all-cause mortality. It also turns out that the cheaper first-generation antipsychotic (perphenazine) worked about as well and was tolerated about as well as the newer antipsychotics. And clozapine, another first-generation antipsychotic, showed nearly a threefold increase in time until drug discontinuation compared to the three new antipsychotics olanzapine, risperidone, and quetiapine. These researchers state, "This study strongly confirms what we have seen before, that clozapine is our most effective drug for schizophrenic psychosis" (Tamminga, 2006). The results of the CATIE clarify a great deal now about the pharmacologic treatment for the real-world schizophrenic patient. Clearly, the one essential finding is that any new treatment modality, especially one without side effects, now must be pursued rigorously and vigorously for the treatment of schizophrenia.

The reviews by Buckley et al. (2009) and Weber et al. (2009), along with the CATIE trial results, make it abundantly clear that much greater attention must be given to finding new ways to prevent the onset and mitigate the severity of the course of schizophrenia, especially using treatments without side effects, and this suggests finding therapies that may reduce the need for drugs for treating this complex and comorbid condition. It is this author's opinion that the Kundalini yoga protocol in Chapter 2 that is specific for schizophrenia, along with the additional adjunctive options for that protocol, will become an appealing and effective approach for treating all stages of the disease. It is also likely that when patients exhibit prodromal symptoms, these techniques will become very useful in helping to prevent or minimize the severity and course of this difficult-to-treat disease. Kundalini yoga has a rich history for improving health and as a therapeutic modality for treating many different psychiatric disorders (Shannahoff-Khalsa, 2006). In fact, "Kundalini yoga as taught by Yogi Bhajan" is the parent science and the integrated format for all of the other branches of yoga. In addition, much of what is otherwise taught today as yoga is a commercialized product compared to the original teachings. The case histories in Chapter 2 and the rich single case history in Chapter 5 of a multimorbid and complex young adult female initially diagnosed with schizophrenia, bipolar disorder, and both borderline and narcissistic personality disorders may inspire further study and implementation with this schizophrenia-specific protocol and the related meditation techniques. It is worth noting that a specific 11-part Kundalini yoga meditation protocol has been shown to significantly outperform other meditation techniques in a randomized controlled clinical trial for the treatment of OCD, usually considered to be the most difficult-to-treat psychiatric disorder (Shannahoff-Khalsa, 1997, 2006; Shannahoff-Khalsa et al., 1999). In fact, that OCD-specific Kundalini yoga meditation protocol showed a greater mean group improvement rate (71% over 12 months) using the gold standard for OCD treatment efficacy (the Yale-Brown Obsessive Compulsive Scale) than any other treatment modality to date.

There is both a high prevalence rate and a real need to find new and better ways to both prevent and treat the 10 different personality disorders. However, it is important to first note one expert's insight into the treatment of the personality disorders. "Most psychiatrists ignore axis II pathology" (Gabbard, 2005), referring to the 10 different personality disorders as defined by the *Diagnostic and Statistical Manual of Mental Disorders,* 4th edition, text revision (*DSM-IV-TR*) (APA, 2000). According to the World Health Organization (WHO) World Mental Health Surveys, the estimated worldwide incidence rate for the personality disorders is 6.1% for any personality disorder, and 3.6%, 1.5%, and 2.7% for Clusters A, B, and C, respectively (Huang et al., 2009). These rates do not reflect comorbidity; however, we know that the personality disorders are highly comorbid with Axis I disorders (Huang et al., 2009).

According to the WHO World Mental Health Surveys, "Over half (51.2%) of people with a personality disorder also meet criteria for at least one Axis I disorder. This overlap is higher for Clusters B (74.1%) and C (64.3%) than A (44.1%)" (Huang et al., 2009). But only 16.5% of individuals with an Axis I disorder have one or more personality disorders, and the rate of this comorbidity is 27.6% for the disruptive or externalizing disorders (conduct disorder, oppositional-defiant disorder, attention-deficit/hyperactivity disorder), 23.6% for the mood disorders, 19.9% for the anxiety disorders, and 18.8% for the substance use disorders (Huang et al., 2009). "The odds ratio for having three or more Axis I disorders (v. none) and a personality disorder are 9.7 for Cluster A, 49.3 for Cluster B, 34.8 for Cluster C and 21.1 for any personality disorder" (Huang et al., 2009). Thirty-seven percent of people with a personality disorder received treatment for a mental disorder in the United States, and this treatment was primarily for an Axis I disorder (Huang et al., 2009). However, these researchers also noted that "people with personality disorders seek help largely for Axis I disorders even though most of the impairments associated with personality disorders are not due to comorbid Axis I disorders." They also noted that the prevalence rates in their surveys for the individual personality disorders were somewhat lower than in other studies (see Chapter 3), and that this discrepancy may be the result of different survey instruments, methods of calculation, and a downward bias for detection in several countries (China and Nigeria).

When considering some of the problems due to the personality disorder patient population, one study with 1,740 patients (mean age 33.9 years, range 18–67, 35.2% male) between March 2003 and March 2006 was conducted in the Netherlands because of the suspected high economic cost to society due to a high demand on psychiatric, health, and social care services. These patients were assessed for their mean total direct and indirect costs over the 12 months prior to the treatment they were seeking in centers specialized for psychotherapy. "The mean costs were 11,126 Euros per patient. Two thirds (66.5%) of these costs consisted of direct medical costs, while the remaining costs were related to productivity losses. Borderline and obsessive-compulsive personality disorders were uniquely associated with increased mean total costs" (Soeteman, Hakkaart-van Roijen, Verheul, & Busschbach, 2008). These researchers also noted that this economic burden is substantially higher than that found in patients with depression or generalized anxiety disorder, and it is comparable to that of patients with schizophrenia. "These high societal costs present a strong argument in favor of prioritizing effective personality disorder treatments in reimbursement decisions." It is not difficult to imagine the burden that the Cluster B (antisocial, borderline, histrionic, and narcissistic) personality disorders cost society both economically and otherwise, especially with the antisocial and narcissistic populations.

While the personality disorders are considered separate from the externalizing (acting-out behavior) disorders, there are clearly high rates of comorbidity between these groups of disorders. When looking at the age of onset (AOO) for any of the psychiatric disorders, it is worth noting that "the impulse-control disorders have the earliest AOO distributions of any disorders studied, with median AOO in middle childhood for attention-deficit/hyperactivity disorder (ADHD), middle-late childhood for oppositional-defiant disorder and conduct disorder, and late childhood to late adolescence for intermittent explosive disorder" (Kessler & Wang, 2008). One might also intuit that childhood psychiatric disorders and criminality in young adults are related. To test this hypothesis, one study "looked at the rates of juvenile psychiatric disorders in a sample of young adult offenders and then tested which childhood disorders best predicted young adult criminal status" (Copeland, Miller-Johnson, Keeler, Angold, & Costello, 2007). They found that 51.4% of young male adult offenders and 43.6% of female offenders had a child psychiatric history. "Childhood psychiatric profiles predicted all levels of criminality. Severe/violent offenses were predicted by comorbid diagnostic groups that included both emotional and behavioral disorders" (Copeland et al., 2007).

This author suggests that it is most important and most cost worthy to attempt to prevent the onset and also to provide treatment in the earliest stages when the signs of the personality disorders begin to exhibit. This also makes sense since the "most seriously impairing and persistent adult mental disorders are associated with child-adolescent onsets and high comorbidity" (Kessler & Wang, 2008). Kessler and Wang also made the point that "increased efforts are needed to study the public health implications of early detection and treatment of initially mild and currently largely untreated child-adolescent disorders." The protocols and some of the individual meditation techniques in this book could be useful therapies toward the prevention and early treatment of the personality disorders. Indeed, case histories are presented here for difficult comorbid patients that have full-blown psychiatric disorders.

Patients with the autism spectrum disorders (ASDs) also commonly exhibit symptoms of other psychiatric disorders. A study looked at 122 adult ASD patients on an outpatient basis with normal intelligence to assess patterns of comorbid psychopathology

(Hofvander et al., 2009). Five patients had autistic disorder (AD), 67 had Asperger's syndrome (AS), and 50 were diagnosed with pervasive developmental disorder not otherwise specified (PDD NOS). They found that a "lifetime psychiatric axis I comorbidity was very common, most notably mood and anxiety disorders, but also ADHD and psychotic disorders. The frequency of these diagnoses did not differ between the ASD subgroups or between males and females. Antisocial personality disorder and substance abuse were more common in the PDD NOS group. Of all subjects, few led an independent life and very few had ever had a long-term relationship" (Hofvander et al., 2009). Forty-three percent of patients with PDD NOS had significantly more symptoms of inattention and hyperactivity/impulsivity compared to subjects with AS, but the categorical diagnosis of ADHD did not differ significantly between the groups (Hofvander et al., 2009). While there were only five patients in the AD group, 80% had at least one other major Axis I disorder, and the AS and PDD NOS subgroups all had at least one comorbid Axis I disorder; 53% had a mood disorder as a lifetime comorbid disorder; 8% had a bipolar disorder; 12% had a psychotic disorder (most often not otherwise specified); 4 had a schizophreniform disorder; 3 had a brief psychotic disorder; 1 a delusional disorder; 15% had been treated with neuroleptics at least once in their lives; and 16% had a substance abuse disorder (Hofvander et al., 2009). The anxiety disorders were the second most common Axis I comorbid disorder, with generalized anxiety disorder at 15%, social phobia at 13%, panic disorder at 11%, specific phobias at 6%, 2 patients with PTSD, and 6% with an impulse control disorder, intermittent explosive disorder being the most prevalent, followed by kleptomania, pyromania, pathological gambling, trichotillomania, and impulse control disorder NOS, all affecting one patient each (Hofvander et al., 2009).

Even though this study included a relatively small population, when they assessed for the rates of comorbid personality disorders, OCPD was significantly more common in the AS group and antisocial personality disorder in the PDD NOS group. The rate of personality disorders did not differ between men and women, with the exception of schizoid personality disorder, which was significantly more common among the female subjects (Hofvander et al., 2009). In part, they concluded, "This study demonstrated the high rates of *DSM-IV* axis I and II disorders, especially depression and ADHD. Differences between men and women were very few. Our results reflect the indistinct demarcations of the adult clinical neurodevelopmental phenotypes and stress the importance of the clinician's attention to a wide spectrum of psychiatric symptoms."

When looking at comorbidities in AS only, it is noted that the information about the neuropsychiatric comorbidities is limited because this disorder has only recently been recognized as a distinct disorder and there "is no established method for clinicians to assess comorbid neuropsychiatric disorders in this population" (Tsai, 2007). One study of 20 AS individuals, 11 to 19 years of age, with normal intelligence, found that 35% met the criteria for generalized anxiety disorder, 10% had a specific phobia, and 30% were comorbid for two or more psychiatric disorders (Green, Gilchrist, Burton, & Cox, 2000). This same study found that the AS patients had more worry, hypochondria, panic, specific fears, and obsessive-compulsive ruminations and rituals when compared to a control group of children and adolescents with conduct disorder. The AS patients also had more physical signs of anxiety and more facial tics compared to the controls. Another study found that the AS patients had higher rates of comorbidity than the AD patients (Klin, Pauls, Schultz, & Volkmar, 2005). When normally developing children are compared to AD and AS children for sleep problems, the results showed a high prevalence of sleep problems with significantly more problems reported in the AD and AS groups (normals = 50%, AD = 73%, and AS = 73%), with no significant differences between groups on the severity or the type of sleep problem, although the AS group was more sluggish and disorientated after waking (Polimeni, Richdale, & Francis, 2005).

In sum, there is no need to make an argument for the importance of finding new methods to treat the pervasive developmental disorders at the earliest possible stage, as would be true with any psychiatric or medical disorder. However, this author would like to make the argument that the highly unique and complex disorder-specific Kundalini yoga meditation techniques and protocols in this book provide a reasonable option for investigating the utility here for treatment at any stage of the disorder. Perhaps the case histories in Chapter 4 will help lend some credence to this argument. In addition, research on the pervasive developmental disorders with the Kundalini yoga techniques published in this book should be considered in light of the relatively poor efficacy evidence of the other treatment modalities that are described in some detail in Chapter 4. This is also true for the variants of the psychoses, details of which are described in Chapter 2, and for the personality disorders described in Chapter 3. There clearly is a great need for improvement in the treatment of all three of these complex categories when the evidence is reviewed for the individual disorder groups.

TWO

Treating Schizophrenia and Other Psychotic Disorders

The greatest miracle is unity.

Yogi Bhajan, date unknown

God is your own Unknown.

Yogi Bhajan, date unknown

In stillness lies the sound which is the creative existence of God. Whoever masters the stillness and the silence, and can read it, that person gets all knowledge which exists.

Yogi Bhajan, date unknown

Definitions, Subtypes, Diagnostic Features, Prevalence, Natural History, and Results Using Conventional Treatment Modalities

Psychosis is a generic term that refers to a mental state where there is a loss of contact with reality. Beer (1996) thoroughly reviewed the rich history of the concept of psychosis and stated that the Austrian psychiatrist Ernst von Feuchtersleben (1845) was the first to use this term as an alternative to insanity and mania (Beer, 1995).

The word originates from the Greek *psyche* (soul) and *-osis* (diseased or abnormal condition). The *Oxford English Online Dictionary* defines psychosis as a "severe mental illness, characterized by loss of contact with reality (in the form of delusions and hallucinations) and deterioration of intellectual and social functioning, occurring as a primary disorder or secondary to other diseases, drug ingestion, etc." In Beer's 1996 review, he included the description used in the *International Statistical Classification of Diseases and Related Health Problems* (10th Revision) (ICD-10) where *psychotic* "simply indicates the presence of hallucinations, delusions or a limited number of several abnormalities of behaviour, such as gross excitement and over activity, marked psychomotor retardation and catatonic behaviour" (WHO, 1992). Those afflicted with psychosis have either delusional beliefs or hallucinations or both and they usually also exhibit one or any of the following to some degree: disorganized thinking, changes in personality, bizarre behavior, difficulties with social interaction, and impairment in daily activities. Jibson, Glick, and Tandon (2004) provided an excellent description of delusions:

> Delusions are false beliefs based on internally generated concepts of reality or on incorrect inferences about actual events. By definition they are not amenable to correction by contrary evidence or persuasive argument. Although they may occur within the context of specific cultural customs or belief systems, they are not shared by others who have a similar background, and they are readily acknowledged by peers to be aberrant. They occur in a wide range of categories, such as persecutory, religious, somatic, grandiose, and so forth. Ideas of reference, the belief that neutral events are uniquely directed to the individual, are of special note because of their frequency. Among such delusions is the belief that messages from the television or radio are directed specifically at the person, that newspaper articles secretly refer to the person, or that conversations among strangers are about the person. Also common is the belief that one's thoughts are being read or controlled by others.

They also provided an excellent description of hallucinations:

> Hallucinations are false perceptions occurring in any sensory modality. Auditory hallucinations, especially voices, are the most common in patients with schizophrenia (Kitamura, Okazaki, Fujinawa, Takayanagi, & Kasahara, 1998). Hallucinatory voices may vary in frequency, intensity, number of speakers, and content. Command hallucinations, voices instructing the patient to do something, may place the patient at risk of acting on the commands. Visual hallucinations, although sometimes associated with substance intoxication or withdrawal, are also common in schizophrenia (Kitamura et al., 1998). Similarly, tactile, olfactory, and gustatory hallucinations may occur in schizophrenia and are not uniquely attributable, as some older texts suggested, to seizures, substance abuse, or other medically identifiable causes. (Jibson et al., 2004)

Delusions occur in 65% of schizophrenic patients (Appelbaum, Robbins, & Roth, 1999; Breier & Berg, 1999), and hallucinations and thought disorganization each occur in approximately 50% of patients. A large majority of patients experience multiple symptoms (Breier & Berg, 1999). Disorganized thinking "is most often noted as bizarre behavior or a disruption of the logical associations of speech" that "is especially disruptive to the routine tasks of life and creates severe problems in social, occupational, and self-care functions" (Jibson et al., 2004). The remaining classic positive schizophrenic symptom is catatonia, which is well described as

> an altered state of motor activity and attention. Lack of movement is common and may be accompanied by either catalepsy (waxy flexibility), in which the person maintains a posture into which he or she has been passively moved by the examiner, or negativism, in which the patient actively resists such attempts by the examiner. Echopraxia refers to the patient's inappropriately mirroring movements of the examiner. Spontaneous movements may be stereotypic and bizarre, or patients may exhibit excessive motor activity

that appears without direction or purpose. Speech may be absent (mutism) or may repeat the examiner's speech in a rigid and stereotypic way (echolalia). The patient may appear stuporous or may be internally preoccupied with other psychotic symptoms. (Jibson et al., 2004)

The term *schizophrenia* was coined by the Swiss psychiatrist and psychologist Paul Eugen Bleuler in 1908, using the Greek roots *schizein*, meaning "to split," and *phren*, meaning "mind," to describe the fragmented thinking of people with this disorder and how they feel removed or split off from an earlier identity, family members, and society. It was not meant to convey the idea of split or multiple personalities, which remains a common public misconception. This disorder was previously called dementia praecox (praecox meaning early), which was the term used by German psychiatrist Emile Kraepelin, regarded by many as the father of descriptive psychiatry. Kraepelin defined dementia praecox in 1893 as the "sub-acute development of a peculiar simple condition of mental weakness occurring at a youthful age" in his fourth German edition of *Lehrbuch der Psychiatrie* (Burgmair, Engstrom, & Weber, 2000–2006). However, Bleuler (1908) realized the condition was neither an organic dementia per se nor always occurring in young people, and therefore he believed it should have a less stigmatizing name. Schizophrenia is considered to be a "pervasive disorder that, it could be argued, changes or molds a person's personality forever" (Lauriello, 2004).

Perhaps Kraepelin's most important scientific contribution came from his study of the long-term course of mental illness as an insightful way of classifying mental disorders, which remains a challenge to this day. "His aim was to generate quantifiable psychological norms that could be used to diagnose mental deviance. . . . He was convinced that careful, longitudinal documentation would enable him to delineate specific disease entities" (Engstrom et al., 2006). Kraepelin viewed the traditional diagnostic criteria of his times as focusing too much on individual symptoms, which he called "symptomatic," whereas his view was based on grouping diseases together based on the classification of syndromes, or common patterns of symptoms.

The definition of schizophrenia and its variants has evolved over time, as researchers attempt to more accurately delineate the respective variants and their causes. Thus classifications are still mostly based on how specific symptoms group together. Currently, the conceptualization of psychosis remains a hotbed of debate. Kroll (2007) stated, "In essence, current thinking views psychotic symptoms along one or several continua, ranging from subclinical phenomena in otherwise 'normal' individuals to nuclear or negative symptom schizophrenia along one axis, and from mood lability and mood congruent hallucinatory-like phenomena in otherwise 'normal' individuals to major affective disorders with mood-incongruent delusions and hallucinations along a different axis, or possibly with both axes themselves overlapping." While the Kraepelinian approach to psychiatry still dominates, there are those who would do away with a half-century of accumulated biological and phenomenological studies. Bentall (2006) is one of those in strong opposition to Kraepelinian psychiatry. Kroll (2007) summarized Bentall's views as being that "there is no clear dividing line between madness and normal functioning, that the traditionally discrete types of severe mental illnesses (schizophrenia and manic depression) fail all empirical tests of their validity, and that the risk of experiencing psychotic complaints is influenced by adverse environmental factors." Furthermore, Kroll stated, "Kraepelinian psychiatry and all that go with it are being assailed by the affective disorder champions on one side, behavioral psychologists and environmentalists on another, and a variety of cross-cultural findings and anthropological attacks about psychoses on a third front. It is unlikely that these issues of classification and the etiology of mental illnesses will resolve anytime soon."

Here we accept the definition of psychosis according to the *Diagnostic and Statistical Manual of Mental Disorders*, 4th edition (*DSM-IV*), where "psychosis is restricted to delusions or prominent hallucinations, with the hallucinations occurring in the absence of insight into their pathological nature" (APA, 1994). This characteristic lack of insight clearly differs from that of an individual with hallucinations after taking a psychedelic substance, where the individual understands that the visual, auditory, or tactile experiences are all in fact the result of an ingested substance.

The classification scheme employed in this chapter for the psychotic disorders is according to the current standard of the American Psychiatric Association (APA), which now lists nine different psychotic disorders, including the following: (1) schizophrenia, (2) schizophreniform disorder, (3) schizoaffective disorder, (4) delusional disorder, (5) brief psychotic disorder, (6) shared psychotic disorder (folie à deux), (7) psychotic disorder due to a general medical condition, (8) substance-induced psychotic disorder, and (9) psychotic disorder not otherwise specified. The APA also lists other disorders with psychotic features, including major depressive disorder with psychotic features, Alzheimer's disease and other forms of dementia, and the psychotic state that can result from degenerative brain disorders, epilepsy, brain tumors, and strokes.

As a prelude to the description of these nine individual disorders as defined by the APA, the following quote is informative:

> The presentation of schizophrenia varies enormously. The current definition of schizophrenia includes distinct symptom domains, each of which may vary independently, as well as diagnostic subtypes. The concept of symptom domains represents a dimensional approach to the disorder, in which positive, negative, cognitive, and affective symptoms, which are present to varying degrees in every patient with schizophrenia, are characterized as separate components of the illness. The subtypes of the disorder represent a categorical approach to symptom description, each defined by the presence or absence of specific symptoms. (Jibson et al., 2004)

The four symptom domains are: (1) positive symptoms that include delusions, hallucinations, thought disorganization, and catatonia; (2) negative symptoms that are characterized by the absence of certain functions that include blunted affect, alogia (a reduction in language production, including both the number of words spoken and the number of ideas communicated by those words), anhedonia (a loss of enjoyment of and satisfaction in productive and recreational activities, even when they are pursued), social isolation, and lack of motivation; (3) cognitive impairment symptoms that include inattention, memory impairment, impaired executive function, and language disturbance; and (4) mood disturbance symptoms that include blunted affect, bizarre or inappropriate affect, and dysphoric mood (Jibson et al., 2004). Clearly, there is some overlap in this four-symptom domain categorization scheme. For example, blunted affect is listed in both the negative symptoms and the mood disturbance categories. It should be noted that cognitive impairment is the most direct cause of functional impairment and that improvements here are the most important for enhancing the quality of life (Breier, Schreiber, Dyer, & Pickar, 1991), and that, not surprisingly, dysphoria with demoralization occurs in approximately 60% of schizophrenic patients (Martin, Cloninger, Guze, & Clayton, 1985), which tends to be most severe immediately after an acute episode.

The five subtypes of schizophrenia according to the APA are the paranoid, disorganized, catatonic, undifferentiated, and residual. However, it is argued that the postulate of stable schizophrenic subtypes mainly depends on the conceptualization of the criteria applied and that their individual prevalence rates are also bound by these criteria (Stompe, Ortwein-Swoboda, Ritter, Marquart, & Schanda, 2005). In addition, it has been argued "that long-term stability of subtypes in schizophrenic disorders is not the rule but the exception" (Deister & Marneros, 1993).

Stompe and colleagues summarized the results of studies on the prevalence rates of schizophrenic subtypes based on the somewhat different conceptualizations and populations. The term *hebephrenic* used below is another term for the disorganized subtype.

Using Bleulerian subtypes, Morrison found 8.5% catatonic schizophrenia, 5.8% hebephrenia, 39.3% paranoid, and 4% simple schizophrenia among a sample of 1243 patients with schizophrenia (Morrison, 1974). Forty two percent did not meet one of these subtypes.
By means of DSM III-R, Deister and Marneros reported 31% paranoid type, 7% disorganized type, 6% catatonic type, 33% undifferentiated type, and 23% residual type (Deister & Marneros, 1993).
Applying ICD-10 criteria on the same sample, they found 48%
paranoid schizophrenia, 7% hebephrenic schizophrenia, 6% catatonic schizophrenia, 28% undifferentiated schizophrenia, and 11%
residual type (Deister & Marneros, 1993). Among 1077 patients,
Leonard described 11.1% affect-laden paraphrenia, 16.0% catapha-
sia, 12.6% periodic catatonia, 17.2% hebephrenias, 24.7% systematic paraphrenias, and 21.5% systematic catatonias (Leonard, 1999;
Stompe et al., 2005).

Stompe and colleagues (2005) also studied a sample of 220
consecutively admitted schizophrenic patients from three different
psychiatric institutions classified according to *DSM-IV*, ICD-10-R,
and Bleuler's and Leonard's criteria. "Especially, the frequency of
catatonic (10%–22%) and hebephrenic (5%–20%) subtypes of
schizophrenia varied within a broad range depending on the diagnostic system applied." Thus it is clear that using various schema
are key to how we understand and break down the prevalence
rates, and even how different populations will exhibit variations in
subtypes.

The following are the current APA (1994) descriptions for the
five subtypes of schizophrenia. The paranoid subtype is marked by
prominent delusions or auditory hallucinations, while maintaining
suitable cognitive functions and mood. The delusional beliefs are
usually thematic and involve those of a persecutory, grandiose, or
jealous nature, and the hallucinations are usually related. The onset
here is relatively later in life without much or any cognitive impairment, and the prognosis tends to be better toward maintaining
autonomy and a career.

The disorganized subtype exhibits with disturbed speech patterns and behavior and either a flat or inappropriate affect (APA, 1994). The speech can include silliness and laughter that is unrelated to what the patient is otherwise trying to communicate. The disturbed behavior leads to difficulties with or the inability to maintain normal hygiene, preparation of foods, and other daily life activities. The delusions and hallucinations are also not organized in coherent themes, and they may be accompanied by facial oddities and abnormal body movements and mannerisms. The onset is usually early and is usually related to a poorly developed personality. The prognosis is comparatively poor.

The catatonic subtype exhibits with at least two of the following: motoric immobility, as evidenced by cataplexy (including waxy flexibility) or stupor; excessive motor activity that is frequently purposeless and not influenced by external stimuli; extreme negativism that can manifest with a rigid posture against attempts to be moved, resistance to all instructions, or even mutism; peculiarities of voluntary movement with inappropriate or bizarre postures, stereotyped movements, prominent mannerisms, or grimacing; or echolalia (parrotlike and apparently senseless repetition of a word or phrase just spoken by another person) or echopraxia (repetitive imitation of movements of another person) (APA, 1994).

The undifferentiated subtype exhibits with two or more of the following: delusions, hallucinations, disorganized speech (frequent derailment or incoherence), grossly disorganized or catatonic behavior, and negative symptoms (e.g., affective flattening, alogia, or avolition), but also the person does not meet criteria for the paranoid, disorganized, or catatonic subtypes (APA, 1994).

The residual subtype is defined as having a previous episode of schizophrenia, but no longer exhibiting any prominent positive symptoms (delusions, hallucinations, or disorganized speech or behavior). However, the negative symptoms continue to exhibit (i.e., an affective flattening, where a person's face appears immobile and unresponsive with poor eye contact and limited body language; alogia, which is poverty of speech with brief, laconic, empty replies; or avolition, which is the inability to start or continue goal-directed activities). If the negative symptoms are not prominent, there can be attenuated positive symptoms. But if delusions or hallucinations are present, they are much reduced and are not accompanied by strong affect. This subtype may be a transition state between a full-blown episode and complete remission or it may exist for many years, with more intermittent full-blown episodes (APA, 1994).

In addition, it is worth pointing out that Cougnard et al. (2007) stated that "low-grade psychotic experiences in the general population are a common but transitory developmental phenomenon and that these subclinical psychoses may evolve into the persistent clinical forms when combined during development with exposure to such risk factors as cannabis, childhood trauma, and urbanicity."

Here, we deal only with the nine primary psychotic disorders as defined by the APA (1994) in the *DSM-IV*. The formal definition will be provided, including the diagnostic features, the prevalence rates, and the results of treatment using the conventional modalities.

1. "Schizophrenia is a disturbance that lasts for at least six months and includes at least one month of active-phase symptoms (i.e., two [or more] of the following: delusions, hallucinations, disorganized speech, grossly disorganized or catatonic behavior, negative symptoms)."
2. "Schizophreniform Disorder is characterized by a symptomatic presentation that is equivalent to schizophrenia except for its duration (i.e., the disturbance lasts from one to six months) and the absence of a requirement that there be a decline in functioning."
3. "Schizoaffective Disorder is a disturbance in which a mood episode and the active-phase symptoms of schizophrenia occur together and were preceded or are followed by at least 2 weeks of delusions or hallucinations without prominent mood symptoms."
4. "Delusional Disorder is characterized by at least one month of

nonbizarre delusions without other active phase symptoms of schizophrenia."

5. "Brief Psychotic Disorder is a psychotic disturbance that lasts more than one day and remits by one month."
6. "Shared Psychotic Disorder (Folie à Deux) is a disturbance that develops in an individual who is influenced by someone else who has an established delusion with similar content."
7. For "Psychotic Disorder Due to a General Medical Condition, the psychotic symptoms are judged to be a direct physiological consequence of a general medical condition."
8. For "Substance-Induced Psychotic Disorder, the psychotic symptoms are judged to be a direct physiological consequence of a drug of abuse, a medication, or toxin exposure."
9. "Psychotic Disorder Not Otherwise Specified is included for classifying psychotic presentations that do not meet the criteria for any of the specific psychotic disorders defined above or psychotic symptomatology about which there is inadequate or contradictory information."

Prevalence and Incidence Rates

One systematic review of the literature that included 18 prevalence and 8 incidence studies found significant differences for 1-year prevalence, lifetime prevalence, and 1-year incidence rates for schizophrenia, with the following respective results for pooled rates: 0.34 per 100, 0.55 per 100, and 11.1 per 100,000, and the authors concluded that the variation in rates between studies was generally between 2- and 5-fold (Goldner, Hsu, Waraich, & Somers, 2002). They stated, "there remains significant heterogeneity of prevalence and incidence rates" and "this strengthens support for the hypothesis that there is real variation in the distribution of schizophrenia around the world." Others stated, "The prevalence of schizophrenia has been estimated at 0.5%–1%, with most estimates approaching 1%" (Jibson et al., 2004). And the most recent review stated, "The point prevalence rate ranges from 2.7/1000 to 8.3/1000, and this range would not be affected greatly if several dozen other studies, available from prior reviews, were included" (Messias, Chen, & Eaton, 2007). They also stated, based on selected studies of the general population in defined geographic areas with a diagnosis made by a psychiatrist, published after 1985, that the range in annual incidence is from 0.11/1,000 per year to 0.70/1,000, and that there is considerable variation in incidence rates around the world, with a variation greater than one order of magnitude, from a low estimate in Vancouver, Canada, of 0.04/1,000 per year to a high estimate in Madras, India, of 0.58/1,000 per year (Messias et al., 2007).

Natural History

When the onset of schizophrenia is defined by the occurrence of the first psychotic episode, it most commonly occurs in young adulthood (Jibson et al., 2004). One classic study in the literature showed that about 50% of patients had an acute onset, and about 50% had a long prodrome (the early phases of the disease, when symptoms and signs are mild or nonspecific) (Ciompi, 1980a, 1980b). This same study showed that about half the subjects had an undulating course, with partial or full remissions followed by recurrences in an unpredictable manner, and that about one third had a relatively chronic unremitting course with poor outcome, and that a small minority had a steady pattern of recovery with good outcome (Ciompi, 1980a). "After the initial hospitalization, about 25% are not rehospitalized even after 15 years. For the sub-group of the cohort with 10 hospitalizations, more than 90% are rehospitalized within 3 years following the tenth episode" (Messias et al., 2007). One fact is intuitively clear: "Although relatively more first-admission patients have a positive course than do multiple admissions patients, the findings confirm the substantial heterogeneity in course and outcome" (Ram, Bromet, Eaton, Pato, & Schwartz, 1992. One study on the prodrome suggests that onset of negative symptoms usually occurs approximately 5 years before the first psychotic episode, and that the positive symptoms occur much closer to the first hospitalization (Hafner, Maurer, & Loffler, 1999).

The following factors have all been listed as frequent components that often lead to the development of schizophrenia: lower IQ, poor attention skills, thought disorder–like symptoms, poor social adjustment, psychiatric symptoms, and that schizophrenics differ from their peers, even in early childhood, in a variety of developmental markers, such as the age of attaining developmental milestones, levels of cognitive functioning, educational achievement, neurological and motor development, social competence, and psychological disturbances (Messias et al., 2007). These authors also stated, "There seem to be no common causal paths linking these developmental markers with schizophrenia. Indeed, individuals who later develop schizophrenia or related disorders already may have experienced a general or pan-developmental impairment early in their childhood." Considerable evidence suggests that schizophrenia results in part from childhood developmental abnormalities that lead to defects in early brain development (Isohanni, Murray, Jokelainen, Croudace, & Jones, 2004; Maki et al., 2005; Murray & Lewis, 1987; Weinberger, 1995).

A Dutch study found that the "risk of schizophrenia was associated with unemployment, low educational attainment, being single, lower wealth status, low income, and being childless. Increased risk was associated with a family history of psychiatric disorders, birth in urban areas, birth outside of Denmark, and having three or more siblings. Increased risk of schizophrenia was associated with parental unemployment and parental lower income, but was not associated with parental wealth" (Byrne, Agerbo, Eaton, & Mortensen, 2004). But uniquely, "risk for schizophrenia was associated with higher education in parents." Other known risk factors are the season of birth (higher for births in the winter months), complications of birth and delivery (with malnutrition, extreme prematurity, hypoxia, or ischemia as the possible causes), parental age (an increased risk with older parents), infections during pregnancy, abnormalities in the immune system (but it is not clear if they are causal or a consequence of the disorder), possible ethnic factors that may result from social pressures, cannabis use (schizophrenics are more likely to have used or be using), and urban residence (those living in the center of cities tend to be more vulnerable than those living in outer zones) (Messias et al., 2007).

Exactly what predicts the outcome for the course of schizophrenics is not clear; however, negative symptoms and a slow onset seem to be the major factors (Ram et al., 1992). A 1992 study compared the patient outcomes after 5 years for chronic psychosis versus no symptoms for England, Denmark, Russia, and the United States as "developed" countries versus India, Columbia, and Nigeria as "developing" countries (Leff, Sartorius, Jablensky, Korten, & Ernberg, 1992). What may be surprising for many is that the prognosis in the developing countries is significantly better. Messias and colleagues (2007) speculated that one reason may be that "the environment of recovery in the developed world is more pernicious, involving harsher economic competition, a greater degree of stigma, and smaller family networks to share the burden of care for persons who have schizophrenia." It is also clear that this disorder is not equally distributed across nations, even though many reports propagate the myth that the incidence rate is about the same for all nations worldwide (Messias et al., 2007). One study showed a median value of 15.2 per 100,000 population and a range of 7.7 to 43 (McGrath et al., 2004). The common myth that schizophrenia equally affects both males and females is also not true. "A review of available data from 31 studies estimates the median male:female ratio to be 1.4:1" (McGrath, 2005).

Results Using Conventional Treatment Modalities

Our best and most valid insight for the treatment effectiveness of schizophrenia using antipsychotic medications comes from a study conducted between January 2001 and December 2004. This multiphase trial included 1,493 patients and was conducted at 57 clinical sites in the United States, at the cost of $45 million, funded by the National Institute of Mental Health, and called the Clinical Antipsychotic Trials for Interventions Effectiveness or CATIE study (Lieberman et al., 2005). The mean patient age was 40.6 years

(74% males). The mean age at the first treatment for any behavioral or emotional problem was 24 years, and the mean time since the first antipsychotic medication was prescribed was 14.4 years at the time of entry into the CATIE study. Among the patients, 28% also had depression, 25% had alcohol dependence or alcohol abuse, 29% suffered from drug dependence or drug abuse, 5% had obsessive-compulsive disorder, and 14% had another anxiety disorder. "These 'real-world' features of the study, which were intended to make the results widely applicable, may account for the differences in results between this and previous studies comparing first- and second-generation antipsychotic agents" (Lieberman et al., 2005). This patient population is typical of the average patient presenting with schizophrenia, whereas pharmaceutical company–funded trials are highly restricted and limited for the additional compounding real-world features and problems that usually affect patients. However, "Patients were excluded if they had received a diagnosis of schizoaffective disorder, mental retardation, or other cognitive disorders; had a history of serious adverse reactions to the proposed treatments; had only one schizophrenic episode; had a history of treatment resistance, defined by the persistence of severe symptoms despite adequate trials of one of the proposed treatments or prior treatment with clozapine; were pregnant or breastfeeding; or had a serious and unstable medical condition" (Lieberman et al., 2005).

Phase 1 of the trial randomly assigned patients to receive olanzapine, quetiapine, risperidone, or perphenazine, under double-blind conditions, and patients were followed for up to 18 months or until treatment was discontinued for any reason. Ziprasidone was later added in January 2002 since it had just received approval by the Food and Drug Administration. Perphenazine was the only first-generation antipsychotic compared in the trial, and all of the other medications are classified as the later second-generation antipsychotic medications. There was no placebo control group. Patients who failed treatment in phase 1 could receive other treatments in phases 2 and 3. "Successful treatment time was defined as the number of months of treatment during phase 1 in which patients had a Clinical Global Improvement Scale score of at least 3 (mildly ill) or a score of 4 (moderately ill) with an improvement of at least two points from baseline" (Lieberman et al., 2005).

However, the most striking results for the numbers of patients dropping out of the first phase of the study are the following: "Seventy-four percent of patients in the intention-to-treat analysis (1061 of 1432) discontinued their assigned treatment in phase 1 before 18 months (median of 6 months treatment time before dropping out)." For each drug specifically, the dropout rates were

> 64 percent of those assigned to olanzapine, 75 percent of those assigned to perphenazine, 82 percent of those assigned to quetiapine, 74 percent of those assigned to risperidone, and 79 percent of those assigned to ziprasidone. The time to the discontinuation of treatment for any cause was significantly longer in the olanzapine group than in the quetiapine ($P < 0.001$) or risperidone ($P = 0.002$) group, but not in the perphenazine ($P = 0.021$) or ziprasidone ($P = 0.028$) group. The times to discontinuation because of intolerable side effects were similar among the groups, but the rates differed ($P = 0.04$); olanzapine was associated with more discontinuation for weight gain or metabolic effects, and perphenazine was associated with more discontinuation for extrapyramidal effects. (Lieberman et al., 2005)

The authors summarized their results as follows:

> In summary, patients with chronic schizophrenia in this study discontinued their antipsychotic study medications at a high rate, indicating substantial limitations in the effectiveness of the drugs. Within this limited range of effectiveness, olanzapine appeared to be more effective than the other drugs studied, and there were no significant differences in effectiveness between the conventional drug perphenazine and the other second-generation drugs. There were no significant differences among the drugs in the time until discontinuation of treatment owing to intolerable side effects.

However, olanzapine was associated with greater weight gain and increases in glycosylated hemoglobin, cholesterol, and triglycerides, changes that may have serious implications with respect to medical comorbidity such as the development of the metabolic syndrome. How clinicians, patients, families, and policymakers evaluate the trade-offs between efficacy and side effects, as well as drug prices, will determine future patterns of use. (Lieberman et al., 2005)

Phase 2 of the CATIE study had a projected 6-month endpoint, and that trial included those patients that failed treatment in the first phase and elected to continue with another antipsychotic medication for treatment. A total of 444 patients entered the double-blind phase 2 treatment and were then treated with a different antipsychotic (olanzapine, quetiapine, risperidone, or ziprasidone) instead of the one they attempted during phase 1. Again, the aim was to determine if there were differences between these treatments in effectiveness measures by time until discontinuation for any reason and with tolerability (Stroup et al., 2006). The authors described their results as follows:

The time to treatment discontinuation was longer for patients treated with risperidone (median: 7.0 months) and olanzapine (6.3 months) than with quetiapine (4.0 months) and ziprasidone (2.8 months). Among patients who discontinued their previous antipsychotic because of inefficacy ($N = 184$), olanzapine was more effective than quetiapine and ziprasidone, and risperidone was more effective than quetiapine. There were no significant differences between antipsychotics among those who discontinued their previous treatment because of intolerability ($N = 168$). (Stroup et al., 2006)

They concluded:

Among this group of patients with chronic schizophrenia who had just discontinued treatment with an atypical antipsychotic, risperidone and olanzapine were more effective than quetiapine and ziprasidone as reflected by longer time until discontinuation for any reason. . . . Medication discontinuation integrates patient and clinician judgments of efficacy, safety, and tolerability into a global measure of effectiveness and signals the need for a new treatment strategy. . . . In phase 2, 74% of the 333 patients in the intent-to-treat cohort (i.e., excluding the 106 patients assigned before the availability of ziprasidone) discontinued treatment before completion of the study. Median treatment duration was 4 months. (Stroup et al., 2006)

A median of 4 months is a rather short time frame for patients tolerating medications. Therefore, since we are acutely aware that schizophrenia can be a lifelong disorder for the majority of patients, these discontinuation times for medication due to intolerability or ineffectiveness are therefore wholly inadequate for a chronic disorder.

For phase 2 of the CATIE study, the adverse events and side effects were summarized thus:

Significantly lower rates of insomnia were seen in patients receiving olanzapine (13%) and quetiapine (16%) relative to patients receiving risperidone (23%) or ziprasidone (31%). Patients receiving risperidone experienced higher rates of adverse effects involving sexual functioning (29%) relative to the other groups (11%–17%). Risperidone was also associated with higher rates of gynecomastia or galactorrhea (5%) relative to the other groups (<1%). More patients receiving quetiapine experienced orthostatic faintness (13%) relative to the other groups (4%–7%). Patients receiving quetiapine also spontaneously reported other adverse events more often than did those in the other treatment groups (34% versus 25%–28%). (Stroup et al., 2006).

There were no differences in the four groups for the incidence of extrapyramidal side effects, akathisia, or abnormal movements. In respect to weight gain and metabolic effects,

Patients receiving olanzapine gained more weight than did patients receiving any of the other drugs, with a mean of 1.3 pounds per month. Patients receiving ziprasidone had a mean loss of 1.7 pounds per month. Those receiving risperidone and quetiapine had negligible mean changes in weight over the course of phase 2. A larger proportion of patients receiving olanzapine gained over 7% of their baseline body weight compared with risperidone, quetiapine, and ziprasidone. No patients receiving ziprasidone discontinued treatment because of weight gain or metabolic side effects as opposed to patients receiving risperidone (5%), olanzapine (8%), or quetiapine (10%). . . . Olanzapine was associated with substantial increases in total cholesterol and triglycerides, whereas risperidone and ziprasidone were associated with decreases in these parameters. (Stroup et al., 2006)

In respect to other adverse events: "The medications exhibited no substantially different effects on the electrocardiographic QTc interval or incidence of new cataracts. Ziprasidone was associated with more serious adverse events other than hospitalizations for schizophrenia than the other treatments (15% versus 6–11%). Although no clear pattern of serious adverse events was noted, there were two completed suicides among patients receiving ziprasidone. The only other completed suicide was in a patient taking risperidone" (Stroup et al., 2006).

Those patients who discontinued treatment with a second-generation (also called atypical) antipsychotic in phase 1 because their symptoms were not adequately relieved also had an option to be randomized to another arm of the study where they would receive either clozapine or a different atypical antipsychotic (olanzapine, quetiapine, or risperidone) that they did not receive in phase 1. This arm of the CATIE study was called the clozapine trial (McEvoy et al., 2006). This arm of the study was only partially blinded. Patients knew if they were randomly assigned to clozapine, but were blinded to the identity of the other three medications. Clozapine is generally considered to be the most effective antipsychotic drug. However, "because of clozapine's burden of serious side effects, it is not known whether multiple trials involving some or all of the newer atypical antipsychotics should be undertaken before treating a patient with clozapine"(McEvoy et al., 2006). Therefore, this arm of the CATIE study was justified for comparing clozapine with olanzapine, quetiapine, or risperidone. Again, patients had the option to enter the trial for clozapine versus one of the other three, or they could go into the arm of phase 2 that only compared olanzapine, quetiapine, risperidone, and ziprasidone, all blindly. Patients were informed about the potential side effects of clozapine and the respective comparison drugs. Out of the patients that elected to enter this arm of phase 2, 99 were "randomly assigned to either open-label treatment with clozapine (N = 49) or blinded treatment with another newer atypical antipsychotic not previously received in the trial (olanzapine [N = 19], quetiapine [N = 15], or risperidone [N = 16])" (McEvoy et al., 2006).

The results were as follows:

> Time until treatment discontinuation for any reason was significantly longer for clozapine (median = 10.5 months) than for quetiapine (median = 3.3), or risperidone (median = 2.8), but not for olanzapine (median = 2.7). Time to discontinuation because of inadequate therapeutic effect was significantly longer for clozapine than for olanzapine, quetiapine, or risperidone. At 3-month assessments, Positive and Negative Syndrome Scale total scores had decreased more in patients treated with clozapine than in patients treated with quetiapine or risperidone but not olanzapine. One patient treated with clozapine developed agranulocytosis, and another developed eosinophilia; both required treatment discontinuation. . . .
>
> Forty-four percent (N = 20) of the clozapine-treated patients, 29% (N = 5) of the olanzapine-treated patients, 7% (N = 1) of the quetiapine-treated patients, and 14% (N = 2) of the risperidone-treated patients continued taking their phase 2 medication for the duration of the trial. Eleven percent (N = 5) of the clozapine-treated patients, 35% (N = 6) of the olanzapine-treated patients,

and 43% ($N = 6$) of both the quetiapine- and the risperidone-treated patients discontinued treatment because of lack of efficacy.

The authors concluded, "For these patients with schizophrenia who prospectively failed to improve with an atypical antipsychotic, clozapine was more effective than switching to another newer atypical antipsychotic. Safety monitoring is necessary to detect and manage clozapine's serious side effects." They also commented, "Despite its therapeutic advantages, clozapine has been underused, perhaps because of the array of serious side effects it may cause; these include agranulocytosis, myocarditis, other inflammatory reactions, seizures, obesity, diabetes mellitus, and other metabolic abnormalities. Extensive monitoring is required to avoid the consequences of these side effects."

The following related comments are from a 2006 editorial titled "Practical Treatment Information for Schizophrenia" published in the *American Journal of Psychiatry* that reviews the highlights of state-of-the-art treatment, status, and the findings of the CATIE study. "Schizophrenia, with its pervasive life impairments and the woeful lack of knowledge regarding its molecular pathophysiology, is a distressing mental illness. Its treatments have been empiric and serendipitously discovered, not rationally understood. Moreover, the treatments are partial, in that psychosis is the treatment-responsive symptom domain, whereas cognition and negative symptoms respond minimally" (Tamminga, 2006). Tamminga noted that the results of phase 1 suggested a superiority of olanzapine in length of time to drug discontinuation. However, "the hope that other new antipsychotics with fewer metabolic side effects might offer a similar effect was not fulfilled. Some have pointed out that older drugs like perphenazine, with their lower costs, may now once again become rational first-line therapies. The memory of patients with tardive dyskinesia still haunts many clinicians, however. The debate over less expensive first-generation drugs obscures the sobering results of phase 1." In addition, "That first report thus also showed once again the stark reality of antipsychotic drugs—their therapeutic limitations and their problematic side effects, especially the metabolic effects." Tamminga also commented on phase 2 of the CATIE trial: "the side effect outcomes are staggering in their magnitude and extent and demonstrate the significant medication burden for persons with schizophrenia." When clinicians are faced with the question of what to do if a new antipsychotic fails, Tamminga answers, "The evidence, clearer than many clinicians might have believed, is that clozapine is the only rational alternative. This answer is only tempered by the significantly greater side effect burden with clozapine, again demonstrated: weight gain, increased metabolic measures, sialorrhea, sedation, and the agranulocytosis that we all know to add in (even though adequate surveillance methodology is now in place). But this is a side effect risk profile that is positively balanced by clozapine's increased efficacy and effectiveness."

When looking at the CATIE trial overall, Tamminga commented, "There has not been a previous set of treatment studies that has so clearly shown the tradeoffs for persons who need antipsychotic medication. There is no clear 'winner' among the second generation of antipsychotics, weighing effectiveness and efficacy against side effects, nor a clear 'loser.' It is only clozapine that is superior, although its side effects are clearly challenging. These data make it abundantly clear that the risks and benefits of any single medication need to be weighed individually with each patient, and that side effect risk needs to be weighed repeatedly during treatment."

While the NIMH-funded CATIE study focused on chronic schizophrenia, another pharmaceutical company–funded large trial studied 498 "first-episode" patients that excluded those with positive symptoms of schizophrenia for more than 2 years, or who had received an antipsychotic medication for more than 6 weeks at any time (Kahn et al., 2008). The patients were between 18 and 40 years with a mean age of 26, which is significantly younger than those in the CATIE study, which had a mean age of 40.6 years, and 40% were women, compared to 26% in the CATIE trial. They were recruited from 50 sites in 14 countries (13 European countries and Israel) where each was highly skilled with treating schizophrenic patients, and 36 sites were university hospitals. Among the patients, 53% were diagnosed with schizophrenia, 40% with schizophreniform disorder, and 7% with schizoaffective disorder.

The objective here was to compare another first-generation antipsychotic (haloperidol) again with second-generation atypical antipsychotics (amisulpride, olanzapine, quetiapine, or ziprasidone). Here haloperidol was given in a relatively low dose, but considered effective for first-episode patients, where higher doses are not generally known to be more effective for this patient group, but higher doses can increase the risk of side effects. While the patients were randomized to their respective groups, they and their psychiatrists were "unmasked for the assigned treatment, since this reflected routine clinical practice, increasing the trial's external validity; it also improved the trial's acceptability for patients and psychiatrists, leading to a more representative group of patients, which further increased the trial's external validity" (Kahn et al., 2008). This awareness by patient and psychiatrist differs significantly compared to the CATIE trial. However, again, no placebo group was included. Participants were randomized to receive daily doses of one of the following: haloperidol 1–4 mg, amisulpride 200–800 mg, olanzapine 5–20 mg, quetiapine 200–750 mg, or ziprasidone 40–160 mg, with a respective mean dose per group of 3.0, 450.8, 12.6, 498.6, and 107.2 mg. The primary outcome of the study was the rate of treatment discontinuation at 1 year, which was defined as the use of a medication dose outside of the range defined above, the use of an additional antipsychotic medication, or complete discontinuation of the medication. Again, compared to most other pharmaceutical company–funded trials with end points of less than or equal to 2 months, the 1-year end point here was most admirable and realistic for treatment efficacy with an illness potentially lasting a lifetime. Secondary outcomes included multiple measures of antipsychotic efficacy and adverse events. Overall discontinuation of treatment before 1 year was less likely with second-generation antipsychotics versus haloperidol. The respective rates of treatment discontinuation for haloperidol, amisulpride, olanzapine, quetiapine, and ziprasidone were 72%, 40%, 33%, 53%, and 45% (Kahn et al., 2008). Comparisons with haloperidol showed lower risks for any-cause discontinuation with amisulpride, olanzapine, quetiapine, and ziprasidone. However, symptom reductions were virtually the same in all the groups, at around 60% (Kahn et al., 2008). Discontinuation of treatment caused by adverse events was lower with olanzapine and quetiapine versus haloperidol. Haloperidol was associated with higher rates of parkinsonism than the second-generation antipsychotics, and haloperidol and ziprasidone increased the rate of akathisia versus the other drugs. The second-generation antipsychotics promoted reduced severity of illness and improved functioning versus haloperidol, but several other measures of treatment efficacy were similar when the second-generation antipsychotics and haloperidol were compared. Rates of hospitalization did not differ between treatment groups. More subjects receiving olanzapine used antidepressants versus the other study medications. The incidence of significant weight gain was high in the study cohort but did not differ between the medications, although olanzapine was associated with the highest mean weight gain, which is again consistent with the CATIE trial. The authors concluded, "We cannot conclude that second-generation drugs are more efficacious than is haloperidol, since discontinuation rates are not necessarily consistent with symptomatic improvement" (Kahn et al., 2008). These results at large tell us the same basic story as the CATIE trial. These are the most reliable trials conducted by highly trained specialists for real-world patients with schizophrenia.

Thus, the conventional medical approach to treatment using medications for the real-world schizophrenic population today, chronic or first episode, is not very hopeful or promising and is fraught with serious concerns for patient well-being, both medically and psychologically. Apparently, a very high percentage of patients suffer side effects from the antipsychotic medications that lead to early termination of treatment even when delusions and hallucinations are reduced. The severity of drug-induced medical problems is simply too great to warrant the continuation of treatment in many cases.

While there have been several theories in recent decades involving neurotransmitter systems and how they might contribute to the cause of this disease, mainly the dopamine hypothesis, today a pharmaceutical cure is not in sight. We only need to remember the comments above about the history of drug intervention: "Its treatments have been empiric and serendipitously discovered, not rationally understood" (Tamminga, 2006). Little has changed in this regard.

In addition, those with the confidence that studies pursuing a genetic basis for the disease, in the form of a DNA sequence variation, with what some researchers call risk genes, candidate genes, or disease-related genes, may be thoroughly disappointed with the most compelling, most recent, and largest study on associations of single-nucleotide polymorphisms (SNP) associated with schizophrenia. This very well-designed study included 1,870 patients with either schizophrenia or schizoaffective disorder, and 2,002 screened comparison control subjects, all of European ancestry. The "study of the association of schizophrenia to DNA sequence variants in 14 of the best supported of these current candidate genes" led to negative findings (Sanders et al., 2008). The study results, published by 23 authors, found that "neither experiment-wide nor gene-wide statistical significance was observed in the primary single-SNP analyses or in secondary analyses of haplotypes or of imputed genotypes for additional common HapMap SNPs. Results in SNPs previously reported as associated with schizophrenia were consistent with chance expectation, and four functional polymorphisms in COMT, DRD2, and HTR2A did not produce nominally significant evidence to support previous evidence for association." They concluded, "It is unlikely that common SNPs in these genes account for a substantial proportion of the genetic risk for schizophrenia, although small effects cannot be ruled out." Confidence in this study, compared to smaller and earlier studies, comes from the fact that the population was very uniform, "whereas most schizophrenia samples are smaller or were assembled from separate studies." Also, this large study "tested dense sets of single nucleotide polymorphisms (SNPs) in each gene (rather than a few), including 'tags' for most known common SNPs, plus additional SNPs in critical gene elements such as those that change amino acid sequence." Therefore, this study is also robust because it is comprehensive for genotyping. Given every possible linkage relationship here that they studied, they stated, "We were unable to detect association of any one SNP with schizophrenia by any of these criteria." The same negative results were obtained when the authors looked only at the population without schizoaffective disorder. Much effort has also been directed in the past decade to finding risk genes with most of the other major psychiatric disorders. This field of neurogenetics has yet to show great promise, where the hope has been to identify novel risk genes for each specific psychiatric disorder. Therefore, it may turn out that the advances for treating schizophrenia and its relatives, in the nearer future, may be found in other approaches to psychiatry.

One other approach is the use of cognitive therapy (CT). "Cognitive-therapy for psychosis focuses on altering the thoughts, emotions, and behaviors of patients by teaching them skills to challenge and modify beliefs about delusions and hallucinations, to engage in experimental reality testing, and to develop better coping strategies for the management of hallucinations. The goals of these interventions are to decrease the conviction of delusional beliefs, and hence their severity, and to promote more effective coping and reductions in distress" (Gould, Mueser, Bolton, Mays, & Goff, 2004). This is a relatively new field for controlled studies with CT. "The relative lag in controlled research on CT for psychosis can be traced to common assumptions that the cognitive deficits of schizophrenia preclude the use of CT approaches or that such approaches, which assume basic reasoning skills, are inappropriate for clients with psychosis" (Gould et al., 2004). A meta-analysis of seven studies, mostly performed in the United Kingdom, was conducted on a total of 340 patients with a mean duration of the disorder of 14.0 years. Nearly 100% were taking psychotropic medications; 70% were male; and the majority were in outpatient settings with a usual breakdown of schizophrenia-spectrum disorders. However, those who rated the changes in therapy were not the providers, but they were also not blinded to which group the patient was allocated to. In summary, "The mean effect size for reduction of psychotic symptoms was 0.65. The findings suggest that cognitive therapy is an effective treatment for patients with schizophrenia who have persistent psychotic symptoms. Follow-up analyses in four (of the seven) studies indicated that patients receiving CT continued to make gains over time (ES = 0.93)" (Gould et al., 2004). The authors also stated, "Further research is needed to determine the replicability of standardized cognitive interventions, to evaluate the clinical significance of cognitive therapy for schizophrenia, and to determine which patients are most likely to benefit from this intervention." To date, by far the most commonly employed therapeutic modality for treatment is the antipsychotic medications, and to a very limited degree the use of CT.

One study examined the efficacy of hatha yoga therapy (YT) as an add-on treatment to ongoing antipsychotic treatment, including 61 moderately ill schizophrenic patients, ages 18–55 years, about 66% male, that were randomly assigned to YT or physical exercise therapy (PT) for 4 months. They were assessed at baseline and 4 months after the start of intervention, by a rater who was blind to their group status. Only patients with Clinical Global Impression Severity Scale scores of 4 or more and who were cooperative for YT were included. Positive and Negative Syndrome Scale for Schizophrenia (PANSS), extrapyramidal symptoms, and quality of life were measured. "Forty-one subjects (YT = 21; PT = 20) were available at the end of 4 months for assessment. Subjects in the YT group had significantly less psychopathology than those in the PT group at the end of 4 months. They also had significantly greater social and occupational functioning and quality of life" (Duraiswamy, Thirthalli, Nagendra, & Gangadhar, 2007). "The subjects in the YT group scored significantly lower in different symptom dimensions (except positive syndrome score) and PANSS total score. . . . In 74% of the subjects medications and their dosages were unchanged for at least 8 weeks before entering the study, and in all subjects there was no change for at least 4 weeks. Medication was changed during the study period in only two patients (one from each group) as they had exacerbation of symptoms. Thus the results are not attributable to changes in antipsychotic medications." There were no serious adverse effects of either YT or PT during the study period. A comprehensive assessment of side effects using scales developed for drug trials was not made. They concluded, "Both non-pharmacological interventions contributed to reduction in symptoms, with YT having better efficacy. . . . This study showed YT is beneficial in schizophrenia as an add-on treatment. This benefit is seen across several dimensions of the schizophrenia outcome. It remains to be established whether the benefits extend to cognitive symptoms and are enduring."

The Yogic View on the Etiology of Schizophrenia and Other Forms of Psychosis

Hallucinations occur in approximately 50% of schizophrenic patients (Breier & Berg, 1999). The yogic insight about hallucinatory events is that when a person is hallucinating, he is experiencing the world of dreams and the world of ordinary waking consciousness at the same time. Hallucinating schizophrenics have lost the ability to differentiate between these two states of consciousness during the event, and, consequently, these two worlds have merged for them during the periods of their hallucinations. Normally, by the time we reach a certain age, we are culturally conditioned to believe that our dreams during sleep are in fact only dreams. Essentially, we are taught that this world of dreams is a nonreality and that only the waking state is real. Thus, we learn to recognize the differences and to separate these experiences in our intellectual framework. One is real and one is not. Unfortunately, the schizophrenic is no longer able to separate dreams from waking reality during a hallucination. The closest that normals come to this merged experience is the fuzzy time when a dream is ending and we begin the transition to the full waking state. Some dreams are more lucid than others and we may or may not give an interpretation to the content. But clearly the dream is frequently multisensory in content and we experience it through our sensory systems of hearing, seeing, touching, smelling, and tasting, much like any event in a waking-state activity. Hallucinating schizophrenics have the same experience where the sensory systems are mixed during the waking event. But they simply cannot differentiate these experiences during the waking state. In time they learn about the incongruence of their world and the world that others perceive, which in addition contributes to their disordered thinking. Their "reality" eventually does not add up when compared to the conventional norm of the waking adult. Consequently, this leads to significant pain and confusion for most patients. This is especially true in societies where reality is strictly defined with more rigid borders, and where there is less tolerance for what others may label as a valid experience of a nonordinary reality, or what some choose to call spiritual or mystical experiences. Different societies have had different levels of tolerance, appreciation, and acceptance throughout the ages for these boundaries of ordinary and nonordinary realty. It is also important to understand here that what a schizophrenic may experience and what a mystic may experience may be similar, but that the mystic can differentiate between the ordinary reality and that of the altered states of consciousness. The mystic can effectively integrate these experiences and has some mastery and control over the many different realms of consciousness. For the most part, I think we can assume that Western psychiatry has a rather firm, rigid, and established boundary for what is termed an acceptable, healthy experience of a waking reality within the norm. However, a further discussion of the worlds of ordinary and nonordinary realities is beyond the scope of this book. But here it is the yogic view that hallucinations are "leaking" into the world of ordinary reality for schizophrenic patients, and that their ability to differentiate the borders has been lost.

How does this leakage of one world into the other happen? First, we must take a quick glimpse at how yogis view the nature of our being. In that view, we are made up of multiple bodies that respectively represent the different layers of our being, which also differentially support the separate functions and levels of conscious experience. These bodies are the physical body, etheric body, subtle body, mental body, auric body, radiant body, and so on. Ordinarily, there is an adequate cohesive strength to keep these bodies "glued" together. However, when a schizophrenic is hallucinating, the bodies are no longer well connected, and the person can then have experiences from more than one realm simultaneously. This can be viewed as a leakage. The hallucinating schizophrenic is in fact living in multiple dimensions at the same time. This of course suggests that when normal individuals are dreaming during sleep that one body dominates over another to support our presence and self. However, during the waking state our ordinary reality is experienced almost exclusively through the physical body. Why do these bodies separate, and why does the glue weaken during the waking state in the schizophrenic patient? The answer is simple. This separation is the cumulative result of trauma, stress, and damage to the nervous system and chakras. The yogic view for the causal factors that influence this break is not significantly different from those discussed above (Messias et al., 2007). However, in my own experience with these patients, I find that drug abuse is the most common factor these days, followed by early trauma from a long, complicated, and difficult birth. Whether the insults to the nervous system or psyche are singular or multiple over time, the result is the same. There is a break in reality and multiple dimensions are experienced simultaneously as a result of the leaking in of dream-like experiences. Multiple factors also come into play that allow for the merging of these two worlds. Schizophrenics rarely hallucinate for 24 hours a day, 7 days a week. Hallucinations wax and wane in severity, as do all natural physiological and psychological phenomena. There are natural endogenous rhythms that govern our psychophysiological states during both waking and sleep (Shannahoff-Khalsa, 2008), and the study of our natural endogenous rhythms in relationship to the tendencies to hallucinate and which phases of these cycles dominate during hallucinations is likely to yield important new findings. It is also the case that our vulnerability to this break and leakage is dependent on external stressors and threats, their additive effects, and our basic mental and physical constitution. It is highly likely that we have rhythms of vulnerability that more easily support the merging of these two worlds.

A Case History of Hallucinations and Biological Rhythms

This case history supports the thesis that biological rhythms and psychophysiological states can allow for and differentially support hallucinations (Shannahoff-Khalsa, 2009). Ms. E smoked tobacco and used alcohol, amphetamines, marijuana, MDMA, LSD, and other psychedelics from the ages of 19 to 25. She quit tobacco at 31. At 24 she was diagnosed with depression and prescribed citalopram. Two weeks later she experienced her first manic episode and was hospitalized and prescribed olanzapine and topiramate and given a series of electroconvulsive shock treatments. After 1 year she stopped all medications because of the unpleasant side effects and soon experienced hallucinations lasting for days or weeks at a time.

At the age of 26 she was diagnosed with bipolar disorder with psychotic features and borderline personality disorder, and prescribed olanzapine and lithium. Later she sought my help with Kundalini yoga techniques for her bipolar disorder, without mentioning the hallucinations or the diagnosis of her personality disorders. I saw her twice over 18 months. She initially reported being stable with only "light mania." However, Ms. E again stopped her medications due to side effects without consulting with her treating psychiatrist, and her hallucinations became severe. During this period of time I too was not consulted, nor did I see the patient.

She was soon admitted to a long-term locked facility and remedicated. However, her hallucinations became increasingly painful, out of control, and occurred for hours on end at essentially the same time every day. Upon restarting her yoga practice without my guidance, her episodes reduced to about twice a week.

After two years, Ms. E's mother requested that I see her daughter again. I was told that she was now diagnosed with schizophrenia and borderline and narcissistic personality disorders and was taking clozapine and fluphenazine and living in a board-and-care facility. Her hallucinations had stabilized to about twice a week but "remained intolerable." I taught her a new series of techniques (see Chapter 5 for an explanation of the protocols). After several weeks her hallucinations were reduced to once a week and the duration of her episodes reduced from 6–10 hours to 2–3 hours. At this point she chose to stop the fluphenazine, again without a professional consult.

Since I knew that she had a strong yogic discipline and interest in the techniques, in January 2009 I suggested that she observe if one of her nostrils was more dominant during her hallucinations (no clues were given about my expectations). Two days later she reported, "Yesterday I experienced mild hallucinations for half an hour after a stressful day. During the hallucinations my breath was left nostril dominant, and as soon as it was over my breath switched to right nostril dominant." I asked her to continue observing her nasal dominance and the periods of her hallucinations. After several months and at least 15 episodes it was clear that she was only left nostril dominant during her hallucinations, but on very rare occasions she started hallucinating during the very brief transition phase where both nostrils are equal leading into left nostril dominance.

After the initial observations I suggested that she practice slow deep breathing through her right nostril during the hallucinations to see if this would reduce the severity and time of the hallucinations. In fact, the right nostril breathing did lead to relief in the severity of content and the duration of the hallucinations. In March

2009, I developed a four-part miniprotocol for helping to terminate hallucinations for her to practice during her hallucinations
and preferably at the immediate onset. The protocol includes the
tuning-in and Victory Breath techniques, a specific four-part right
nostril breathing exercise using the mantra Sa Ta Na Ma, and the
L-form meditation of the Sa Ta Na Ma mantra. The entire protocol
is described in detail at the end of the section on yogic protocols
for treating schizophrenia. This four-part miniprotocol helped Ms.
E to substantially reduce the times and "dread" of her hallucinations. As of October 20, 2009, Ms. E continues her full daily yogic
practice and has had hallucinations lasting for only about 10 minutes to one hour, with events occurring only every 15 to 18 days
for the preceding three months. She remains on 225 mg of clozapine.

The following quotation is from Ms. E describing her experience and use of this four-part miniprotocol after several months of
experience with it.

> In my own experience, when hallucinations start, I would immedi-
> ately begin the Victory Breath, and sometimes the hallucinations
> would stop within the first 11 minutes. The hallucinations are more
> likely to end after 11 minutes of the Victory Breath if the day is
> within a short enough time of the previous episode of hallucina-
> tions—I would say within 3 to 4 days. If the hallucinations do not
> end with 11 minutes of the Victory Breath, I would continue the
> Victory Breath until I can sit some place quiet, and do the entire
> treatment (on days more than 7 days from the previous episode, I
> would go immediately to the whole treatment): Tuning in, Victory
> Breath 11 minutes (if not already done), Sa Ta Na Ma four-part
> right nostril breathing for 11 minutes, Sa Ta Na Ma in the L-form
> meditation for 11 minutes. The hallucinations usually would have
> ceased completely at this point. But if the mini treatment was de-
> layed (I cannot say how long), clarity of mind will resume after first
> practicing the mini-protocol and then laying down on the left side,
> at the most for one hour.

The longer case history and treatment of Ms. E are further described as an example of treating complicated comorbid cases in Chapter 5. What is clearly unique here is that Ms. E only experienced her hallucinations during her left nostril–right hemisphere dominant mode, a psychophysiological state that apparently more readily supports hallucinations. The rhythms of the nasal cycle and alternating cerebral hemispheric dominance have been explained in depth (Shannahoff-Khalsa, 2006, 2007, 2008). To date, it is not clear if all patients will experience their hallucinations only during the left nostril–right hemisphere dominant mode, but the results with Ms. E are suggestive and give us new insight into this mental condition and a powerful tool for treating these horrific episodes.

Now let's turn to the most common positive schizophrenic symptom, the delusions that occur in approximately 65% of schizophrenic patients (Appelbaum et al., 1999; Breier & Berg, 1999). The definition provided above (Jibson et al., 2004) that describes delusions as internally generated false beliefs that are not amenable to contrary evidence or persuasive argument, and that are acknowledged by peers to be aberrant beliefs, is a definition with loose boundaries and one that is open to social and political prerogatives. One might argue that people in positions of power and authority who suffer from grandiosity are somehow not eligible for this diagnosis as a result of their status, or we must concede that we occasionally elect those who are delusional and for some reason we fail to identify their problems. This might also suggest that psychiatric terminology may be more often applied to those who are more vulnerable. History is replete with examples of how societies have used psychiatry as a social weapon. Perhaps the corollary here is "those with the most gold rule" and those with authority have the opportunity to redraw the borders of sanity or at least are not subject to a diagnosis when they are clearly delusional. However, let's restrict ourselves here to the cases of those who believe in some of the more popular and perhaps common delusional extremes, for example, the delusion that one is Jesus Christ, or the new incarnation of Jesus, or Mary Magdalene or the incarnation of Mary, or Cleopatra. There are also numerous other religious and historical personalities that are adopted by individuals in their delusional states. What allows for or gives rise to this form of delusion? Clearly, the patient is choosing a more convenient, acceptable to the self, and pleasant version of reality, rather than the obvious condition that is perceived by others. We could call this a lie and say that it reflects the capacity for self-deceit. We might say that the capacity for delusions is directly proportional to one's character and ability to be honest with oneself. The factor of character here, or lack of values, enters the equation, and the interpretation of reality is obviously aberrantly skewed by including these illusions. The patient first lies to herself, and then to others, directly or indirectly. Usually the patient is in pain but also has a lack of integrity, and therefore chooses an interpretation of history that is much easier to live with rather than the basic bleak facts that have led to her misery, which proves to be so unacceptable. Some people are more prone to self-aggrandizement and illusion than others. However, rarely does the world react to someone who thinks too little of himself, and sometimes the world does not react quickly enough to those who think too highly of themselves. Some lies are more convenient than others. Some individuals enlist others in supporting their delusions by sharing the wealth, and the result is a mutual sociopolitico-financial gain. Therefore, the element of the definition that requires acknowledgment by peers that the beliefs are aberrant does not hold in all circles. The darkness of human character and inherent ignorance is the primary basis for delusions. The issues of psychiatric definitions are indeed complicated and involve many sociopolitical factors. It may be that we have to accept the fact that these descriptions of psychiatric definitions are not always appropriately openly applied in modern societies. Or one might conclude that the shared psychotic disorder (folie à deux) is more common than once believed. However, in part, these issues are subject to what is considered extreme or aberrant in any given social context, by the one who is making the diagnosis. Nonetheless, the yogic view is not a complex issue. The situation reduces to the fact that we are all subject to illusions and delusions, and some of us are more able than others to evade the label of delusional. The nature of reality and illusion is not a black-and-white matter with definitive borders. Until we can agree on what constitutes the ingredients (and not just the aberrations) of a healthy character, and who is manifesting that character, the word *delusional* and who is or is not delusional will be the subject of much controversy. However, each society seems to choose its own standards and borders, which may or may not shift over time.

In addition, the yogic view includes another important dimension of the psychotic person that must be considered in both our understanding and treatment of the patient. Usually before the onset of the condition, the psychotic patient has a deep sense of self and a reverence for this deep sense, but the world rejects it and this becomes part of the underlying problem. The patient wants others to revere his deep self, and in addition, the patient is afraid of his own deep self, but only because the patient sees the world reacting negatively to his experience of self. These factors play a vital role in the therapy of the patient, which is described in the next section.

The Yogic Protocols for Treatment

The psychotic disorders are the most nuanced and complex category of the three major groups described in this book. While these patients have a deep sense of self, they also have a variety of fears that tend to increase as the day progresses. It is natural with these patients to have fears accumulate and create a sort of critical mass during the waking hours. It is also true that the real events that trigger these fears tend to increase over the course of the day. In an effort to combat this strong tendency, patients will make the best progress if they practice some exercises at least three times per day or even five times per day when necessary. This frequency for treatment is also dependent on patients' ability to self-administer the techniques and the availability of someone to help guide them and also to practice the techniques along with them. However, the first step in therapy with these patients is to investigate whether they have the desire to self-heal. Not all do. If they have the desire, then patients are either directly taught the techniques as one would teach any yoga student, or it may be necessary for the coordinator to first model and practice the techniques so that they can first observe and then agree to experiment either immediately or at some mutually acceptable time later. Since these patients have a reverence for their own deep selves, which they believe is not honored by others, it is very important and a key to therapy for these patients to be joined in practice by the coordinator. This shared mutual experience is recognized by patients as a tribute to and recognition of their own deep selves. This helps provide a holy respect for self that patients are missing and it also helps provide a greater level of comfort for them when they face their fears. With time, the mutual practice of breathing and chanting together continues for protracted periods. It plateaus with a defined level of achievement, and then it can become more intense as the patient progresses. This increasing intensity and the depth of experience directly honors the patient's deep self. All of the exercises, whether combined as in the multipart exercise set below that is to be followed by the two respective meditation techniques, or not, must end with the patient inhaling deeply and extending his or her arms up at a 60-degree angle while stretching back behind the body with a full expansion of the chest. This must be repeated at least three times. This movement symbolizes the extension of the deep self that is now reaching out into the world and welcoming and grasping life itself with a much greater capacity. While this step sounds trivial, it is critical for the patient's progress in therapy.

A Protocol for Treating the Variants of Schizophrenia*

This protocol has four major components: (1) the essential practice called tuning in; (2) a 10-part exercise set specific for schizophrenics called True Glue, which helps to realign the spiritual bodies for treating and preventing psychotic episodes, followed by a 10-minute rest; (3) a meditation technique called Gan Puttee Kriya; and (4) a meditation technique to help combat delusions and to help stabilize a healthy sense of self-identity. The practice of all four parts in this sequence represents the ideal regimen and protocol for psychotic patients as a whole. However, much depends on the patient's initial abilities and will to progress. Some patients have youth, vitality, and a marked enthusiasm to overcome their disorder, while others may be older, less capable, and less enthusiastic about experimenting. Some patients at first are only willing to attempt the tuning-in technique, and this may be an excellent starting point for them. When this is the case, the technique can be practiced for much longer times with the participation of the coordinator, even for periods of 11–15 minutes. Every patient is different, and each patient must be respected according to his or her own ability and desire to experiment and to heal. Patients' progress is also often determined by the feeling of love and respect that they receive from their coordinator. This is often a key component to their willingness to proceed and to progress. They must feel an affinity with the coordinator and know that the coordinator feels an affinity with them. The ideal scenario is that a patient wants to practice the entire exercise set, followed by the meditation technique called Gan Puttee Kriya, and then the final meditation technique to help combat delusions and to help stabilize a healthy sense of self-identity. The bottom line for compliance for most patients over time is their new sense of clarity, stability, inner peace, rejuvenation, reduced fears, and the reduced length and frequency of their hallucinations. They quickly learn that this work is not easy, but it is

*Copyright © David Shannahoff-Khalsa, 2008. No portion of this protocol may be reproduced without the express written permission of the author.

much preferred to living with their suffering, fear, dread, confusion, depression, and anxiety.

1. Technique to Induce a Meditative State: Tuning In

Description of technique (see Figure 2.1): Sit with a straight spine and with the feet flat on the floor if sitting in a chair. Put the hands together at the center of the chest in prayer pose—the palms are pressed together with 10–15 pounds of pressure between the hands (a mild to medium pressure, nothing too intense). The area where the sides of the thumbs touch rests on the sternum with the thumbs pointing up (along the sternum), and the fingers are together and point up and out with a 60-degree angle to the ground. The eyes are closed and focused at the "third eye" (imagine a sun rising on

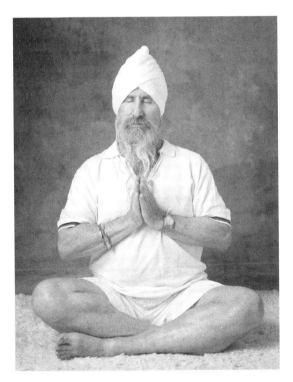

Figure 2.1
Technique to Induce a Meditative State: Tuning In

the horizon or the equivalent of the point between the eyebrows at the origin of the nose). A mantra is chanted out loud in a 1½ breath cycle. Inhale first through the nose and chant "Ong Namo" with an equal emphasis on each word. Then immediately follow with a half-breath inhalation through the mouth and chant "Guru Dev Namo" with approximately equal emphasis on each word. (The *o* in Ong and Namo are both long *o* sounds; Dev sounds like *Dave*, with a long *a* sound.) The practitioner should focus on the experience of the vibrations these sounds create on the upper palate and throughout the cranium while letting the mind be carried by the sounds into a new and pleasant mental space. This should be repeated a minimum of three times. This technique helps to create a protected meditative state of mind and is always used as a precursor to the other techniques.

2. An Exercise Set Specific for Schizophrenics Called True Glue— This Set Helps to Realign the Spiritual Bodies for Treating and Preventing Psychotic Episodes

All of the exercises below include a 1-minute relaxation period between each exercise.

1. Flex the spine as in the elementary spine flex exercise, which is also taught in Chapter 3 as technique 2 for the three cluster A, B, and C protocols, but here the arms are extended straight up over the head with the hands facing forward and with the fingers spread wide for 2 minutes (see Figures 2.2 and 2.3). This technique can be practiced while sitting either in a chair or on the floor in a cross-legged position. If you are in a chair, sit with both feet flat on the ground. Begin by pulling the chest up and slightly forward, inhaling deeply at the same time. Then exhale as you relax the spine down into a slouching position. Keep the head up straight, as if you were looking forward, without allowing it to move much with the flexing action of the spine. This will help prevent a whip action of the cervical vertebrae. All breathing should only be through the nose for both the inhalation and exhalation. The eyes are closed as if you were looking at a central point on the horizon, the third eye.

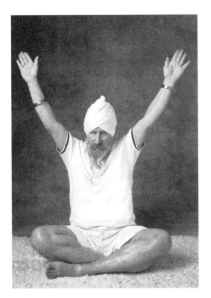 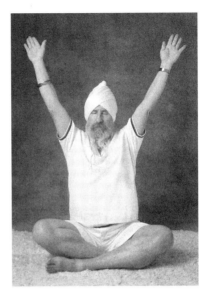

Figures 2.2 and 2.3
Spine-Flexing Exercise in Slouch Position and with a Straight Spine

Your mental focus is kept on the sound of the breath while listening to the fluid movement of the inhalation and exhalation. Begin the technique slowly while loosening up the spine. Eventually, a very rapid movement can be achieved with practice, reaching a rate of 1 to 2 times per second for the entire movement. Two minutes here is the maximum time. Food should be avoided for several hours if possible prior to this exercise set. When finished, inhale and hold the breath while stretching the arms straight over the head and stretching up the spine, then slowly exhale. Then repeat the inhale, hold and stretch, and exhale procedure two more times.

2. The hands are held in the posture called "gyan mudra," where the tip of the index finger and the tip of the thumb are touching and the other fingers are held straight up from the hand, and the arms are up with the elbows and forearms forming 90-degree angle and the spine, torso, and arms are twisted to the left with the inhalation and to the right with the exhalation. This movement is continued for 2 minutes (see Figure 2.4).

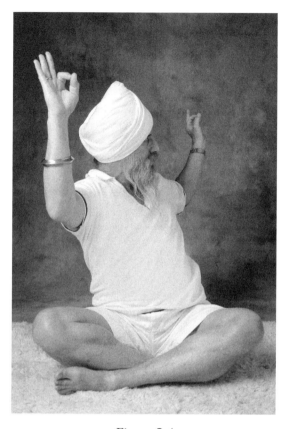

Figure 2.4
Spine Twist Exercise with Hands in Gyan Mudra

3. Lay flat on the ground and extend the arms out straight behind the head and the legs are out straight. Inhale through the nose and simultaneously raise the arms and legs up 90 degrees and perpendicular to the floor. Exhale and then lower both the arms and legs to their original position. Continue for 1 minute (see Figure 2.5).

4. Inhale through the nose and rise up on the knees with the arms extended above the head (see Figure 2.6), then exhale through the nose and squat on the heels and the knees with the arms extended straight out in front of the body with the palms down. Continue this movement for 2 minutes (see Figure 2.7).

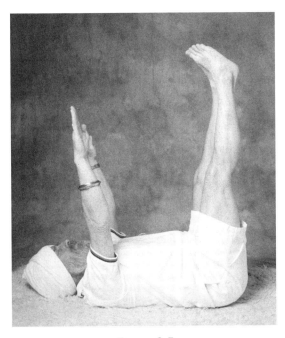

Figure 2.5
Leg and Arm Raise Exercise With Legs and Arms up at 90 Degrees

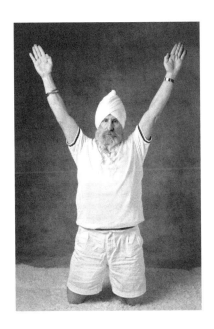

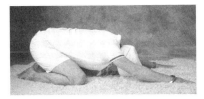

Figures 2.6 and 2.7
Exercise up on Knees With Arms
Over Head and With Arms Extended
Straight Sitting on Heels

5. Inhale through the nose and come up into camel pose with the head hanging back (see Figure 2.8), then exhale and lower the body into baby pose (see Figure 2.9). Continue for 2 minutes.

6. Stand up straight and inhale through the nose while twisting to the left with the left arm extended out and swinging toward the back as far as possible with the right arm then crossing in front of the chest (see Figure 2.10). Then exhale through the nose while reversing the posture and twisting around to the right with the right arm then extended back and out toward the back as far as possible and the left arm then coming across the chest. The head also turns with the torso. Keep the hands in lightly closed fists, and continue the movement for 2 minutes.

7. Get down on the hands and knees and start by extending the left arm directly out in front of the body. The right leg is then also extended out straight back behind the body (see Figure 2.11). Make a right angle with the extended hand so that you appear to be pushing against the wall, and also maintain a right angle at the ankle with the extended foot. The head is raised up and the eyes are open. Visually focus on a point directly out in front of the body and stare at a point off in the "infinite horizon." Either do Breath of Fire through the nose (see explanation below), or do long slow

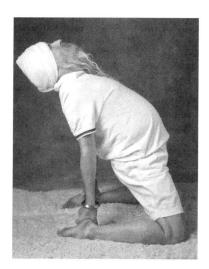
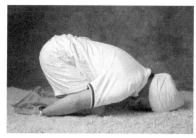

Figures 2.8 and 2.9
Camel Pose and Baby Pose

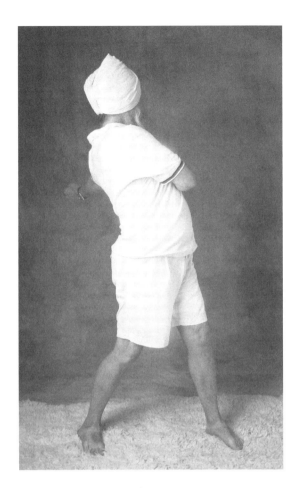

Figure 2.10
Side Twisting Exercise

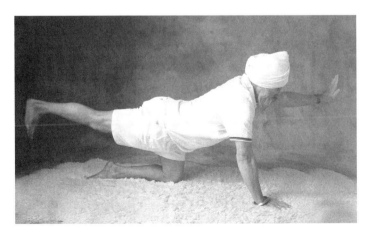

Figure 2.11
Exercise With Opposite Leg and Arm Extended

61

deep breathing through the nose. Maintain the posture perfectly without bending either limb, or losing balance, and continue holding this posture with the breathing for 2 minutes. Rest briefly (1 minute or less) and then reverse sides and continue everything for 2 additional minutes. Note that the opposite arms and legs are extended in the first part and then they are reversed for the second part.

Breath of Fire is practiced where the air is pulled in and pumped out very quickly and rhythmically at a rate of about 2 to 3 times per second, just like pumping a bellows, at the navel point. Make an effort to avoid holding any tension in the muscles of the chest, rib cage, or shoulders, which remain relaxed throughout the breath. The only tension felt is a mild effort by the abdominal muscles when the breath is quickly forced out. Every effort is made so that the sound of the inhale and exhale become nearly equal and indistinguishable and where very little work is being done. The easiest way to understand how to do Breath of Fire is to imagine that you have dirt in your nose and you make the effort to rapidly exhale through the nose to push the dirt out using the breath. When doing this, you need to briefly tighten the abdominal muscles at the navel and force the breath out through the nose. Then the inhalation happens naturally. So this can be one way to help develop the rhythm correctly.

8. Sit with a straight spine and inhale only through the nose while extending the arms directly out to the sides parallel to the ground while maintaining a lock at the elbows. The hands are maintained with the fingers spread wide and loose. In this position the eyes are closed (see Figure 2.12). Then quickly bring the hands toward each other meeting about 6 inches apart directly in front of the body without letting the hands touch, and this movement is made while exhaling through the nose. The eyes are opened when the hands come close together (4–6 inches apart) (see Figure 2.13). Continue to rapidly repeat the movement for 2 minutes and make sure that the eyes and breathing phases are correctly synchronized with the movement of the arms. The pace of the complete move-

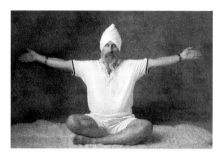
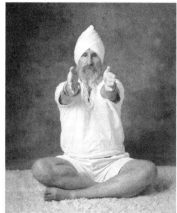

Figures 2.12 and 2.13
Exercise With Arms Extended Out to Sides and
With Arms 6 Inches Apart in Front

ment can approach one cycle every 1 to 2 seconds. This is a brain exercise that mimics the opening and closing of a camera shutter, which helps to coordinate the brain and increases the mental focus.

9. Stand up with the arms extended and raised directly above the head as if reaching for the sky, and inhale when coming up. Then slowly bend forward at the waist without bending the knees and with the head coming toward the ground in front of the body. When the head comes down, the arms swing up behind the body as if reaching up toward the sky. The exhalation through the nose is produced in this phase of the exercise. Start slowly and eventually speed up the pace. Continue for 2 minutes.

10. Sat Kriya is the final exercise in this set. It is practiced by sitting on the heels with the knees brought together in front, and the tops of the feet are then flat on the ground under the buttocks (see Figure 2.14). It is also possible to do Sat Kriya sitting in a chair. The arms are positioned straight up over the head with the upper arms pressed lightly against the sides of the head. The elbows are locked in an effort to keep the arms straight, and the hands are brought together and the fingers of the right and left hands are in-

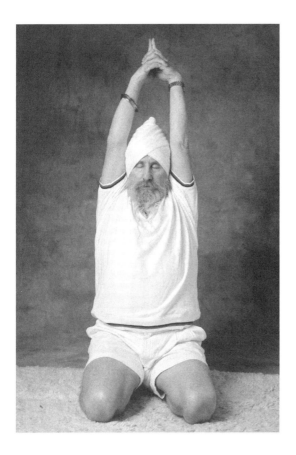

Figure 2.14
Sat Kriya

terlocked with only the two index fingers pointing straight up. For males, the right thumb crosses over the left thumb in the interlacing of the fingers and the left little finger is the last finger on the outside with this interlock. For females, the interlacing is reversed, with the right little finger on the outside and the left thumb dominating over the right thumb. The eyes are closed and focused at the third eye point where the eyebrows meet at the root of the nose. The bij mantra Sat Nam is chanted out loud with this exercise. While maintaining this position, the navel point is pulled in toward the back of the spine and simultaneously the muscle between the rectum and sex organ is tightened in what is called root lock. When the navel point is pulled in, the effort will also lead to what is called diaphragm lock. During the simultaneous pulling of the navel point and tightening of the lower muscle, the sound "Sat" is chanted quickly, almost like a cracking sound, and then the abdominal muscles and muscle between the sex organ and rectum are briefly relaxed while the sound "Naam" is chanted quickly. Yogi Bhajan helped to clarify the fine details of this practice by explaining: "Often when you try to do Sat Kriya from the Navel Point, you incorrectly try to apply one of the locks instead of starting with the navel. If you do Sat Kriya and just apply the root lock you temporarily raise your blood pressure. If you do Sat Kriya just with the diaphragm lock, you temporarily lower the blood pressure. Actually in Sat Kriya the locks come from an automatic involvement" (personal communication, date unknown). So the Corrective guiding statement is "Do Sat Kriya only from the Navel Point and the two locks should become little helpers automatically in balance." When chanting "Sat" the mantra sounds more like "Sut." When the sound "Sat (Sut)" is chanted mentally visualize healing energy and light coming in the navel point and traveling up the spine to the center of the head. While chanting "Nam," visualize the energy and light traveling out from the center of the head and out through the third eye point. This entire exercise is fairly rapid and rhythmic and is repeated eight times in 10 seconds. It should not be chanted faster or slower and there can be a tendency to either chant too fast or too slowly. Be careful not to flex the spine during the exercise, although sometimes the shoulders will rise up slightly during the practice. The practice time here is 2 minutes. Frequently a student will ask about when to inhale and exhale. The best answer here is that the breath regulates itself and it is not necessary to focus on the breath. By pulling and releasing the navel rhythmically, the breath will join in to support the process. Trying to focus on the breath only leads to confusion on how to practice this exercise. Also, it is important to note that the spine stays still and straight. The rhythmic contraction and relaxation produces waves of energy that circulate, energize, and heal the body. This is neither a spinal flex nor a pelvic thrust. The practitioner should remain firmly seated on the heels throughout the motions of this exercise. To end the practice at 2 minutes, inhale and gently squeeze the muscles from the buttocks all the way up along the spine. Hold the muscles tight for 5–10 seconds as you concentrate on the top of the head. Then exhale completely. Inhale, exhale totally, and hold the breath out as you contract the lower pelvis, lift the diaphragm, lock the chin to straighten the cervical vertebrae, and squeeze all the muscles from the buttocks up to the neck. Hold the breath out for 5 to 20 seconds according to your comfort and capacity. Then inhale and relax, and immediately proceed to the rest, exercise 11. If this technique is practiced by itself, then one should also rest and relax on the back for two times the practice time. Sat Kriya can also be practiced for longer times—11, 31, or 62 minutes, or the maximum time of 2 hours and 31 minutes. When there is an effort to practice for longer times, focus your attention on perfecting the form, rhythm, and the visual and mental concentration efforts. When building up the time, start with rotation cycles of 3 minutes of Sat Kriya with 2 minutes of relaxation. This 3 minute–2 minute cycle can be repeated 3 to 5 times and then the cycle can be increased to 5 minutes of Sat Kriya and 5 minutes of rest. Then times of 3 to 5 minutes can more easily be added to the kriya, depending on the practitioner's ability. Sat Kriya is the master exercise in Kundalini yoga. It works to heal the nervous and glandular systems, and it helps to correct, open, and balance all eight chakras. The ultimate result of this technique is that it can lead to "a nervous system that is as strong as steel and steady as stone" when practiced consistently for the 31 minute and greater times. This is an excellent technique for people who are trying to recover from the ravaging effects of substance abuse and addiction, which have a destructive effect on the nervous system and the chakras.

11. When finished with Sat Kriya, relax on the back while maintaining the arms relaxed by the sides with the palms facing up and both legs straight out in front of the body with the heels kept together. This posture is called corpse pose or shavasana. Deeply relax in this posture for 10 minutes.

*3. Gan Puttee Kriya: A Technique to Help Eliminate Negativity
From the Past, Present, and the Future*

Sit with a straight spine, either on the floor or in a chair. The backs of your hands are resting on your knees with the palms facing upward. The eyes are nine tenths closed (one tenth open, but looking straight ahead into the darkness at the third eye point, not the light below). Chant from your heart in a natural, relaxed manner, or chant in a steady relaxed monotone. Chant out loud the sound "Sa" (the *a* sounds like "ah"), and touch your thumb tips and index finger tips together quickly and simultaneously with about 2 pounds of pressure. Then chant "Ta" and touch the thumb tips to the middle finger tips. Chant "Na" and touch the thumb tips to the ring finger tips. then chant "Ma" and touch the thumb tips to the little finger tips. Chant "Ra" and touch your thumb tips and index finger tips. Chant "Ma" and touch the thumb tips to the middle finger tips. Chant "Da" and touch the thumb tips to the ring finger tips. Chant "Sa" and touch the thumb tips to the little finger tips. Chant "Sa" and touch your thumb tips and index finger tips. Chant "Say" (sounds like the word *say* with a long *a*) and touch the thumb tips to the middle finger tips. Chant "So" and touch the thumb tips to the ring finger tips. Chant "Hung" and touch the thumb tips to the little finger tips.

Chant at a rate of one sound per second. The thumb tip and fingertips touch with a very light 2 to 3 pounds of pressure with each connection. This helps to consolidate the circuit created by each thumb-finger link. Start with 11 minutes and slowly work up to 31 minutes of practice. To finish, remain in the sitting posture and inhale, holding the breath for 20 to 30 seconds while you shake and move every part of your body with the hands and arms extended over your head. Exhale and repeat this inhale, hold, and shaking two more times to circulate the energy and to break the pattern of tapping, which affects the brain. Then immediately proceed with focusing the eyes on the tip of the nose (the end you cannot see) and breathe slowly and deeply for 1 minute.

The sounds used in this meditation are each unique, and they have a powerful effect on the mind, both the conscious and subconscious mind. The sound "Sa" gives the mind the ability to expand to the infinite. "Ta" gives the mind the ability to experience the totality of life. "Na" gives the mind the ability to conquer death. "Ma" gives the mind the ability to resurrect. "Ra" gives the mind the ability to expand in radiance (this sound purifies and energizes). "Da" gives the mind the ability to establish security on the earth plane, providing a ground for action. "Say" gives the totality of experience. "So" is the personal sense of identity, and "Hung" is the infinite as a vibrating and real force. Together, "So Hung" means "I am Thou." The unique qualities of this 12-syllable mantra help cleanse and restructure the subconscious mind and help heal the conscious mind to ultimately experience the superconscious mind. Thus, all the blocks that result from an extreme traumatic event are eliminated over time with the practice of Gan Puttee Kriya.

4. A Meditation to Help Combat Delusions and to Help Stabilize a Healthy Sense of Self-Identity

This meditation was first taught by Yogi Bhajan on April 19, 2000, in Espanola, New Mexico, and is identified as #NM0342. Yogi Bhajan taught this technique for those who have an overloaded subconscious mind and for those who get stuck in their neuroses and psychoses, and where one result is that a haunting thought remains in the conscious mind. He said this technique is useful when "fantasy overextends to the point that you start believing it, and finally you become that. When reality, earth and the heavenly fantasies do not meet together, we get in trouble." In that condition, he said, "What is keeping you bound down to your lower self? It is your neurosis. You are stuck in your neuroses. You are trapped. You love your ego more than your identity. In God I trust, is what you have to learn." This is a perfect meditation technique for people who are lost in their neurosis and psychosis and with their sense of self and identity—the condition that manifests when a person becomes delusional. This technique helps to establish a healthy state of mental stability and is most appropriate for the schizophrenic with a weakened identity who is questioning the deep self.

This technique can be practiced while sitting in a chair and maintaining a straight spine, or while sitting on the floor and maintaining a straight spine. Both arms are raised out to the sides (see Figure 2.15) and the elbows are bent at 90 degree angles so that the forearms are pointing straight up. The hands face forward. The eyes are open and focused at the tip of the nose (the end point that you cannot see). The mantra "Humee Hum Brahm Hum" is chanted. The mantra is most effective when it is chanted to the rhythm in a CD (*Humee Hum and Peace and Tranquillity*, Kaur, Nirinian.). In rhythm with the mantra, touch the top of your head with the left hand (see Figure 2.16) while chanting "Humee Hum" and blessing yourself. Then return to the original position while chanting "Brahm Hum." The meditation is continued for 11 minutes. To end the technique, inhale through the nose, hold the breath, and tighten the spine, and also stiffen only the left hand. Pull the energy of the spine into the left hand. Then exhale and repeat the breath holding and tightening two more times, and then relax. In part, the intention with this technique is to also learn to become kind, humble, helpful, and compassionate.

Additional Meditation Techniques for Schizophrenics

Other meditation techniques in this book would also be most useful for helping to treat patients with the nine variants of the psychoses. There are two techniques in Chapter 3 for treating the personality disorders that would be appropriate: (1) the multipart meditation to release pressure from the subconscious mind and overcome compulsive behavior patterns, and (2) a meditation technique to help overcome all psychological weaknesses. Five techniques in Chapter 4 for treating the pervasive developmental disorders would also be most beneficial, including (1) the meditation to balance and synchronize the cerebral hemispheres, (2) the meditation for balancing the brain hemispheres, (3) a meditation to balance the western hemisphere of the brain with the base of the

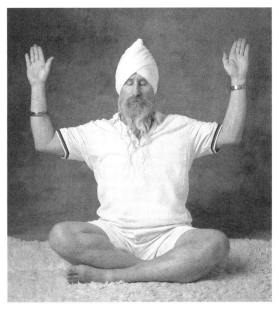

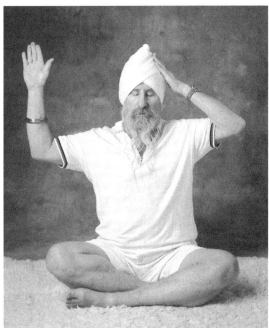

Figures 2.15 and 2.16
Meditation to Help Combat Delusions and to Help Stabilize
a Healthy Sense of Self-Identity

eastern hemisphere, (4) the meditation to balance the two brain hemispheres and to correct any spiritual, mental, and physical imbalance, and (5) a meditation to correct language and communication disorders—Ad Nad Kriya. These seven meditation techniques would be best as single additions to the Protocol for Treating the Variants of Schizophrenia. To date, that protocol, including the True Glue exercise set, Gan Puttee Kriya, and a meditation to help combat delusions and to help stabilize a healthy sense of self-identity, has been the most widely tested and it has always been successful for treating schizophrenic patients. It is also a very balanced and comprehensive protocol and should be appropriate for all patients with any of the nine variants of the psychoses. In some cases, it may also be more beneficial to add one of these seven additional meditation techniques. All seven are completely balanced as individual techniques and they will only add to the positive and more rapid treatment for this patient population. They are not overstimulating, nor are they likely to take the patient too far into the etheric realms if they are practiced with the initial suggested treatment times.

One caution must be taken with schizophrenic patients, and that is they should not practice techniques that are too powerful and specifically meant to exclusively and directly open chakras five through eight. However, none of the techniques that are described in this chapter, or referred to as possible substitutions in the other chapters, are too powerful for the psychotic patient when they are practiced for the specified length of time.

A Four-Part Miniprotocol for Helping to Terminate Hallucinations*

This protocol is best applied as soon as the patient begins to experience any hallucinations or has any prodromal symptoms of onset that he or she can detect based on past experience. The evidence to date suggests that the best and quickest results are achieved if the patient can begin the practice within the first 10 minutes or earlier. While the intent here is to have the patient sit down and practice the entire protocol, the first two steps can be started if the patient is not in a place where this is possible, and it is not possible for the patient to close his or her eyes or openly practice any meditation techniques. The four-part protocol is as follows.

1. Technique to Induce a Meditative State

Use the tuning in technique (see the description and Figure 2.1 for a Protocol for Treating the Variants of Schizophrenia).

2. Technique for Meeting Mental Challenges: The Victory Breath

This technique can be used at any time (Shannahoff-Khalsa, 1997, 2003, 2005, 2006). It does not require that the practitioner is sitting. It can be employed while driving a car, while participating in a conversation, or while taking a test. This technique can be applied anytime the patient is beginning to experience stress or has any prodromal signs of a hallucination, or of course while having an episode of hallucinations. The eyes can be open or closed, depending on the situation.

Take a nearly full breath through the nose. Hold this breath without straining or tensing the stomach muscles for exactly 3 to 4 seconds and only during this hold phase mentally say to yourself the three separate sounds *vic, tor, y*, then exhale. Mentally creating the three separated sounds should take 3 to 4 seconds, no longer or less. The entire time of each repetition should take about 8 to 10 seconds. The breath should not be exaggerated to the extent that anyone would even notice that you are taking a deep breath. While it can be employed multiple times until you achieve the desired relief when it is not being practiced in the four-part protocol, the practice times here for the protocol are 5 to 11 minutes. Sitting with a straight spine with the eyes closed will help to maximize the benefits. There is no upper time limit for its practice.

3. The Right Nostril Four-Part Breath
Using the Mantra Sa Ta Na Ma

Sit in a chair with the feet flat on the ground or in an easy cross-legged pose and maintain a straight spine. The left hand is raised up in front of the face and the left thumb tip is used to block the end of the left nostril. The remaining fingers point straight up and the palm faces toward the right. The elbow of the left hand is relaxed by the side to help avoid producing tension in the left arm and shoulder. The right hand is relaxed in the lap with the palm facing up, and the tip of the right index finger is touching the tip of the right thumb, forming the mudra called gyan mudra. The eyes are closed. The breath pattern is exclusively practiced through the right nostril even if it is slightly congested and if it feels completely blocked. It is still possible to breathe through a congested nostril, and with a little practice the congestion usually reduces. The inhalation and exhalation phases are both broken into four approximately equal steps where the first step involves inhaling to fill the lungs approximately to one-fourth volume, and then the second part fills the lungs to approximately one-half lung volume, and the third step to approximately to three-fourths capacity, and the final step to full capacity. However, in practice the lungs are never stretched to full capacity. The above description is meant to help provide an understanding that each part of the breath is about one-fourth of the lung volume. No strain is required here and it is not mandatory to fill the lungs to full capacity. However, the breath should be somewhat forceful, and it is definitely not a light, timid, or weak breath effort. The same pattern is repeated in four parts when emptying the lungs with equal force. The rate of the full breath cycle should take about 5 seconds to complete the inhalation and exhalation phases. This pattern is called a four-part breath. Instead of counting the four parts using numbers, the mantra Sa Ta

Na Ma is mentally recited with each of the four sounds paired to each of the four breath parts on both the inhalation and exhalation phases. This then includes two cycles of the Sa Ta Na Ma mantra per breath cycle. The mantra is repeated through once on the inhalation and once on the exhalation. This mantra is called the Panj Shabd, which means the five primal sounds of the universe. The sound Sa gives the mind the ability to expand to the infinite. Ta gives the mind the ability to experience the totality of life. Na gives the mind the ability to conquer death. Ma gives the mind the ability to resurrect. A fifth sound is the *ah* sound that is common to all four sounds here. This technique is practiced for 11 minutes.

4. The Silent L-Form Meditation Technique Using the Mantra Sa Ta Na Ma

This technique is practiced immediately after doing step 3. The spine remains straight and the patient now sits with both hands resting on the knees with the palms facing up, and the tips of the index fingers are touching the tips of the thumbs on the respective hands. The eyes are kept closed with this technique and the patient mentally visualizes the four separate syllables of the Sa Ta Na Ma mantra in what is called the L-form meditation. The patient visualizes a white or gold light and healing energy coming in through the top center of the head while mentally hearing the sound of *S* as it comes down to the middle of the head, and then the *ah* sound is heard as it exits out through the third eye region (the point where the eyebrows meet and where the nose has its origin). This is the use of the sound Sa but where it is more clearly differentiated with the two parts. Note, the mantra is heard silently; the mantra is not chanted out loud. The healing light is visualized as the light comes in and goes out. The same process is practiced for the three remaining sounds of Ta, Na, and Ma, where each sound is slightly broken into its respective two components. The entire cycle for the four-part mantra takes about 3 to 5 seconds. This is practiced for 11 minutes. The breath is not regulated here.

Case Histories of Treatment

Case History 1: A Case of First-Episode Schizophrenia and a History of Substance Abuse

Eric presented in 1993. He was an 18-year-old Caucasian male attending his senior year in high school. He was from a wealthy divorced family. His mother had sole legal and physical custody, and he had irregular and only occasional visits with his father during holidays. Eric's mother was a corporate executive and worked extended hours. His parents had divorced when he was 12 years old. He had one sister, age 21, living away from home and attending college. When I asked Eric's mother about any unusual and significant stressors in Eric's life, she reported that her labor with him had lasted 30 hours and the delivery was much more difficult than when she delivered her daughter. She added that during the marriage the father was inattentive to all family members, and especially to the children. He traveled frequently for work, often for 1 to 2 weeks at a time. She reported that Eric's father was a "problem drinker," frequently angry, and she suspected that he had had a series of extramarital affairs. Eric's scholastic skills were mediocre. During Eric's adolescent years, he had several good friendships with male peers; however, he did not date nor did he have significant female friends. He began experimenting with alcohol and cannabis at age 12. At age 16 he began experimenting with psychedelic drugs (LSD, mescaline, and ecstasy or MDMA). In his senior year, Eric began having extended flashbacks that he found troubling and disruptive. He then started skipping school. His mother was notified of his absenteeism, whereupon he and his mother met with the school counselor. Eric then admitted to his early extensive cannabis and alcohol use, and that he been experimenting with psychedelic drugs for the previous 2 years. He also said that he was now experiencing intermittent but aggravating flashbacks that he found to be "too disruptive" in his life. His hallucinations included time distortions, visual distortions of people's faces and other ob-jects, and the "undulating-like" movement of the ground. He also recalled hearing voices of people that he knew, and at other times these were the voices of strangers.

His mother knew about my research with Kundalini yoga and that I worked privately with people that had psychiatric disorders. She was not interested in having Eric medicated with antipsychotic drugs, and she decided to bring him to me to see if I could teach him something to help him overcome his hallucinations. Fortu-nately, Eric realized that he had to end his psychedelic drug use once he started having hallucinations. When I first saw Eric, he was having hallucinations almost every day. Sometimes they would last for 2 to 3 hours at a time, and this had been going on for at least a month. While he thought he could hide his inner world from those around him, he also knew that he could no longer man-age his schoolwork.

Eric was the first adolescent psychotic patient that I treated using the True Glue exercise set. At that time I had not yet learned Gan Puttee Kriya or a meditation to help combat delusions and to help stabilize a healthy sense of self-dentity. Eric started coming for private 1-hour yoga classes three times per week. Fortunately, he enjoyed the effects of the exercise set the very first time. He commented on how much "calmer and more stable" he felt after the set. While he was originally hesitant, he also knew he had to do something to help himself, and he too was not keen on taking med-ications. The first time I saw him was a Friday afternoon, and he said that he also felt calmer and more stable the next day and that he only had minimal visual distortions. On Sunday he again started having some hallucinations, but they were not nearly as intense or as long as they had been previous to his yoga class. He was eager to continue attending, although he did not find the interest to prac-tice on his own at home for the first 2 weeks. During this time, however, he remarked that his hallucinations had become much less severe and that they had lasted for much shorter time periods, and sometimes only for periods of 10 to 15 minutes. After 2 weeks of therapy he thought he might try to do some of the exercises on his own at home. After 1 month of therapy he noticed a major shift and change in his life and that he was no longer having hallucinations. I saw him for a total of 6 weeks, three times per week. Eric decided to give up using drugs and alcohol and realized that they had almost destroyed his life. After 5 weeks of therapy he returned to school and graduated after attending extra classes in the summer session.

Case History 2: A Simple Case of First Episode Schizophrenia

The following is a short case history for a patient in São Paulo, Brazil, who was treated under my supervision by Rodrigo Yacubian Fernandes, MD, a physician and Kundalini yoga teacher who requested my guidance in treatment. Daniel is a single male, 21 years of age. He had worked as an office boy, cashier, and salesperson in a bookstore since the age of 15. His employment was concurrent with his attendance in high school. He also played soccer and participated in local theater. He had good friendships during his elementary and high school years, and he had a girlfriend for 3 years during high school. However, he became very sad when his girlfriend terminated their relationship, which also coincided with the end of high school. At the same time his grandmother, to whom he had a very deep and loving connection, died. After her death, he was raised in a "nonsolid" family situation. His father and mother argued all of the time and they started to have serious relationship problems. They were divorced in 2005. This was a very difficult and stressful time for Daniel. In addition to the stress of his family relationships, he attempted to endure the stress of passing the test to get into a university. The test was difficult and he made several unsuccessful efforts to pass over a 3-year period.

Daniel started to be delusional in June 2008, when he started to exhibit very abnormal behavior. He became aggressive toward others, which was very uncharacteristic of his personality and behavior. He was hospitalized beginning in June 2008 for 39 days in a psychiatric ward in a major hospital in São Paulo. After several days of observation, the doctors diagnosed him with schizophrenia. During his hospitalization he was started on Risperdal 6 mg per day. The attending psychiatrist requested that Dr. Fernandes attempt to teach him Kundalini yoga as a possible adjunctive therapy. Initially, while in the hospital, he was taught to use the mantra for tuning in (Ong Namo Guru Dev Namo), spine flexes, shoulder shrugs, Gan Puttee Kriya, and Sat Kriya. He was not inclined to practice the entire multipart True Glue exercise set. Daniel commented, "I am practicing every day. It is helping me to find my equilibrium." He later said, "After my stay at the psychiatric hospital and starting to practice Kundalini yoga, I could start to see the world in a different and more aware way."

After Daniel's release from the hospital, he started to practice the entire True Glue protocol, and he eventually achieved the ability to practice Sat Kriya for 7–11 minutes. He also increased his time with Gan Puttee Kriya to 31 minutes almost every day. He started to "feel better and better." From early October 2008 to the last week of November, his Risperdal was reduced from 6 mg to 1 mg. After the first week of December, he was both free of medication and free of all symptoms. As of February 2009, he remained asymptomatic and medication free, and he says he now feels very confident in himself. In early January 2009 he got a new job at a music store in São Paulo that he enjoys, and he also plans to renew his studies for gaining entrance to the university. In the beginning of January 2009 he also ended his Kundalini yoga practice for some months, but later decided to again resume the practice, but not because of any renewal of symptoms. Daniel still holds the aspirations to attend a university.

One can also suggest that in Daniel's case the medication alone was the source of his recovery, and that was all he needed along with an opportunity to relax in the hospital while escaping from the stress and strain of his personal life. But he also had a firm conviction of the therapeutic benefits of the techniques that he practiced because he also claimed that he benefitted on a daily basis when he practiced the techniques.

Case History 3: A Case of Schizophreniform Disorder, Depression, and Post-Traumatic Stress Disorder

Monica presented at age 21 in 2007 with a diagnosis of schizophreniform disorder, depression, and post-traumatic stress disorder (PTSD). Her child and adolescent years were unremarkable, with the exception that her parents went through a bitter and expensive divorce when she was 16 years of age. Her mother remarried 3 years later to a physician who had two older children from a previous marriage, both of whom were married. At the time of Monica's parents' divorce, she had two older siblings, a brother aged 20 and a sister aged 22, attending universities out of state. Monica also started attending a university out of state after high school. While both of her older siblings had pursued an education in law, to follow in their father's footsteps as a highly successful criminal attorney, Monica was undecided about her future career, with the exception that she knew that she did not want to go into law. During her freshman year she passed her courses with average grades. In the beginning of her second year she decided that apartment living was more likely to give her the active social life that she missed during her freshman year. She attended more off-campus parties and found herself engaging in frequent weekend binge drinking with her cohorts. While she had an occasional date with college men during her sophomore year, she had no stable or romantic relationships. In the middle of her sophomore year she became the victim of a date rape drug while attending a fraternity party. She chose not to report the event to the university or to the local police. She was dreadfully ashamed, felt guilty, and tried to hide the incident because she feared the terrible stigma that she knew it would carry. She did not want to become known on campus as "the girl that got raped." She started binge drinking in a frenzy, her class attendance dropped, and her grades plummeted. She became very anxious and depressed and began to isolate herself in her apartment. She attempted to manage her fears, anxiety, and moods by self-medicating with illegally obtained benzodiazepines and amphetamines. She had fears of being raped again and fears of retribution by her unknown assailant. While she could see an image of him in her mind, she could not see his face. She soon started hearing voices of people that were not there along with nightmares of the initial event and having it reoccur. She stopped talking with men because she was afraid that at any time her rapist might attack her again. She did not know who he was and thought that being reclusive might help keep her safe. Realizing that she was in a downward spiral and not able to get back to her studies, she finally sought help with the psychological counseling services at her university. The psychologist advised her to return to her mother's home and take a break from school until she recovered. The school psychiatrist prescribed daily citalopram (40 mg), risperidone (2 mg), and alprazolam (0.5 mg) on an as-needed basis.

Monica's mother had previously seen me for her own stress management and anxiety, and she realized that I might be able to help her daughter. When I first saw Monica, her hallucinations were mostly controlled by her medications, but she also had some numbing, dissociation, intermittent generalized and situational hyperarousal, anxiety, depression, and fears of a recurrent event. She understood that she had classic symptoms of PTSD. The alprazolam helped to reduce some of her anxiety symptoms when they became severe. However, she also felt too lethargic after taking it and knew that it was not a long-term solution. She was afraid of becoming addicted to it, and her desire was to ultimately regain her life free of medication. She had been athletic during most of her adolescent years, with private training in modern dance and gymnastics during high school. While she had never tried yoga, she was open to it and she trusted in her mother's opinion. She believed that it might be a good option for her.

At our first meeting, Monica's primary and most severe symptoms were related to her PTSD, anxiety, and depression. Her hallucinations, although very disturbing, were less frequent. Therefore, since she identified what hurt most, I decided that her initial introduction to Kundalini yoga should be with the eight-part meditation protocol for PTSD (Shannahoff-Khalsa, 2006). Her mother also attended the appointment and participated in the practice. Monica was still not willing to be alone with men. At the end of the practice, her mother remarked, "This is the first time that I have seen you smile since you have been home." At that point they both gave each other a big hug. I saw both of them again twice a week for the next 6 weeks. After the first week, Monica stopped using the alprazolam altogether. After the first month I taught them the True Glue exercise set prior to the PTSD protocol and followed that with a meditation to help combat delusions and to help stabilize a healthy sense of self-identity. Since the PTSD protocol has Gan Puttee Kriya in it, I thought that maintaining that multipart protocol would help to be completely comprehensive for her comorbidities. These classes took about 2.5 hours, but both of them thought that it was worth the time and effort, and they were hopeful that Monica would achieve a full recovery. They were also very appreciative of the bonding that came from their joint efforts in class and how this was helping them to build a much closer mother-daughter relationship. They both noticed over time how Monica's mood and anxiety levels were improving and how she was beginning to be more open with non-family members. She was also no longer having any hallucinations or dissociative events, and her numbing and reactivity were substantially reduced. Eventually, Monica decided that she could see me by herself. Her mother had encouraged this as an important step for her in therapy. I continued to see Monica twice a week for two more months. During the first month she decided to attempt to discontinue her Risperdal. Her psychiatrist agreed to her decision. She reduced it to 1 mg per day for 2 weeks without any renewal of symptoms, and she then discontinued it completely after another 2 weeks. In the second month she reduced her citalopram to 20 mg, again without a renewal of symptoms. After those 2 months, I saw her once every 2 weeks for two more months. Shortly thereafter she reentered the university. However, she decided that the party life was no longer an option for her and for the time being, she did not want to have close male friends. She decided to major in psychology, and she continued to practice Kundalini yoga on her own as a form of stress management.

Case History 4: A Complex Case With Severe Hallucinations and Delusions, Bipolar Disorder, and Narcissistic and Borderline Personality Disorders

This case is presented in Chapter 5 as a unique example of a multimorbid and very complex case with successful treatment. The case of Elizabeth is a lengthy patient self-described case history. Elizabeth has been my most difficult, problematic, and complex case to date.

THREE

Treating the Personality Disorders

Paranoid, Schizoid, Schizotypal, Histrionic, Narcissistic, Antisocial, Borderline, Avoidant, Dependent, and Obsessive-Compulsive Personality Disorders

On the tombs of kings you will find pigeon droppings
And on the tombs of saints you will find candles lit.
Yogi Bhajan, date unknown

If there is a purpose other than compassion in the
relationships in your life, you will also find pain in those
relationships.
Yogi Bhajan, date unknown

Subtypes and Diagnostic Features, Prevalence, and Results Using Conventional Treatment Modalities

The modern study of personality disorders in the West began with that of antisocial behavior in the early 19th century by the French psychiatrist Philippe Pinel, who is regarded by many as the father of modern psychiatry (Weiner, 1999). Pinel coined the phrase *manie sans delire* (insanity without delusions) to describe the psychopathic personality (Pinel, 1801). Today these patients are diagnosed as having an antisocial personality disorder. Specifically, Pinel described these patients as lacking in impulse control. They often rage when frustrated and are prone to outbursts of violence, but are not subject to delusions. Pinel's overall goal was to isolate, identify, and classify mental illnesses, which he divided into five major categories: melancholia, nondelirious furor, delirium, dementia, and idiocy. Pinel is also well known for his pioneering humanistic treatment efforts for removing the chains from patients at the Paris Asylum for insane women, and also for the use of "moral [psychological] treatment" with the insane. Shortly after Pinel's publication, independently, the famous American physician Benjamin Rush described a similar condition that he called "moral derangement" or "anomia," that is, ethical derangement (Rush, 1812). These patients were morally deranged, yet had intact intellectual and reasoning abilities and engaged in socially disruptive behaviors and deception from early in life and did not show remorse, guilt, or preoccupation with the negative consequences of their actions.

"Increasingly, cases of insanity became known where the patients did not seem to dwell in some delusive state. They displayed deep sullenness, unmitigated fury, utter shamelessness, seemingly without either purpose or motivation" (Augstein, 1996). Here, Augstein refers to the work of British physician James Cowles Prichard, who published his famous *Treatise on Insanity, and Other Disorders Affecting the Mind*, in 1835 wherein he endeavored to explain this derangement of one's mental faculties and poor moral faculty, which he labeled a "moral insanity." Prichard described this moral insanity as "a morbid perversion of the natural feelings, affections, inclinations, temper, habits, moral dispositions, and natural impulses without any remarkable disorder or defect of the intellect or knowing or reasoning faculties and in particular without any insane delusion or hallucination." Prichard also described the psychopathic personality: "A propensity to theft is sometimes a feature of moral insanity and sometimes it is its leading if not sole characteristic. When however such phenomena are observed in connection with a wayward and intractable temper with a decay of social affections, an aversion to the nearest relatives and friends formerly beloved—in short, with a change in the moral character of the individual, the case becomes tolerably well marked." Prichard also described at least partial characteristics of what the APA defines as a Cluster A personality disorder (see definition below): "Eccentricity of conduct, singular and absurd habits, a propensity to perform the common actions of life in a different way from that usually practiced, is a feature of many cases of moral insanity but can hardly be said to contribute sufficient evidence of its existence."

Fifty years later, the English physician Henry Maudsley used the phrase "moral insanity" to describe a patient: "Having no capacity for true moral feeling—all his impulses and desires, to which he yields without check, are egoistic, his conduct appears to be governed by immoral motives, which are cherished and obeyed without any evident desire to resist them" (Maudsley, 1874; Pinel & Maudsley, 1977). But Maudsley also disapproved of the term "moral insanity" and said, "It is a form of mental alienation which has so much the look of vice or crime that many people regard it as an unfounded medical invention" (Maudsley, 1874).

At the end of the 19th century, the German doctor J. L. Koch published *Die Psychopatischen Minderwertigkeiter*, where he made an effort to classify the condition scientifically rather than morally, and he coined the phrase "psychopathic inferiority" to replace the phrase "moral insanity" (Koch, 1891). Psychopathic inferiority was later changed to "psychopathic personality" in an effort to overcome the poor choice and stigma of the word *inferiority* (Millon & Davis, 2000). After the turn of the century, Emile Kraepelin, who had been influenced by Prichard's view of the morally insane and Koch's work on personality disorders, wrote in his famous book series *Psychiatrie: Ein Lehrbuch* about psychopathic personalities (Kraepelin, 1913), and he described six psychopathic personality types that were not attributable to any specific clinical syndrome or disease process (Herve & Yuille, 2007). These six psychopathies were called the born criminals, the unstables, the morbid liars, the pseudo-querulants (i.e., self-centered and egocentric individuals with subclinical forms of paranoia), the excitables, the impulsives, and the eccentrics (Herve & Yuille, 2007).

In 1950, the German psychiatrist Kurt Schneider published *The Psychopathic Personality* and proposed an extensive list of 10 psychopathic personalities (Schneider, 1958). While Kraepelin used value-laden terminology, Schneider's focus was on using descriptions defining how the individual or society would suffer. Herve and Yuille (2007) summarized this list with clear descriptions:

> the *hyperthermic* (i.e., cheerful, overly optimistic, and boastful individuals with elevated moods who constantly start new projects but lack endurance in their activities); the *depressive* (i.e., pessimistic individuals characterized by predominantly depressed mood); the *insecure* (i.e., anxious individuals with high standards, inner uncertainty, and feeling of insufficiency); the *fanatic* (i.e., individuals with prevailing, or overvalued, ideas which control and confine them); the *attention-seeking* (i.e., entitled, boastful, and dramatic individuals who, in their quest to appear better than they are, are prone to manipulate and deceive those around them); the *labile* (i.e., individuals with labile and reactionary emotions, especially depressive ones); the *explosive* (i.e., impulsive individuals with violent affective outbreaks to seemingly innocuous situations); the *affectionless* (i.e., callous, remorseless, deceptive, and incorrigible individuals with emotional dullness towards others and a propensity to engage in criminal activities); the *weak-willed* (i.e., shallow, chameleon-like individuals who appear to have few motivations of their own and, consequently, are at the whim of their environment); and the *asthenic* (i.e., highly nervous and anxious individuals who are prone to psychosomatic complications.

Herve and Yuille (2007) noted that the clinical construct of psychopathy by Pinel, Rush, Prichard, Kraepelin, Schneider, and others in the 19th and early 20th centuries did not lead to one definition. This left psychiatry in a state of confusion regarding the diagnostic boundaries of the term *psychopathy*, and they concluded that this led to the "wastebasket effect" for clinical syndromes and personality disorders, and too often a wrongful diagnosis based on value judgments rather than sound clinical observations.

Herve and Yuille also summarized at length the significant contributions of others (Partridge, Henderson, Karpman, Arieti, McCord, Cleckley, and Hare) toward the earlier perspectives on psychopathic personalities, as well as commentary on the first *Diagnostic and Statistical Manual of Mental Disorders* (*DSM*) that included the term *sociopathy*. However, sociopathy is no longer in the *DSM*. Clearly, the earliest major works on personality disorders focused on antisocial personality disorder (Herve & Yuille, 2007). It is important to note, however, that the common meaning of the word *psychopath* today refers exclusively to the personality aberration of the extreme antisocial personality, an individual that wreaks havoc on society.

Today, the APA's *Diagnostic and Statistical Manual of Mental Disorders*, 4th edition, text revision (*DSM-IV-TR*) defines the much broader and all-inclusive group of 10 personality disorders as "an enduring pattern of inner experience and behavior that deviates markedly from the expectations of the individual's culture, is pervasive and inflexible, has an onset in adolescence or early adulthood, is stable over time, and leads to distress or impairment" (APA, 2000).

The APA ranks psychiatric disorders by levels or axes that include the different aspects of the disorder or disability. The first level, or Axis I disorders, includes the major mental as well as developmental and learning disorders and thus includes the anxiety disorders, depression, bipolar disorders, attention-deficit/hyperactivity disorder (ADHD), and schizophrenia. Axis II includes the personality disorders as well as mental retardation. Here is where all 10 different personality disorders are listed. Axis III is for any acute medical and physical condition including brain injuries. Axis

IV is for psychosocial and environmental factors contributing to the disorders, and Axis V is for the rating of the global assessment of functioning for children under age 18 (APA, 2000).

The systematic categorization of the personality disorders has evolved over time compared to the work of Kraepelin and others, but the current listing of 10 disorders has striking similarities to Schneider's list of 10 distinct disorders. For patients to satisfy the diagnostic criteria of a specific personality disorder, they must satisfy the following more general criteria and a certain number of the specific criteria listed for any one of the 10 unique personality disorders.

Besides the general but brief APA definition stated above, the APA also more clearly delineates the following six diagnostic features and their respective criteria (A through E) and states:

> The essential feature of a Personality Disorder is an enduring pattern of inner experience and behavior that deviates markedly from the expectations of the individual's culture and is manifested in at least two of the following areas: cognition, affectivity, interpersonal functioning, or impulse control (Criterion A). This enduring pattern is inflexible and pervasive across a broad range of personal and social situations (Criterion B) and leads to clinically significant distress or impairment in social, occupational, or other important areas of functioning (Criterion C). The pattern is stable and of long duration and its onset can be traced back at least to adolescence or early adulthood (Criterion D). The pattern is not better accounted for as a manifestation or consequence of another mental disorder (Criterion E) and is not due to the direct physiological effects of a substance (e.g., a drug of abuse, a medication, exposure to a toxin) or a general medical condition (e.g., head trauma) (Criterion F). (APA, 1994)

While children and adolescents are usually not diagnosed with a personality disorder, if they are, the symptoms must be present for at least 1 year. However, by definition, antisocial personality disorder cannot be used to label those under the age of 18 years.

The APA in the *DSM-IV* currently groups the 10 personality disorders into three separate groups or clusters; cluster A disorders are termed "odd-eccentric," cluster B disorders "dramatic-emotional," and cluster C disorders "anxious-fearful." This is because the disorders in each cluster have shared characteristics. Cluster A includes three separate disorders called respectively paranoid, schizoid, and schizotypal personality disorders. Cluster B includes four separate disorders called antisocial, borderline, histrionic, and narcissistic personality disorders. Cluster C includes the three called avoidant, dependent, and obsessive-compulsive personality disorders.

Cluster A Personality Disorders (Odd or Eccentric)

Paranoid Personality Disorder

According to the *DSM-IV-TR* (APA, 2000), the essential diagnostic criteria are as follows.

A. A pattern of pervasive distrust and suspiciousness of others such that their motives are interpreted as malevolent, beginning by early adulthood and present in a variety of contexts, as indicated by four (or more) of the following:

1. Suspects, without a sufficient basis, that others are exploiting, harming, or deceiving him or her.
2. Is preoccupied with unjustified doubts about the loyalty or trustworthiness of friends or associates.
3. Is reluctant to confide in others because of unwarranted fear that the information will be used maliciously against him or her.
4. Reads benign remarks or events as threatening or demeaning.
5. Persistently bears grudges, i.e., is unforgiving of insults, injuries, or slights.
6. Perceives attacks on his or her character or reputation that are not apparent to others and is quick to react angrily or to counterattack.
7. Has recurrent suspicions, without justification, regarding fidelity of spouse or sexual partner.

B. Does not occur exclusively during the course of Schizophrenia, a Mood Disorder with Psychotic Features, or another Psychotic Disorder and is not due to the direct physiological effects of a general medical condition. (APA, 2000)

Schizoid Personality Disorder

A. A pervasive pattern of detachment from social relationships and a restricted range of expression of emotions in interpersonal settings, beginning by early adulthood and present in a variety of contexts, as indicated by four (or more) of the following:

1. Neither desires nor enjoys close relationships, including being part of a family.
2. Almost always chooses solitary activities.
3. Has little, if any, interest in having sexual experiences with another person.
4. Takes pleasure in few, if any, activities.
5. Lacks close friends or confidants other than first-degree relatives.
6. Appears indifferent to the praise or criticism of others.
7. Shows emotional coldness, detachment, or flattened affectivity.

B. Does not occur exclusively during the course of Schizophrenia, a Mood Disorder with Psychotic Features, another Psychotic Disorder, or a Pervasive Developmental Disorder and is not due to the direct physiological effects of a general medical condition. (APA, 2000)

Schizotypal Personality Disorder

A. A pervasive pattern of social and interpersonal deficits marked by acute discomfort with, and reduced capacity for, close relationships as well as by cognitive or perceptual distortions and eccentricities of behavior, beginning by early adulthood and present in a variety of contexts, as indicated by five (or more) of the following:

1. Ideas of reference (excluding delusions of reference).
2. Odd beliefs or magical thinking that influences behavior and is inconsistent with subcultural norms (e.g., superstitiousness, be-

lief in clairvoyance, telepathy, or "sixth sense"; in children and adolescents, bizarre fantasies or preoccupations).

3. Unusual perceptual experiences, including bodily illusions.
4. Odd thinking and speech (e.g., vague, circumstantial, metaphorical, overelaborate, or stereotyped).
5. Suspiciousness or paranoid ideation.
6. Inappropriate or constricted affect.
7. Behavior or appearance that is odd, eccentric, or peculiar.
8. Lack of close friends or confidants other than first-degree relatives.
9. Excessive social anxiety that tends to be associated with paranoid fears rather than negative judgments about self.

B. Does not occur exclusively during the course of Schizophrenia, a Mood Disorder with Psychotic Features, another Psychotic Disorder, or a Pervasive Developmental Disorder. (APA, 2000)

Cluster B Personality Disorders (Dramatic or Emotional)

Antisocial Personality Disorder

A. There is a pervasive pattern of disregard for and violation of the rights of others occurring since age 15 years, as indicated by three or more of the following :

1. Failure to conform to social norms with respect to lawful behaviors as indicated by repeatedly performing acts that are grounds for arrest.
2. Deceitfulness, as indicated by repeatedly lying, use of aliases, or conning others for personal profit or pleasure.
3. Impulsivity or failure to plan ahead.
4. Irritability and aggressiveness, as indicated by repeated physical fights or assaults.
5. Reckless disregard for safety of self or others.
6. Consistent irresponsibility, as indicated by repeated failure to sustain consistent work behavior or honor financial obligations.
7. Lack of remorse, as indicated by being indifferent to or rationalizing having hurt, mistreated, or stolen from another.

B. The individual is at least age 18 years.

C. There is evidence of Conduct Disorder with onset before age 15 years.

D. The occurrence of antisocial behavior is not exclusively during the course of Schizophrenia or a Manic Episode. (APA, 2000)

Borderline Personality Disorder

The diagnostic criteria are defined as:

A pervasive pattern of instability of interpersonal relationships, self-image and affects, as well as marked impulsivity, beginning by early adulthood and present in a variety of contexts as indicated by five (or more) of the following:

1. Frantic efforts to avoid real or imagined abandonment. [Not including suicidal or self-mutilating behavior covered in Criterion 5.]

2. A pattern of unstable and intense interpersonal relationships characterized by alternating between extremes of idealization and devaluation.

3. Identity disturbance: markedly and persistently unstable self-image or sense of self.

4. Impulsivity in at least two areas that are potentially self-damaging (e.g., promiscuous sex, eating disorders, binge eating, substance abuse, reckless driving). [Again, not including suicidal or self-mutilating behavior covered in Criterion 5.]

5. Recurrent suicidal behavior, gestures, threats, or self-mutilating behavior such as cutting, interfering with the healing of scars, or picking at oneself.

6. Affective instability due to a marked reactivity of mood (e.g., intense episodic dysphoria, irritability, or anxiety usually lasting a few hours and only rarely more than a few days).

7. Chronic feelings of emptiness, worthlessness.

8. Inappropriate anger or difficulty controlling anger (e.g., frequent displays of temper, constant anger, recurrent physical fights).

9. Transient, stress-related paranoid ideation, delusions or severe dissociative symptoms. (APA, 2000)

Histrionic Personality Disorder

The diagnostic criteria are:

A pervasive pattern of excessive emotionality and attention seeking, beginning by early adulthood and present in a variety of contexts, as indicated by five (or more) of the following:

1. Is uncomfortable in situations in which he or she is not the center of attention.
2. Interaction with others is often characterized by inappropriate sexually seductive or provocative behavior.
3. Displays rapidly shifting and shallow expression of emotions.
4. Consistently uses physical appearance to draw attention to self.
5. Has a style of speech that is excessively impressionistic and lacking in detail.
6. Shows self-dramatization, theatricality, and exaggerated expression of emotion.
7. Is suggestible, i.e., easily influenced by others or circumstances.
8. Considers relationships to be more intimate than they actually are. (APA, 2000)

Narcissistic Personality Disorder

The diagnostic criteria are:

A pervasive pattern of grandiosity (in fantasy or behavior), need for admiration, and lack of empathy, beginning by early adulthood and present in a variety of contexts, as indicated by five (or more) of the following:

1. Has a grandiose sense of self-importance (e.g., exaggerates achievements and talents, expects to be recognized as superior without commensurate achievements).
2. Is preoccupied with fantasies of unlimited success, power, brilliance, beauty, or ideal love.
3. Believes that he or she is "special" and unique and can only be understood by, or should associate with, other special or high-status people (or institutions).

4. Requires excessive admiration.

5. Has a sense of entitlement i.e., unreasonable expectations of especially favorable treatment or automatic compliance with his or her expectations.

6. Is interpersonally exploitative, i.e., takes advantage of others to achieve his or her own ends.

7. Lacks empathy: is unwilling to recognize or identify with the feelings and needs of others.

8. Is often envious of others or believes others are envious of him or her.

9. Shows arrogant, haughty behaviors or attitudes. (APA, 2000)

Cluster C Personality Disorders (Anxious or Fearful)

Avoidant Personality Disorder

According to the *DSM-IV-TR*, the essential diagnostic criteria are defined as:

pervasive pattern of social inhibition, feelings of inadequacy, and hypersensitivity to negative evaluation, beginning by early adulthood and present in a variety of contexts, as indicated by four (or more) of the following:

1. Avoids occupational activities that involve significant interpersonal contact, because of fears of criticism, disapproval, or rejection.

2. Is unwilling to get involved with people unless certain of being liked.

3. Shows restraint initiating intimate relationships because of the fear of being shamed, ridiculed, or rejected due to severe low self-worth.

4. Is preoccupied with being criticized or rejected in social situations.

5. Is inhibited in new interpersonal situations because of feelings of inadequacy.

6. Views self as socially inept, personally unappealing, or inferior to others.

7. Is unusually reluctant to take personal risks or to engage in any new activities because they may prove embarrassing. (APA, 2000)

Dependent Personality Disorder

According to the *DSM-IV-TR*, the essential diagnostic criteria are defined as

pervasive and excessive need to be taken care of that leads to submissive and clinging behavior and fears of separation, beginning by early adulthood and present in a variety of contexts, as indicated by five (or more) of the following:

1. Has difficulty making everyday decisions without an excessive amount of advice and reassurance from others.
2. Needs others to assume responsibility for most major areas of his or her life.
3. Has difficulty expressing disagreement with others because of fear of loss of support or approval (this does not include realistic fears of retribution).
4. Has difficulty initiating projects or doing things on his or her own (because of a lack of self-confidence in judgment or abilities rather than a lack of motivation or energy).
5. Goes to excessive lengths to obtain nurturance and support from others, to the point of volunteering to do things that are unpleasant.
6. Feels uncomfortable or helpless when alone because of exaggerated fears of being unable to care for himself or herself.
7. Urgently seeks another relationship as a source of care and support when a close relationship ends.
8. Is unrealistically preoccupied with fears of being left to take care of himself or herself. (APA, 2000)

Obsessive-Compulsive Personality Disorder

According to the *DSM-IV-TR*, the essential diagnostic criteria are defined as

A pervasive pattern of preoccupation with orderliness, perfection-ism, and mental and interpersonal control, at the expense of flexi-bility, openness, and efficiency, beginning by early adulthood and present in a variety of contexts, as indicated by at least four (or more) of the following traits:

1. Is preoccupied with details, rules, lists, order, organization, or schedules to the extent that the major point of the activity is lost.
2. Shows perfectionism that interferes with task completion (e.g., is unable to complete a project because his or her own overly strict standards are not met).
3. Is excessively devoted to work and productivity to the exclusion of leisure activities and friendships (not accounted for by obvi-ous economic necessity).
4. Is over conscientious, scrupulous, and inflexible about matters of morality, ethics, or values (not accounted for by cultural or religious identification).
5. Is unable to discard worn-out or worthless objects even when they have no sentimental value.
6. Is reluctant to delegate tasks or to work with others unless they submit to exactly his or her way of doing things.
7. Adopts a miserly spending style toward both self and others; money is viewed as something to be hoarded for future catastro-phes.
8. Shows rigidity and stubbornness. (APA, 2000)

The *DSM-IV-TR* also includes "personality disorder not other-wise specified" (PD-NOS), a diagnosis that may be given when no other personality disorder defined in the *DSM* fits the patient's syndrome. The previous version of the *Diagnostic and Statistical Manual of Mental Disorders*, 3rd edition, revised (*DSM-III-R*) also included passive-aggressive personality disorder, which was defined as a pattern of negative attitudes and passive resistance in interper-sonal situations. It also included self-defeating personality disorder, which was characterized by behavior that consequently under-mines the person's pleasure and goals, and sadistic personality disorder, which was defined as a pervasive pattern of cruel, demeaning, and aggressive behavior (APA, 1987). However, the latter two disorders were only included in the appendix section with a call for further study. However, these three disorders are not included in *DSM-IV* or *DSM-IV-TR* since the APA questioned whether they are indeed separate disorders.

The *International Statistical Classification of Diseases and Related Health Problems*, 10th Revision (ICD-10) also lists and defines the personality disorders in Chapter 5 ("Mental and Behavioural Disorders"), in a section called "Disorders of Adult Personality and Behaviour" (WHO, 2007). This list includes the following eight specific personality disorders and three broader categories at the end, respectively: paranoid personality disorder; schizoid personality disorder; dissocial personality disorder (the same as antisocial, psychopathic, or sociopathic personality disorders); emotionally unstable personality disorder (the same as borderline personality disorder); histrionic personality disorder; anankastic personality disorder (the same as obsessive-compulsive personality disorder); anxious (avoidant) personality disorder; dependent personality disorder; other specific personality disorders (including the eccentric, *haltlose* type, immature, narcissistic, passive-aggressive, psychoneurotic); personality disorder not otherwise specified (NOS) (character neurosis NOS, pathological personality NOS); and mixed and other personality disorders. This last category is intended for personality disorders that are often troublesome but do not demonstrate the specific pattern of symptoms that characterize the previously described disorders. As a result they are often more difficult to diagnose than the initial list of eight disorders. They may include mixed personality disorders with features of several of the eight listed disorders, but without a predominant set of symptoms that would allow a more specific diagnosis, or troublesome personality changes, not previously classifiable, that are regarded as secondary to a main diagnosis of a coexisting affective or anxiety disorder (WHO, 2007). The APA and WHO lists of personality disorders are remarkably similar; however, some differences remain.

The classification of the personality disorders is further complicated by the dimensional factors that reflect the severity of the disorders and the apparent subtypes. Oldham (2005) discusses at length the current controversy surrounding the dilemma of categorical versus dimensional classifications and the problems with the current APA diagnostic system, the overlapping nature of the categories, and especially how many patients can meet criteria for more than one disorder. The *DSM-IV* also brings light to this issue of category versus dimensional perspective. "Personality Disorders represent maladaptive variants of personality traits that merge imperceptibly into normality and into one another" (APA, 1994). So, clearly, compared to most psychiatric disorders, the boundaries here are not so black and white. A British study looked at the most commonly diagnosed personality disorder, borderline personality disorder, and its homogeneous subtypes based on the nine APA criteria for the disorder and an association with stressful life events (Shevlin, Dorahy, Adamson, & Murphy, 2007). Their results find four discrete classes that make up the borderline continuum, "ranging from a class with a low probability of showing any borderline personality disorder symptoms to a class whose members had a relatively high probability of endorsing all criteria. Severity of borderline personality disorder was associated with higher comorbidity and higher stressful life-events" (Shevlin et al., 2007), as one might expect. When comparing several of the personality disorders with depression for impairment, "patients with schizotypal personality disorder and borderline personality disorder were found to have significantly more impairment at work, in social relationships, and at leisure than patients with obsessive-compulsive disorder or major depressive disorder; patients with avoidant personality disorders were intermediate" (Skodol et al., 2002). More research efforts have gone into the study of the borderline condition compared to the other personality disorders, probably for two reasons. First, this disorder ranks number two in prevalence, with obsessive-compulsive personality disorder ranking number one, and, second, the high incidence of harm to self and others.

Prevalence of Personality Disorders

Lenzenweger and colleagues analyzed the data from the National Comorbidity Survey Replication, which is a highly reliable and nationally representative face-to-face household survey that was taken between February 2001 and December 2003. This survey included 9,282 adults with ages of 18 or greater as representatives of the general population in the continental United States (Lenzenweger, Lane, Loranger, & Kessler, 2007). They found prevalence estimates of 5.7% for Cluster A disorders; 1.5% for Cluster B disorders, with estimates for antisocial at 0.6% and borderline at 1.4%; 6.0% for Cluster C disorders; and 9.1% any personality disorder. Using a smaller subset of the population with only 214 adults, they found prevalence estimates for the individual personality disorders at 2.3% for paranoid, 4.9% for schizoid, 3.3% for schizotypal, 1.0% for antisocial, 1.6% for borderline, 0% for histrionic, 0% for narcissistic, 5.2% for avoidant, 0.6% for dependent, 2.4% for obsessive-compulsive, and 1.6% for personality disorder NOS. In this smaller subset they also found a prevalence estimate of 11.9% for any personality disorder. However, they stated, "the prevalence estimates across individual personality disorders is imprecise, owing to the small size," and this is obvious given the 0% prevalence estimates for the histrionic and narcissistic personality disorders, which through other procedures they estimate to be at 1.3%. They also find that co-occurrence of the personality disorders is common and that co-occurrence is higher within clusters compared to between clusters. In respect to sociodemographic correlations, they founnd, "Gender, race-ethnicity, family income, and marital status are not significantly related to any of these personality disorder measures, although there is a notable trend for antisocial personality disorder to be less prevalent among women than men. Age and education are inversely related to Cluster B. Unemployment is positively related to borderline personality disorder" (Lenzenweger et al., 2007).

They also found that all three clusters were significantly associated with a wide range of *DSM-IV* Axis I disorders (major mental, developmental, and learning disorders) and that the associations of personality disorders with functional impairment were largely accounted for by Axis I comorbidity. They concluded, "Strong Axis I comorbidity raises questions about the somewhat arbitrary separation of personality disorders from Axis I disorders in the *DSM* nomenclature. The impairment findings suggest that the main public health significance of personality disorders lies in their effects on Axis I disorders rather than in their effects on functioning" (Lenzenweger et al., 2007). They also reported that 39.0% of individuals in the survey with a personality disorder "reported receiving treatment for problems with their mental health or substance use at some time in the past 12 months" and that "the percent in treatment was a good deal higher for Cluster B (49.1%) than either Cluster A (25.0%) or Cluster C (29.0%)."

A Norwegian study using *DSM-III-R* criteria for personality disorders with 2,053 adults between the ages of 18 and 65 found a prevalence for any personality disorder of 13.4%, with Cluster C disorders the most common (9.4%), Cluster A second (4.1%), and Cluster B the least common (3.1%), without finding any sex differences for any cluster (Torgersen, Kringlen, & Cramer, 2001). In a two-stage national screening of 8,886 British subjects, where 638 subjects were later screened based on the first-stage analysis, they found a 10.1% prevalence rate for any personality disorder including personality disorder NOS (Coid, Yang, Tyrer, Roberts, & Ullrich, 2006). For Cluster A, B, and C they found comparable prevalence rates of 1.6%, 1.2%, and 1.6%, respectively, with the most frequent diagnosis of personality disorder NOS at 5.7%. They also found Cluster B, but not Cluster A or C, to be significantly more common in women than men.

Lenzenweger (2008) summarized these recent and most reliable to-date epidemiological studies in different populations and stated that they "yield remarkably consistent estimates for any personality disorder as defined by the *DSM* system and assessed using a validated structured clinical interview in the hands of experienced diagnosticians. The median prevalence rate for any personality disorder across these studies is 10.56% and the mean prevalence rate is 11.39%. Despite variation in methods and instrumentation, these data indicate that approximately 1 in every 10 persons suffers from a diagnosable personality disorder."

Most recently, the prevalence estimates and correlates of personality disorders were measured in the Mexican population using the International Personality Disorder Examination with a somewhat smaller but representative sample of the Mexican adult urban population (n = 2,362) as part of the Mexican National Comorbidity Survey (Benjet, Borges, & Medina-Mora, 2008). Prevalence estimates for Cluster A were 4.6%, 1.6% for Cluster B, and 2.4% for Cluster C. There was a 6.1% prevalence for any personality disorder, and "all personality disorders clusters were significantly comorbid with *DSM-IV* Axis I disorders": "one in every five persons with an Axis I disorder in Mexico is likely to have a co-morbid personality disorder, and almost half of those with a personality disorder are likely to have an Axis I disorder" (Benjet et al., 2008).

In the most recent large study, called the National Epidemiologic Survey on Alcohol and Related Conditions (NESARC) Part 1, which was not included in Lenzenweger's summary, Pulay and colleagues (2008) examined personality disorders in 43,093 subjects that were nationally representative of the general U.S. population. The *DSM-IV* prevalence ratings for Part 1 did not include values for schizotypal, borderline, or narcissistic personality disorders due to time and space constraints, although borderline and narcissistic personality disorders were later reported in Part 2 (Grant et al., 2008; Stinson et al., 2008). The prevalence estimates for Part 1 showed, for Cluster A, paranoid at 4.4%, schizoid at 3.1%; for Cluster B, antisocial at 3.6%, histrionic at 1.8%; and for Cluster C, 2.4% for avoidant, 0.5% for dependent, and 7.9% for obsessive-compulsive. In Part 2 of the NESARC, this group of researchers found a lifetime prevalence rate for narcissistic personality disorder of 6.2%, with rates greater for men (7.7%) than for women (4.8%) (Stinson et al., 2008). They also found narcissistic personality disorder to be significantly more prevalent among black men and women and Hispanic women, younger adults, and separated, divorced, or widowed and never-married adults, and that it is also associated with greater mental disability among men but not women (Stinson et al., 2008). In addition, they found high co-occurrence rates of substance use, mood, and anxiety disorders and other personality disorders. "With additional comorbidity controlled for, associations with bipolar I disorder, post-traumatic stress disorder, and schizotypal and borderline personality disorders remained significant, but weakened, among men and women. Similar associations were observed between narcissistic personality disorder and specific phobia, generalized anxiety disorder, and bipolar II disorder among women and between narcissistic personality disorder and alcohol abuse, alcohol dependence, drug dependence, and histrionic and obsessive-compulsive personality disorders among men."

In the NESARC Part 2, these researchers estimated a lifetime prevalence rate of borderline personality disorder of 5.9%, with no significant sex differences in the rates of men at 5.6% and women at 6.2% (Grant et al., 2008). This disorder was "more prevalent among Native American men, younger and separated/divorced/widowed adults, and those with lower incomes and education and was less prevalent among Hispanic men and women and Asian women." This disorder was also associated with "substantial mental and physical disability, especially among women. High co-occurrence rates of mood and anxiety disorders with borderline personality disorder were similar. With additional comorbidity controlled for, associations with bipolar disorder and schizotypal and narcissistic personality disorders remained strong and significant (odds ratios > or = 4.3)." They concluded, "Borderline personality disorder is much more prevalent in the general population than previously recognized, is equally prevalent among men and women, and is associated with considerable mental and physical disability, especially among women. Unique and common factors may differentially contribute to disorder-specific comorbidity with borderline personality disorder, and some of these associations appear to be sex-specific." Most recently, the prevalence, correlates, disability, and comorbidity of schizotypal personality disorder (SPD) have been reported from the Wave 2 NESARC, which targeted a nationally representative sample of the adult civilian population of the United States aged 18 years and older. The results are the following:

> Lifetime prevalence of SPD was 3.9%, with significantly greater rates among men (4.2%) than women (3.7%) ($p < .01$). Odds for SPD were significantly greater among black women, individuals with lower incomes, and those who were separated, divorced, or widowed; odds were significantly lower among Asian men (all $p < .01$). Schizotypal personality disorder was associated with substantial mental disability in both sexes. Co-occurrence rates of Axis I and other Axis II disorders among respondents with SPD were much higher than rates of co-occurrence of SPD among respondents with other disorders. After adjustment for sociodemographic characteristics and additional comorbidity, associations remained significant in both sexes between SPD disorder and 12-month and lifetime bipolar I disorder, social and specific phobias, and posttraumatic stress disorder, as well as 12-month bipolar II disorder, lifetime generalized anxiety disorder, and borderline and narcissistic personality disorders (all $p < .01$). (Pulay et al., 2009)

In part, the authors concluded, "Schizotypal personality disorder is a prevalent, fairly stable, highly disabling disorder in the general population" (Pulay et al., 2009). Raine (2006) suggested that the base population rate for schizotypal personality disorder is 2%. The *DSM-IV* lists a base rate at 3%. Raine also reviewed other studies, with one estimate ranging from 0.7% to 3% (Kotsaftis & Neale, 1993), and another with slightly higher rates of 3% to 5% (Weissman, 1993). Raine claimed that "most studies appear to be reporting a base rate in the 2%–3% range, but a low community rate of 0.6% from Norway has been reported (Torgersen et al., 2001) as opposed to a rate of 4.6% in a representative U.S. community sample (Johnson, Smailes, Cohen, Brown, & Bernstein, 2000)" (Raine, 2006). Torgersen also summarized the prevalence rates for all personality disorders from eight separate studies of various sizes with populations ranging from 229 to 2,053 subjects. He stated, "The prevalence of any personality disorder varies between 3.9% and 22.7%. If the small samples of 303 and under are disregarded, the variation is much less, from 10.0% to 14.3%. The median prevalence of all the studies for any personality disorder is 11.55%, and the pooled prevalence is 12.26%" (Torgersen, 2005).

The remaining personality disorder category is personality disorder NOS, which is the third most diagnosed personality disorder when a structured interview is used, and the most frequently diagnosed personality disorder when a structured interview is not used (Verheul & Widiger, 2004). Structured interviews for the general population give estimates of the prevalence as between 3% and 6%, and the rate in clinical populations is claimed to range from 8% to 13% according to four cited studies (Wilberg, Hummelen, Pedersen, & Karterud, 2008). In a single large clinical study with 1,516 patients from the Norwegian Network of Psychotherapeutic Day Hospitals, employing the *DSM-IV* criteria, 17% of the total sample and 22% of those with personality disorders had a diagnosis of a personality disorder NOS, with an average of nine personality disorder criteria per patient that came from any of the 10 basic personality disorders (Wilberg et al., 2008). These patients were heterogeneous with respect to the types of personality disorder criteria, and 41% were not subthreshold; that is, they fulfilled the minimum criteria on at least one specific personality disorder. These patients were also intermediate with the number of fulfilled criteria between patients with specific personality disorders and those with no personality disorder. However, these patients have relatively less severe psychosocial impairment compared to patients with specific personality disorders (Wilberg et al., 2008).

When comparing the general U.S. population to a clinical population, borderline personality disorder is also the most common personality disorder in any clinical population. It is significantly higher and is estimated to occur in 15% (Gunderson, 2001) to 25% of patients (McGlashan et al., 2000). One study, called the Collaborative Longitudinal Personality Disorders Study, measured the oc-currence rates of representative personality disorders and their co-occurrence with the Axis I disorders. Besides borderline personality disorder as noted above, the baseline occurrence rates for selected personality disorders in this clinical population of 668 patients were paranoid personality disorder, 14.2%; schizoid, 3.2%; and both antisocial and dependent disorders, 8.6%. The co-occurrence rates of selected personality disorders and Axis I disorders are pre-sented in Chapter 5.

In an effort to understand the prevalence of personality disor-ders worldwide, one group estimated prevalence across 13 coun-tries (China, Nigeria, South Africa, Colombia, Mexico, the United States, Lebanon, Belgium, France, Germany, Italy, the Netherlands, and Spain) using a total population of 21,162 (Huang et al., 2009). They found a prevalence estimate of 6.1% for any personality dis-order, 3.6% for Cluster A, 1.5% for Cluster B, and 2.7% for Cluster C disorders. They also found that personality disorders are signifi-cantly higher for males; Cluster C disorders are higher for those who have been previously married or unemployed; and Clusters A and B are higher for younger people and the poorly educated. They concluded, "Personality disorders are relatively common disorders that often co-occur with Axis I disorders and are associated with significant role impairments beyond those due to comorbidity." The ranking for severity across the countries was the following for any personality disorder: Colombia (7.9%), United States (7.6%), South Africa (6.8%), Lebanon (6.2%), Mexico (6.1%), China (4.1%), Nigeria (2.7%), and the Western European grouping (2.4%). Co-lombia scored highest for the Cluster A (5.3%) and Cluster B (2.1%) disorders, and the United States was highest for Cluster C (4.2%).

To complicate matters further, it is worth noting that at least one group has studied borderline personality disorder for any po-tential homogeneous subtypes or distinct classes when assessing subgroup associations with impairment. Using "latent class analy-sis," researchers in Great Britain have classified 8,590 patients, ages

16–74, that either have or do not have borderline personality disorder (Shevlin et al., 2007). They found four personality severity categories when using the nine *DSM-IV* diagnostic borderline-specific criteria. The four categories are (1) no personality disorder, (2) subthreshold personality disorder, (3) simple personality disorder, and (4) complex personality disorder. They concluded that this class analysis scheme suggests "that four discrete classes make up the borderline continuum." However, other classification schemes may lead to other subgroupings. Of course, Shevlin et al. also found that "severity of borderline personality disorder was associated with higher co-morbidity and higher stressful life-events." In addition, they reported on the prevalence rates of the nine *DSM-IV* disorder-specific criteria (see Cluster B listings for borderline personality disorder for a more detailed description for each criterion) for this large population. They found the following percentage occurrence rates for the respective nine criteria:

1. Frantic efforts to avoid real or imagined abandonment, 21.5%
2. A pattern of unstable and intense interpersonal relationships, 20.5%
3. Identity disturbance, 1.5%
4. Impulsivity in at least two areas that are potentially self-damaging, 44.3%
5. Recurrent suicidal or self-mutilating behavior, 2.4%
6. Affective instability due to a marked reactivity of mood, 14.2%
7. Chronic feelings of emptiness, 18.0%
8. Inappropriate, intense anger or difficulty controlling anger, 7.8%
9. Transient, stress-related paranoid ideation or severe dissociative symptoms, 6.1% (Shevlin et al., 2007)

There are indeed many possible ways to study the prevalence rates of these 10 specific personality disorders and the more loosely defined category of personality disorder NOS. There is more discussion about co-occurrence and other factors that complicate treatment in Chapter 5.

Treating Personality Disorders Using Conventional Modalities

Given the marked prevalence as well as the individual and social burden of the personality disorders, it will surprise anyone to hear that "most psychiatrists ignore axis II pathology" (Gabbard, 2005a), which in fact accounts for the vast majority of people with axis II disorders. Furthermore, "personality disorders are often relegated to diagnostic oblivion because they are deemed unfathomable or untreatable by psychiatrists and third party payers alike. Many insurance companies and managed care organizations will shamelessly assert that they do not cover treatment for axis II conditions. If there is no reimbursement for the treatment, clinicians are less likely to make the diagnosis and think about treatment. Yet these conditions are ubiquitous in psychiatric practice and must be taken into account if optimal outcomes are desired" (Gabbard, 2005a).

To further emphasize the importance of treatment here, and the absurdity of ignoring these disorders, it must be noted that some claim that the personality disorders occur in more than 80% of psychiatric outpatients (Alwin et al., 2006). Would we ignore a case of severe hypertension when treating a patient for diabetes, or ignore a case of AIDS in a patient who presented with the shingles? It is also worth noting that depression has a comorbidity with Cluster B and C disorders at the 50% level (Dolan-Sewell, Krueger, & Shea, 2001). Substance abuse has comorbidity at the 50% level with Cluster B disorders (Oldham et al., 1995). And the anxiety disorders have a comorbidity with Cluster C disorders at the 25% level (Dyck et al., 2001). Additionally, one study claimed that 60% of male prisoners have antisocial personality disorder (Moran, 1999). Others have claimed that 50% to 78% of adult prisoners meet criteria for at least one or more of the personality disorders, and even higher prevalence estimates have been reported among young offenders (Alwin et al., 2006). Therefore, the costs of the personality disorders to society may be the greatest burden of all, perhaps second only to that of natural disasters. This is undoubtedly the case when we consider that history is replete with psychopathic personalities that have waged senseless wars and other crimes and atrocities against humanity. More recently, we can only wonder about those who have committed the white collar crimes that have led to the horrendous financial tragedies for investors and the loss of jobs when major industries have failed due to wanton greed and corruption. Would these individuals merit a diagnosis of narcissistic personality disorder?

In making the case for treatment, it is worth noting that California has the third largest penal system in the United States, with 161,000 inmates. The 2008–2009 budget for supporting the corrections and rehabilitation systems was $10.29 billion, or 7.3% of state expenditures. These figures do not include the California jails, which have approximately one half as many inmates behind bars. According to the latest annual report by the Justice Department's Bureau of Justice Statistics, the jail and prison population in this country is increasing at a rate of more than a thousand per week. The total number of people behind bars in the United States at the end of June 2007 was 2,186,230, up more than 56,000 compared to 2006. Once again, the United States retains its title as the world's most prison-crazy nation, holding onto first place in both prisoners per capita and the total number of people imprisoned. If we need another argument for why it is a necessity to consider the importance of the treatment for these Axis II disorders, we only need to consider that substance abuse and antisocial personality disorders are highly correlated. "In the prison systems the percentage of prisoners with a mental health problem is 56% for state prisoners, 45% for federal prisoners, and 64% for jail inmates, and 74% of state prisoners who had a mental health problem and 56% of those without were dependent on or abused alcohol or drugs" (James & Glaze, 2006). In addition, it has been claimed that 50% of the recent increases in the male prison population in the United States, and 42% of the female, have resulted from methamphetamine-related offenses. One can only conclude that the neglect of Axis II disorders leads to a huge societal and individual cost.

However, the key question remains. Are there effective ways to treat (or prevent) antisocial, narcissistic, borderline, and the other personality disorders using conventional modalities? First, it is worth noting that there are several barriers that make personality disorders some of the most difficult psychiatric disorders to treat. Rarely do these patients self-refer for treatment unless they are seeking help for a troubling comorbid disorder. It is simply not the case that narcissists, borderline, or antisocial personality disorder patients, or even those with the other categories, complain about their primary Axis II symptoms. In fact, these people find it very difficult to disclose anything that suggests that they have a character deficit. They also find it difficult to maintain a close and lasting relationship with a therapist. They are profoundly sensitive to what they perceive to be criticism and they have highly reactive and impulsive personalities that often lead to a sudden decision to stop therapy. Other common examples of complications with therapy are that those with avoidant personality disorder avoid group sessions, borderline individuals may have great difficulties dealing with family members, histrionics may complain excessively about medication side effects, and all of these complications also affect the success rates for treating the Axis I disorders (Gunderson, Gratz, Neuhaus, & Smith, 2005).

When it comes to treatment, there are four standard levels of care with the conventional approaches, and four therapeutic goals for personality disorder patients. The four levels of care, by decreasing intensity, are 24-hour hospitalization, partial hospitalization (2–8 hours/day and 3–5 days/week), intensive outpatient care (3–6 hours/week), and outpatient care (1–5 hours/week). The four therapeutic goals are to treat the patient's subjective distress and maladaptive behavior, make interpersonal changes, and make intrapsychic changes. These four goals are usually also the expected sequence of the benefits when therapy-induced changes occur, respectively (Gunderson et al., 2005).

There are at least 11 different conventional approaches to therapy that are now described for use with personality disorder patients, not including the use of medication. These approaches are psychoanalysis, psychodynamic psychotherapies, schema therapy, dialectical behavior therapy, interpersonal therapy, supportive psychotherapy, group therapy, family therapy, psychoeducation, somatic treatments, and mixed or collaborative treatments (Oldham, Skodol, & Bender, 2005). The efficacy of all of these approaches with their respective clinical trial results is discussed later. However, family therapy and psychoeducation are not covered here since the range of therapies for family therapy and approaches to psychoeducation are too varied, and the evidence-based outcome data in the literature remains scant. In addition, both family therapy and psychoeducation are frequently integral components of various treatment packages and are thus difficult to isolate and study for their respective therapeutic value. Family therapy for personality disorder patients has been addressed in some depth (Sholevar, 2005), and so has psychoeducation (Hoffman & Fruzzetti, 2005).

Glen Gabbard, one of the leading authorities on using psychoanalysis with personality disorders, stated in respect to the personality disorders, "Randomized, controlled trials of psychoanalysis for personality disorders do not exist" (Gabbard, 2005b). He also commented on a review conducted by the Research Committee of the International Psychoanalytical Association on studies conducted in North America and Europe (Fonagy, Kächele, Krause, Jones, & Perron, 2002): "The existing studies have significant limitations, including failure to use standardized diagnoses, failure to control for selection biases and sampling, the absence of analyses of subjects who joined the study but later dropped out (intent to treat), inadequate description of treatment procedures, little homogeneity in patient groups, the use of inexperienced therapists, the lack of random assignment, the lack of treatment manualization, and the lack of statistical power" (Gabbard, 2005b). He further stated that this report included 66 investigations, and "whenever effectiveness is fairly assessed, psychoanalysis produces effect sizes equal to those of other therapeutic approaches." However, in all fairness to the difficulty of this research, Gabbard also noted that a suitable control for a treatment that lasts several years is highly problematic; the sheer cost of a study over so many years would be prohibitive, and the dropout rate due to natural life events would likely have disastrous effects on the statistical power of a long-term study.

Gabbard's statement that "randomized, controlled trials of psychoanalysis for personality disorders do not exist" refers to the strict one-to-one therapist-to-patient studies for treatment with psychoanalysis. However, there was a study for borderline personality disorder patients worth noting that used psychoanalytic psychotherapy in a randomized controlled trial that included multiple components in a partially hospitalized group where psychoanalysis was a primary component. This study included 38 patients with 19 patients (13 females) in the primary four-part treatment group and 19 patients (9 females) in the comparison group (mean age 30.3, *SD* 5.86) consisting of standard psychiatric care (mean age 33.3, *SD* 6.60). The primary treatment group program consisted of (1) once-weekly individual psychoanalytic psychotherapy, (2) three times per week group analytic psychotherapy (1 hour each), (3) once per week expressive therapy oriented toward psychodrama techniques (1 hour), and (4) a weekly community meeting (1 hour), all spread over 5 days (Bateman & Fonagy, 1999). Patients in this group also had a meeting with the case administrator (1 hour) and a medication review by the psychiatry resident. Treatment was organized in accordance with the psychoanalytic model of borderline personality disorder as a disorder of attachment, separation tolerance, and mentalization (the capacity to think about oneself in relation to others and to understand others' state of mind) (Fonagy, 1998). Trained nurses without formal psychotherapy qualifications administered all treatments. The average length of stay for patients was 1.45 years, with an attendance rating of 62% for the program's psychotherapy sessions. The control group's standard treatment consisted of "1) regular psychiatric review with a senior psychiatrist when necessary (on average, twice per month); 2) inpatient admission as appropriate (admission rate = 90%, average stay = 11.6 days), with discharge to nonpsychoanalytic psychiatric partial hospitalization focusing on problem solving (72% were partially hospitalized, with an average length of stay of 6 months); followed by 3) outpatient and community follow-up (100%, every-2-week visits by a community psychiatric nurse) as standard aftercare. Members of the control group received no formal psychotherapy" (Bateman & Fonagy, 1999). The medication profiles at entry and during treatment were similar for both groups. However, it is clear that the control group did not receive the same amount of professional attention as the partially hospitalized group. The two groups were compared for the frequency of suicide attempts, self-harm, the duration of inpatient admissions, the use of psychotropic medication, and self-report measures of depression, anxiety, general symptom distress, interpersonal function, and social adjustment. "Patients who were partially hospitalized showed a statistically significant decrease on all measures in contrast to the control group, which showed limited change or deterioration over the same period. An improvement in depressive symptoms, a decrease in suicidal and self-mutilatory acts, reduced inpatient days, and better social and interpersonal function began at 6 months and continued until the end of treatment at 18 months." The authors concluded that psychoanalytically oriented partial hospitalization is superior to standard treatment for patients with borderline personality disorder. In a follow-up to this 18-month study, the authors found that "patients who completed the partial hospitalization program not only maintained their substantial gains but also showed a statistically significant continued improvement on most measures in contrast to the patients treated with standard psychiatric care, who showed only limited change during the same period" (Bateman & Fonagy, 2001).

When it comes to whether psychoanalysis is thought to be a useful choice of treatment for the various personality disorders, Gabbard (2005b) gave the following indications: paranoid (rarely indicated), schizoid (may be indicated in exceptional circum-stances), schizotypal (contraindicated), borderline (generally con-traindicated except for a small group with exceptional strengths), narcissistic (strongly indicated), antisocial (contraindicated), histri-onic (only occasionally indicated), avoidant (indicated for cases not responding to cognitive-behavioral or behavior therapy), depen-dent (likely to do well if motivated), and obsessive-compulsive (strongly indicated). Of course, these indications are only valid if the patient does not have a mixed type, which may disfavor the psychoanalytical method. Gabbard (2005b) concluded, "Psycho-analysis is a long and expensive treatment, but because of its inten-sity and duration, it may be capable of far-reaching changes that briefer therapies cannot approach. Defense mechanisms and repre-sentations of self and other may tenaciously resist change, and for some patients, only a systematic working through of these resis-tances will allow for structural, long lasting changes."

Like psychoanalysis, psychodynamic psychotherapy is also con-sidered a depth psychology and is one of the most commonly used methods of psychotherapy. It includes treatment modalities that operate on a continuum of the supportive-interpretive psychother-apeutic interventions. But it is usually briefer, less intense, and em-ploys a more eclectic range of techniques for revealing the uncon-scious content of the patient's psyche, all in an effort to eliminate the psychic tension that is believed to be the root of the patient's problems with the self and world. Thus, the unconscious mind is considered to be the source for supporting a poorly adapted living strategy that primarily develops in the earlier years of life. The psy-chodynamic psychotherapist first attempts to relieve the discom-fort that results from the patient's poorly adapted living skills, then helps the patient recognize these deficiencies, and ultimately helps the patient build new and more effective living skills. Another commonality with psychoanalysis is the importance of the thera-pist-patient relationship and the challenges with transference and countertransference. It is generally believed that patients with the less severe personality disorders (obsessive-compulsive, hysterical, avoidant, dependent, and narcissistic) are better suited to treatment with psychodynamic psychotherapy (Gabbard, 2001).

The decision to recommend psychodynamic psychotherapy instead of psychoanalysis for Cluster A, antisocial, and borderline personality disorders can be difficult (Yeomans, Clarkin, & Levy, 2005). Much is based here on whether the patient is motivated for "deep change influencing all areas of his or her life versus more specific relief from anxiety or resolution of problems in certain areas" (Yeomans et al., 2005). Other factors include "psychological mindedness, capacity for transference work, propensity to regress, impulse control, frustration tolerance, and financial resources." Yeomans and colleagues also stated that borderline patients with a high level of narcissistic, paranoid, and antisocial traits are the most challenging to treat, and that antisocial personality disorder patients may be beyond the reach of psychodynamic or any form of psychotherapy. They also stated that the more severe cases may be responsive to modified and highly structured forms of psychodynamic treatment.

As noted above, randomized controlled trials have previously been nonexistent for psychoanalysis in any of its forms. However, a year-long outpatient trial has been conducted with 90 borderline personality disorder patients (83 women, 7 men; ages 18–50, mean 30.9 years, SD 7.85) that randomly compared a supportive treatment (emotional support and advice on daily problems where the therapist follows and manages the transference but does not use interpretations) with dialectical behavior therapy and a psychodynamic psychotherapy called transference-focused psychotherapy (Clarkin, Levy, Lenzenweger, & Kernberg, 2007). Patients were recruited from New York City and the adjacent tristate metropolitan area. They were assessed at a university-affiliated hospital, and patients were treated by community practitioners in their private offices. Patients were excluded from the study if they had comorbid psychotic disorders, bipolar I disorder, delusional disorder, delirium, dementia, and/or amnestic as well as other cognitive disorders, and any active substance dependencies. This study included 12 variables for improvement that measured changes in depression, anxiety, global functioning, suicidality, social adjustment, irritability, anger, verbal assault, direct assault, and Barratt factors 1, 2, and 3, which are all measures of impulsive personality traits. All patients received medication when necessary, and at the beginning of treatment 70% of the patients in the dialectical behavior therapy group were medicated; 65% of those in supportive treatment group were medicated; and 52% of those in transference-focused psychotherapy group were medicated. The authors stated that the percentage of patients receiving medication remained relatively constant throughout the 1-year treatment trial. They also claimed, "Any difference in the percentage of patients receiving medication in the three treatment cells cannot be attributed to symptom severity, since there were no significant differences between the three groups of patients at time 1 on the domain measures" (Clarkin et al., 2007). Baseline measures were compared with 4-month interval measures using blinded raters for suicidal behavior, aggression, impulsivity measures, anxiety, depression, and social adjustment. Transference-focused psychotherapy predicted significant improvement in 10 of the 12 variables; dialectical behavior therapy predicted improvement in 5 of the 12 variables; and supportive treatment predicted improvement in 6 of the 12 variables. "Patients in all three treatment groups showed significant positive change in depression, anxiety, global functioning, and social adjustment across 1 year of treatment. Both transference-focused psychotherapy and dialectical behavior therapy were significantly associated with improvement in suicidality. Only transference-focused psychotherapy and supportive treatment were associated with improvement in anger. Transference-focused psychotherapy and supportive treatment were each associated with improvement in facets of impulsivity. Only transference-focused psychotherapy was significantly predictive of change in irritability and verbal and direct assault." The authors also performed an intent-to-treat analysis that compared the population that started the trial with those that finished the trial, and found that the results did not differ in terms of the patterns of findings from those obtained through the completer analysis. Nor did the pattern of results appear to be different for medicated patients compared to the whole group. The authors concluded, "Patients with borderline personality disorder respond to structured treatments in an outpatient setting with change in multiple domains of outcome. A structured dynamic treatment, transference-focused psychotherapy was associated with change in multiple constructs across six domains; dialectical behavior therapy and supportive treatment were associated with fewer changes." For ethical reasons, the authors chose not to use a no-treatment control group in this study due to the potential harm that can come to the borderline personality disorder population, which has a high propensity for suicide and self-destructive behavior.

Randomized controlled trials have yet to be conducted using psychodynamic psychotherapy for the remaining nine personality disorders and personality disorder NOS. Borderline personality disorder remains the most studied single personality disorder to date.

However, a study with 66 patients (mean age 27.4 years; 84% women) employing psychodynamic psychotherapy was conducted in Denmark in a day unit for personality disorder patients. The study group were primarily borderline personality disorder patients but also included avoidant, dependent, NOS, narcissistic, histrionic, and schizoid patients, and 28% of the patients were also comorbid for an anxiety disorder. About 10% of the population had depression and a similar percentage had an eating disorder. These patients were also categorized in the severe range for the "global assessment of functioning" scale, which indicated a high level of psychopathology and low psychosocial functioning. The design of the trial did not include a randomization of the patients, but included the first 38 patients to be admitted. The remaining 28 patients were then allocated to a waiting list with treatment as usual (TAU). The intervention group received 5 months of therapy, which included an 11-hour weekly psychotherapy program where patients received five different components of the program: "1) twice weekly psychodynamic small-group and large-group therapy; 2) weekly cognitive group therapy, body awareness group therapy, psycho-educational group and music or art group therapy; 3) individual psychotherapy; 4) a key person helping patients meet regularly for therapy, usually contacting the patients by phone when they failed to attend treatment and encouraging the patients to meet with community workers; 5) when needed patients received a medication review by the consulting psychiatrist" (Petersen et al., 2008). The program was designed to achieve three things: "1) create an alliance to keep patients in therapy; 2) reduce symptoms of acute illness (hospitalizations and suicide attempts) and maintain social functioning; and 3) reduce the symptom burden and improve interpersonal functioning." The authors stated that the "leading treatment principles were elements from modern psychodynamic and cognitive theories, primarily mentalization-based therapy and schema therapy." The TAU group involved seeing patients only if they were in a crisis or had poor motivation. In this case, the patient attended support and motivation sessions with a team member. These meetings were said to have "two main purposes: 1) to keep patients on the waiting list and 2) to prepare them for day treatment in groups." On average, the patients in the TAU group involved one session per month and the patients had their medication adjusted and were hospitalized when necessary.

Regarding the outcome of the study, 7 of the 38 patients in the treatment group terminated early and were not available for further analysis. This is very typical of borderline personality disorder patients, where dropout rates are known to reach 43% (Gunderson et al., 1989; Kelly et al., 1992). In this study, 71.1% of patients in the intervention group were borderline patients, and 98.7% in the wait-listed group were borderline patients. The authors stated that the "intervention group was significantly less hospitalized and the percentage of patients attempting suicide was significantly lower compared with the comparison group. During treatment, there was one suicide attempt and in three cases it was necessary to take a patient to the psychiatric emergency unit (on average for 1.5 day) because of suicide risk or aggravated symptoms. None was admitted to the psychiatric hospital during the intervention period. In the comparison group, a high number of patients experienced acute symptoms: 12 patients (42.8%) went to the psychiatric emergency room for an average stay of 2 days. Four patients (14.3%) were admitted to the psychiatric hospital for 17 days on average" (Petersen et al., 2008). There were no dropouts from the wait-listed group. Nonblinded raters were used in the study for each group. When each group was compared against itself using the various psychiatric scales, the intervention group experienced a significant result on six of seven scales, and the TAU wait-listed group showed no significant changes. However, when a between-groups analysis was employed, the intervention group showed a significant improvement on only four of the seven scales compared to the wait-listed group. The authors also commented, "A treatment period of only 5 months was not sufficient to achieve clinically valid results for core personality problems in the severely impaired sample with low mentalizing capacity. This short-term intervention should therefore be considered a means for establishing a secure environment, which is known to be a major achievement in the treatment of severe personality disordered patients." This 5-month study is indicative of the recalcitrant nature of the personality disorders, where the prognosis has been traditionally pessimistic, yet it also provides some sense of optimism.

Schema therapy is another approach that has been developed and applied in recent decades for treating the personality disorders and other patients with severe and chronic psychological disorders. This form of psychotherapy combines elements from the schools of cognitive-behavioral therapy, Gestalt therapy, object relations, attachment, constructivist, and psychoanalytic (Young, 1999; Young & Klosko, 2005; Young, Klosko, & Weishaar, 2003). Young and Klosko (2005) describe this therapy:

> Schema therapy addresses the core psychological themes that are characteristic of patients with personality disorders. We call these core themes early maladaptive schemas. The model traces these

schemas from early childhood to the present, with emphasis on the patient's interpersonal relationships. The therapist allies with patients in fighting their schemas using cognitive, affective, behavioral, and interpersonal strategies. When patients repeat dysfunctional patterns based on their schemas, the therapist emphatically confronts them with the reasons for changes. Through limited reparenting, the therapist supplies patients with a partial antidote to their unmet childhood needs.

A 5-year study was conducted in the Netherlands that involved 88 patients in four centers testing the comparative value of schema-focused therapy (SFT) with transference-focused psychotherapy (TFP) for patients with borderline personality disorder. Treatment was twice a week for 50 minutes for 3 years and included baseline and 3-month assessments. The researchers measured changes in the patients with the Borderline Personality Disorder Severity Index, fourth version, score; quality of life; general psychopathologic dysfunction; and measures of SFT/TFP personality concepts (Giesen-Bloo et al., 2006). The sociodemographic and clinical characteristics of the groups were similar at baseline. Patients were between 18 and 60 years of age. Patients were excluded from the study if they had any of the following: psychotic disorders (except short, reactive psychotic episodes), bipolar disorder, dissociative identity disorder, antisocial personality disorder, ADHD, addiction of such severity that clinical detoxification was indicated (after which entering treatment was possible), psychiatric disorders secondary to medical conditions, and mental retardation. These disorders were excluded. Medication use and comorbid Axis I disorders were allowed.

> Survival analyses revealed a higher dropout risk for TFP patients than for SFT patients ($P = .01$). Using an intention-to-treat approach, statistically and clinically significant improvements were found for both treatments on all measures after 1-, 2-, and 3-year treatment periods. After 3 years of treatment, survival analyses demonstrated that significantly more SFT patients recovered (rela-

tive risk = 2.18; P = .04) or showed reliable clinical improvement (relative risk = 2.33; P = .009) on the Borderline Personality Disorder Severity Index, fourth version. Analysis showed that they also improved more in general psychopathologic dysfunction and measures of SFT/TFP personality concepts ($P \leq .001$). Finally, SFT patients showed greater increases in quality of life than TFP patients (P = .03 and $P \leq .001$). (Giesen-Bloo et al., 2006)

The authors concluded that SFT is more effective than TFP for all measures and they hypothesized that "the effective ingredients of SFT for patients with borderline personality disorder may be (1) the model's transparency, (2) the therapist's 'reparenting' attitude on the attachment issues of patients with borderline personality disorder, (3) the many hands-on techniques/strategies that offer a patient structure and control, and (4) the opportunity to contact the SFT therapist (within limits) between sessions."

In a follow-up study, the authors mentioned that both treatments aimed at achieving a full recovery, unlike other therapies, and that both forms of therapy succeeded in reducing disorder-specific and general psychopathologic dysfunction and improving health-related quality of life, with SFT being more effective on all measures. "However, the most effective treatment is not necessarily the most cost-effective treatment. In the context of healthcare budget constraints, an economic evaluation can inform decisions concerning which healthcare services to offer to patients. Therefore, a cost-effectiveness analysis was performed comparing these two forms of therapy" (van Asselt et al., 2008). The mean 4-year bootstrapped costs were 37,826 Euros for SFT and 46,795 Euros for TFP. The percentages of patients who recovered were 52% and 29%, respectively. The SFT intervention was less costly and more effective than TFP. However, the authors also noted a slightly better quality of life for the TFP patient group. They concluded, "Despite the initial slight disadvantage in Quality of Life years, there is a high probability that compared with TFP, SFT is a cost-effective treatment for borderline personality disorder."

A more recent study of women only (ages 22–52) tested the effectiveness of adding a SFT group receiving thirty 90-minute sessions over 8 months to TAU individual psychotherapy for borderline personality disorder patients (Farrell, Shaw, & Webber, 2009). Note that this study was run with six patients in a group with two therapists per group as opposed to individual-based therapy. The patients required a referral from a psychotherapist. Patients were told that they would be randomly assigned to the group treatment added to their individual psychotherapy, or would remain in their individual psychotherapy. The authors described the treatment goals as follows: "1) establishing a positive therapeutic alliance through therapist validation and education that establishes the usefulness of the treatment, 2) increasing emotional awareness, so that patients can notice pre-crisis distress and have some understanding of their emotional experience, 3) developing an effective individualized distress management plan, and 4) helping patients become free enough of maladaptive schemas to be able to use their healthy adult coping skills" (Farrell et al., 2009).

Patients were excluded if they had an "axis I diagnosis of a psychotic disorder or a below average IQ (89), as measured by the Shipley Institute of Living Scale. IQ was made an exclusion criterion because of the cognitive and reading demands of the program. Patients were stabilized on their psychotropic medications before randomization, limiting the likelihood of a confounding effect from drug treatment. Pharmacotherapy was limited to first generation antipsychotics, selective serotonin reuptake inhibitors, tricyclic antidepressants and/or benzodiazepines. All patients had a history of suicide attempts and self-injury in the two-year period before the study began."

This study had 32 patients randomly assigned to SFT-TAU and TAU alone. There was a 0% dropout rate for SFT and 25% for TAU. The authors stated that there were "significant reductions in borderline personality disorder symptoms and global severity of psychiatric symptoms, and improved global functioning with large treatment effect sizes were found in the SFT-TAU group. At the end of treatment, 94% of SFT-TAU compared to 16% of TAU no longer met BPD diagnosis criteria ($p < .001$). This study supports group SFT as an effective treatment for BPD that leads to recovery and improved overall functioning." The authors also stated that SFT can be effectively adapted to the group modality and that the large and significant treatment effects demonstrate that SFT is a cost-effective treatment option for borderline personality disorder patients where these patients can achieve both a symptom reduction and improved global functioning and quality of life.

One of the most popular therapies in use today for treating personality disorders is dialectical behavior therapy (DBT). Marsha Linehan and colleagues developed a comprehensive principle-driven treatment program for suicidal and self-injuring individuals with borderline personality disorders (Linehan, 1987, 1993; Linehan, Armstrong, Suarez, Allmon, & Heard, 1991). Today, DBT is also being used for personality disorder patients with Axis I diagnoses such as eating disorders (Stanley & Brodsky, 2005), borderline patients that do not exhibit self-harm (Robins, Ivanoff, & Linehan, 2001), and other significant problems of behavioral and emotional dyscontrol (Stanley, Bundy, & Beberman, 2001). One of the biggest problems with borderline patients is their trait of withdrawing from therapy, and a primary reason for this is that "these patients tend to experience an almost exclusive focus on change as criticism and invalidation of their suffering rather than its intent as helpful. In attempting to tackle this problem DBT explicitly emphasizes the need to balance change strategies with acceptance and validation techniques" (Stanley & Brodsky, 2005). Therefore, a critical step in therapy is the concept of acceptance as a substitute for the otherwise rigid and locked state where patients believe "it should not have happened" (Stanley & Brodsky, 2005). DBT involves both individual and group therapy and combines the key elements of standard cognitive-behavioral techniques for emotion regulation and reality testing for interpersonal effectiveness with concepts of mindfulness meditation awareness, distress tolerance, and acceptance largely derived from Buddhist meditative practices. Stanley and Brodsky described the four primary skills that are the aim of DBT:

1. The mindfulness practice focuses on the moment and awareness without judgment.
2. Distress tolerance focuses on crisis survival strategies and radical acceptance of reality.
3. Emotion regulation focuses on identifying emotional states, validating and accepting one's emotions, and decreasing the vulnerability to negative emotions while increasing the experience of positive emotions.
4. Interpersonal effectiveness focuses on assertiveness training, cognitive restructuring, and balancing objectives while maintaining relationships and self-esteem.

DBT was first tested in a year-long randomized controlled trial for borderline patients, and it was compared to TAU (Linehan et al., 1991). The study compared 22 females (aged 18–45 yrs) with parasuicidal borderline personality disorder treated with DBT and 22 matched females with parasuicidal borderline disorder with TAU. To be included in the study, patients had to have at least two incidents of parasuicide in the last 5 years, with one during the last 8 weeks, with an age of 18 to 45. Patients admitted to the DBT group could not be involved in additional individual psychotherapy. They were excluded from the trial if they met criteria for schizophrenia, bipolar disorder, substance dependence, or mental retardation. The DBT group met weekly for both individual therapy (1 hour/week) and group therapy (2.5 hours/week) for 1 year. Telephone contact with the individual's primary DBT therapist was allowed as needed. Patients in the TAU group were given alternative therapy referrals from which they could choose.

The patients were assessed at baseline and at 4, 8, and 12 months after the initiation of treatment. They found a significant reduction in the DBT group in the frequency and medical risk of parasuicidal behavior compared to those with TAU. There were 1.5

parasuicidal acts for the DBT group for the year compared to 9 acts for the TAU group. The DBT patients showed a retention rate of 83.3%, compared to a rate of 42% for TAU patients. DBT patients received an average of 8.46 inpatient hospital days for the year compared to an average of 38.86 days for the TAU group. However, the DBT group did not show significantly better results for improving patients' depression, hopelessness, suicidal ideation, or reasons for living (Linehan et al., 1991). On follow-up, 39 of the patients in the above study were assessed again at 6 and 12 months after the study. The DBT patients had significantly better social adjustment scores. "During the initial 6 months of the follow-up, DBT subjects had significantly less parasuicidal behavior, less anger, and better self-reported social adjustment. During the final 6 months, DBT subjects had significantly fewer psychiatric inpatient days and better interviewer-rated social adjustment" (Linehan, Heard, & Armstrong, 1993). But apparently the parasuicidal behavior for the two groups for the latter 6 months was not significantly different. However, the authors concluded, "In general, the superiority of DBT over TAU, found in previous studies at the completion of 1 year of treatment, was retained during a 1-year follow-up."

The first study showing the efficacy of DBT to be replicated and published in a journal by a group independent of Linehan and colleagues was a small pilot study (Koons et al., 2001). A European group also published a randomized controlled 12-month clinical trial, again showing positive results (Verheul et al., 2003). In the latter study, 64 women patients were eligible for the trial. DBT was compared to TAU. There were 31 patients in the DBT group and 33 in the TAU group. Again, the DBT protocol devised by Linehan and colleagues was used, involving individual and group therapy totaling about 3.5 hours per week. But here the "TAU consisted of clinical management from the original referral source (addiction treatment centres $n = 11$, psychiatric services $n = 20$). Patients in this group attended generally no more than two sessions per month with a psychologist, a psychiatrist or a social worker" (Verheul et al., 2003). The patients here were ages 18–70 and lived near Amsterdam. They were only eligible for treatment if the referring therapist was willing to sign an agreement committing to 12 months of TAU if the patient was randomized to the TAU control group. The exclusion criteria were a diagnosis of bipolar disorder or (chronic) psychotic disorder, insufficient command of the Dutch language, and severe cognitive impairments. The biggest difference from the trial conducted by Linehan and colleagues (1991) was that the patients were primarily clinical referrals from both addiction treatment and psychiatric services, and patients were not required to have shown recent parasuicidal behavior.

These researchers found that DBT resulted in better retention rates (DBT = 63% versus TAU = 23%) and greater reductions of self-mutilation. "At the week 52 assessment, 57% of the TAU patients reported engaging in any self-mutilating behavior at least once in the previous 6-month period (median 13 times), against 35% of DBT group (median 1.5 times)" (Verheul et al., 2003). This result was more evident for those with a history of frequent self-mutilation. In terms of self-damaging impulsive behaviors, patients in the DBT group showed more improvement than the TAU group for the interaction term of time by treatment condition, but not for the treatment condition alone. However, the difference in frequency and course of suicidal behavior was not statistically significant between the two groups over the 12 months. The authors also reported, "The greater improvement in the DBT group could not be explained by greater or other use of psychotropic medications by these patients. In both conditions, three-quarters of the patients reported use of medication from one or more of the following categories: benzodiazepines, selective serotonin reuptake inhibitors (SSRIs), tricyclic antidepressants, mood stabilizers and neuroleptics. Use of SSRIs was reported by 14 (52%) of the DBT patients and 19 (61%) of TAU patients. These findings eliminate the possibility of confounding by medication use." They concluded that

DBT is superior to usual treatment in reducing high-risk behaviors in patients with borderline personality disorder (Verheul et al., 2003).

While Linehan and colleagues developed DBT primarily as a therapy for outpatient use with chronically suicidal patients, one group hypothesized that the course of therapy could be accelerated and improved in an inpatient setting for this patient group, who would then undergo long-term outpatient care (Bohus et al., 2000). These researchers conducted an uncontrolled 3-month DBT program with 24 female patients. "The primary goal of the 3-month treatment is improvement of behaviors in 4 priority target areas: suicidal behaviors, nonsuicidal self injury, treatment interfering behaviors, and behaviors that prolong hospitalization." Measures were compared at baseline admission to the hospital and at 1 month after discharge. They found significant improvements in ratings of depression, dissociation, anxiety, and global stress scores, and a "highly significant decrease in the number of parasuicidal acts was also reported." However, as the authors noted, this study did not include a control group.

The same group later conducted a controlled trial with 50 females with borderline personality disorder in another 3-month DBT inpatient treatment program (Bohus et al., 2004). However, patients were not randomized to groups. They described their treatment allocation procedure as the following: "all patients fulfilling inclusion criteria and agreeing to participate at the study were placed on the waiting list. Admission to DBT inpatient treatment happened consecutively and so, any experimenter or referral bias regarding group assignment can be excluded. However, we cannot rule out an alternate hypothesis that individuals who got on the waiting list first and, thus, had a better chance of getting into the DBT group differed in some significant way from those who did not apply for treatment early enough to get into treatment." All patients were required to have one suicide attempt or a minimum of two nonsuicidal self-injurious acts within the last 2 years, and the exclusion criteria were a lifetime diagnosis of schizophrenia, bipolar I disorder, current substance abuse, or mental retardation. They measured changes from baseline to 4 months after baseline (i.e., 4 weeks after discharge for the DBT group) on 10 measures of psychopathology and the frequency of self-mutilation. The 10 psychopathology measures were Lifetime Parasuicide Count, Symptom Checklist 90–Revised, Hamilton Anxiety Scale, State-Trait Anxiety Inventory, Beck Depression Inventory, Hamilton Depression Scale, State-Trait Anger Inventory, Dissociative Experiences Scale, Global Assessment of Functioning Scale, and the Inventory of Personal Problems. In all, 31 patients were in the DBT group, and 19 patients were in a waiting-list TAU group. The groups were the same on demographic variables: ages, DBT = mean 29.1, range 18–44; TAU = mean 29.5, range 19–38; number of psychiatric hospitalizations, DBT = mean 5.5, range 0–29; TAU = 4.9, range 0–14; number of lifetime suicide attempts, DBT = mean 4, range 0–25; TAU = mean 4.7, range 0–11; Axis I comorbid disorders, anxiety disorders, DBT = 70%, TAU = 94%; eating disorders, DBT = 22.6%, TAU = 26.3%; major depression and dysthymia, DBT = 53%, TAU = 61%. The DBT group met criteria for significantly fewer borderline personality criteria than did the waiting-list (TAU) group (DBT: mean 6.81, range 4–9; WL-TAU: mean 7.63, range 6–9).

The pretherapy and posttherapy comparisons "showed significant changes for the DBT group on 9 of 10 psychopathological variables and significant reductions in self-injurious behavior. The waiting list group did not show any significant changes at the four-month's point. The DBT group improved significantly more than participants on the waiting list on seven of the nine variables analyzed, including depression, anxiety, interpersonal functioning, social adjustment, global psychopathology and self-mutilation" (Bohus et al., 2004). Of the DBT group 62% abstained from self-mutilation compared to 31% of the TAU-WL group. They concluded, using specific criteria, "that 42% of those receiving DBT had clinically recovered on a general measure of psychopathology. The data suggest that three months of inpatient DBT treatment is significantly superior to non-specific outpatient treatment. Within a relatively short time frame, improvement was found across a broad range of psychopathological features. Stability of the recovery after one month following discharge, however, was not evaluated and requires further study." They also stated, "there is strong evidence that about 50% of female borderline disorder patients completing the three-month DBT inpatient treatment improve at a clinically relevant level."

The same group followed the patients in this trial to see if the effects of DBT were sustained once patients returned to their usual lives. They looked at 31 patients for an observation period of 21 months after discharge from the DBT program. They found that the improvements persisted over the follow-up period with a steady rate of remitted patients and in a broad range of psychopathology. The short-term treatment response predicted remission after 2 years follow-up. They concluded, "The effects of inpatient dialectical behavior therapy seem to persist after patients returned to their usual lives" (Kleindienst et al., 2008). They also noted one limitation of the study: "the lack of a control group during the follow-up period. For ethical reasons, patients originally assigned to the waitlist condition were not precluded from DBT treatment for another 20 months. In absence of a control group, it is not possible to definitely attribute the observed persistence of treatment effects to inpatient DBT treatment per se. Alternative explanations, such as spontaneous improvements over time, or unmonitored use of treatment might account partially for the persistence of treatment effects. It is also difficult to know what the course of psychopathology is among BPD patients who have not been treated with DBT, given the paucity of published data in this area."

In an uncontrolled trial, DBT was used to treat eight women with borderline personality disorder and eating disorders. Five women had a binge eating disorder, and three had bulimia nervosa. The patients had 6 months of weekly skills group, individual DBT, therapist consultation team meeting, and 24-hour telephone coaching (Chen, Matthews, Allen, Kuo, & Linehan, 2008). Measures of disorders were taken at baseline, after 6 months of treatment, and at 6 months follow-up. The researchers found at the 0-month and 6-month measures that there were large effect sizes for objective binge eating and global adjustment, and that the effect sizes were medium for the non–eating disorder Axis I disorders, suicidal behavior, and self-injury. Also, they found that from 0 to 6 months of follow-up that the effect sizes were large for all these outcomes. They concluded, "This provides promising pilot data for larger studies utilizing DBT for binge-eating disorder and bulimia nervosa and borderline personality disorder" (Chen et al., 2008). They also noted that two major limitations of this study were that the population size was very small and that there was no randomization to a control group. Some patients in the trial were medicated on psychotropics while others were not, and there was minor attrition by the 6-month treatment point, with one patient dropping out, leaving seven patients, and with another patient dropping out prior to the 6-month follow-up point.

There is also interest in why patients drop out of in-patient DBT. Sixty women with borderline personality disorder were admitted for DBT in a German hospital. Those who failed to complete treatment "had higher experiential avoidance and trait anxiety at baseline, but fewer life-time suicide attempts than completers. There was a trend for more anger-hostility and perceived stigma among non-completers. Experiential avoidance and anxiety may be associated with dropout in inpatient DBT. Low life-time suicidality and high anger could reflect a subtype at risk for discontinuation of inpatient treatment" (Rusch et al., 2008). They also acknowledged that their findings cannot be generalized to men or to outpatient populations.

A double-blinded study compared the effects of the antipsychotic olanzapine and whether it could augment DBT in reducing anger and hostility in women with borderline personality disorder (Linehan, McDavid, Brown, Sayrs, & Gallop, 2008). Twenty-four patients were randomized to receive either low-dose olanzapine (allowed dosage range of 2.5–15 mg/day, mean daily dose of 4.46 mg) or placebo. Both groups received DBT for 6 months. Using the strict assessment analysis with an intention-to-treat analysis, both treatment conditions resulted in significant improvements in irritability, aggression, and depression, with a near but not significant result for self-inflicted injuries for each group. "Irritability and aggression scores tended to decrease more quickly for the olanzapine group than for the placebo group. Self-inflicted injury tended to decrease more for the placebo group than for the olanzapine group" (Linehan et al., 2008). However, given the low sample sizes, and perhaps the lack of a real difference due to medication, it is not possible to conclude that olanzapine improves upon DBT for women with borderline personality disorder.

DBT has achieved prominence because Linehan and colleagues have made a treatment manual and workbook available, and there are numerous training workshops in the United States and Europe. Managed care companies in the United States employ DBT, and it has also been recommended as a treatment for borderline personality disorder by the American Psychiatric Association. One key factor in DBT treatment is the use of mindfulness meditation. However, a meta-analysis of mindfulness-based stress reduction (MBSR) on the symptoms of anxiety and depression in a range of clinical populations was conducted on studies published in peer-reviewed journals that used a control group, and that reported outcomes related to changes in depression and anxiety (Toneatto & Nguyen, 2007). The authors found 15 studies where depression and anxiety were measured as outcome variables for a broad range of medical and emotional disorders. They stated, "Evidence for a beneficial effect of MBSR on depression and anxiety was equivocal. When active control groups were used, MBSR did not show an effect on depression and anxiety. Adherence to the MBSR program was infrequently assessed. Where it was assessed, the relation between practicing mindfulness and changes in depression and anxiety was equivocal." The authors concluded, "MBSR does not have a reliable effect on depression and anxiety." Therefore, it is likely that DBT is very dependent on all the factors included in the program, and that the mindfulness component is only a minor player. Nonetheless, DBT remains the primary therapy of choice with substantial data to demonstrate efficacy with women with borderline personality disorder. How effective DBT is with the other personality disorders and men, in both inpatient and outpatient settings, remains to be determined. Again, it is clear that borderline personality disorder remains the most studied personality disorder.

Another form of psychotherapy that has been used to treat the personality disorders is called interpersonal psychotherapy, and this approach employs many of the common factors of psychotherapy to form a supportive, therapeutically optimistic alliance. Markowitz and colleagues differentiate it from cognitive-behavioral therapies by stating that it is "considerably less structured; that treatment focuses on affect and interpersonal responses, rather than on cognitions; that interpersonal psychotherapists do not assign homework, although the resolution of the interpersonal focus (e.g., role transition) is the overarching task of treatment" (Markowitz, Skodol, & Bleiberg, 2006). While interpersonal psychotherapy is "a time-tested, diagnosis-focused, empirically tested treatment" for patients with nondelusional major depression (Weissman, Markowitz, & Klerman, 2000), the use of interpersonal psychotherapy for treating patients with personality disorders "requires examination in—as yet undone—controlled clinical trials" (Markowitz, 2005. In a more recent publication, the authors stated, "It is early to consider why Interpersonal Psychotherapy may help borderline personality disorder patients; we first need to determine whether it does" (Markowitz et al., 2006. These authors have developed an Interpersonal Psychotherapy Outcome Scale to measure patient progress with these disorders.

However, more recently a randomized controlled trial was conducted in Norway with 54 patients given outpatient interpersonal psychotherapy, compared to 60 patients given 18 weeks of day hospital treatment (psychodynamic and cognitive-behavioral group therapies), delivered by therapists without formal training on these methods, that was followed by long-term conjoint group and individual therapy. The therapists for the outpatient interpersonal psychotherapy had a mean work experience as psychotherapists of 20 years. The mean age for all patients in the trial was 31 years and 74% were female. The array of personality disorders included: borderline (46%), avoidant (40%), personality disorder NOS (21%), paranoid (15%), obsessive-compulsive (9%), dependent (7%), narcissistic (2%), and schizoid (1%). "The patients had a mean of 3.4 symptom disorders: 74% with major depression, 37% with dysthymia, 8% with bipolar II disorder, 46% with panic disorder, 47% with social phobia, 12% with obsessive compulsive disorder, 48% with GAD, 27% with substance misuse disorders, and 14% with eating disorder. There were no statistically significant differences in diagnostic distribution between patients in the two treatment conditions" (Arnevik et al., 2008). The exclusion criteria were schizotypal and antisocial personality disorder, current alcohol or drug dependence, psychotic disorders, bipolar I disorder, untreated ADHD (adult type), pervasive developmental disorder (e.g., Asperger's syndrome), organic syndromes, and being homeless. The main outcome measures were attrition rate, suicide attempts, suicidal thoughts, self-injury, psychosocial functioning, symptom distress, and interpersonal and personality problems. "The study showed a low dropout rate and a moderate improvement on a broad range of clinical measures for both treatments. However, there was no indication of the superiority of one treatment over the other. Neither was there any indication that day hospital treatment was better for the most poorly functioning patients" (Arnevik et al., 2008).

Much work employing randomized controlled clinical trials remains to be done to test whether interpersonal psychotherapy is an effective therapy for the Cluster A, B, and C personality disorders. There are two primary reasons that interpersonal and other forms of psychotherapy have not been tested for the treatment of personality disorders. The first reason is that the major governmental funding has gone toward the study of pharmacotherapy for Axis I disorders over 12–20 weeks of treatment. While short-term psychotherapy has also been tested for the Axis I disorders, "the longer treatment trials that Axis II personality disorders are anticipated to need make such research more expensive and complicated" (Markowitz, 2005).

Supportive psychotherapy is also used in the treatment of patients with personality disorders, and it is considered to be the most prevalent form of psychotherapy employed for treating psychiatric disorders in general (Tanielian, Marcus, Suarez, & Pincus, 2001). The 1998 National Survey of Psychiatric Practice showed that 36% of patients treated by psychiatrists received supportive psychotherapy, while only 19% of patients were treated with insight-oriented therapy, 6% received cognitive-behavioral therapy, and only 1% received psychoanalysis (Tanielian et al., 2001). Supportive psychotherapy is used to reinforce a patient's defenses, but in this form of therapy the therapist avoids the deep intensive probing of emotional conflicts that is basic in psychoanalysis and intensive psychotherapy. It is commonly used to achieve behavioral or attitudinal change, and it employs suggestion, persuasion, education, reassurance, and insight. Given the wide and long-standing use of supportive psychotherapy, Douglas (2008) stated, "supportive therapy has not been sufficiently well defined in a manual or tested in controlled clinical trials to be considered evidence based." However, psychiatry residency training in the United States now requires competency in the area of supportive psychotherapy. Hellerstein and Markowitz (2008) suggested, "Perhaps now is the time to complete the process of establishing supportive psychotherapy as an evidence-based treatment. As the most common psychotherapy, supportive psychotherapy should receive high research priority and be developed, applied, and evaluated as rigorously as cognitive behavior therapy or interpersonal psychotherapy."

The only randomized controlled trial that implemented supportive psychotherapy was described in the discussion above on the use of DBT for treating borderline personality disorder patients, where supportive psychotherapy was compared against DBT and transference-focused psychotherapy in 99 randomly assigned patients for a year-long trial (Clarkin et al., 2007). Blind raters assessed the domains of suicidal behavior, aggression, impulsivity, anxiety, depression, and social adjustment. "Patients in all treatment groups showed significant positive change in depression, anxiety, global functioning, and social adjustment across 1 year of treatment. Both transference-focused psychotherapy and DBT were significantly associated with improvement in suicidality. Only transference-focused psychotherapy and supportive treatment were associated with improvement in anger. Transference-focused psychotherapy and supportive treatment were each associated with improvement in facets of impulsivity. Only transference-focused psychotherapy was significantly predictive of change in irritability and verbal and direct assault" (Clarkin et al., 2007). The authors concluded in their comparison of the three treatments, "A structured dynamic treatment, transference-focused psychotherapy was associated with change in multiple constructs across six domains; dialectical behavior therapy and supportive treatment were associated with fewer changes."

Group treatment is also used to help treat patients with personality disorders. However, there are too many different group therapies to cover in depth here. A useful discussion of group treatment in general and its utility for treating personality disorder patients has been presented (Piper & Ogrodniczuk, 2005). There are also complications to employing group therapy for personality disorder patients. "Some patients with personality disorders resent sharing the therapist and feel neglected and deprived. In the group situation, regressive behavior such as emotional outbursts, aggressive actions, or suicidal threats are more difficult to manage and contain than in individual therapy. Groups are prone to scapegoating; patients with personality disorders provide many provocations" (Piper & Ogrodniczuk, 2005). These patients also find groups to be difficult because of a loss of control, individuality, understanding, privacy, and safety. Piper and Ogrodniczuk also stated that specific features of this population facilitate group therapy. This includes their strong tendency to openly demonstrate interpersonal psychopathology through behavior in the group and that they tend to value the connections in the group. But the authors also stated,

"Many behaviors characteristic of those with personality disorders complicate group treatment. Because these behaviors are often offensive to members of the group, they tend to weaken cohesion and distract members from working." They listed other antitherapeutic behaviors as minimal disclosure, excessive disclosure, scapegoating, extra-group socializing, absenteeism, lateness, and premature termination.

Piper and Ogrodniczuk also made the following recommendations for this population in groups. For the Cluster A disorders, schizoid patients can definitely benefit but difficulties can involve passivity and silence, which may irritate others; schizotypal patients may benefit and increase socialization skills, but difficulties can arise if the patient's peculiarities are bizarre and difficult for others, and their prolonged silence can be a problem. Paranoid patients usually do not do well. For Cluster B patients, group therapy can be extremely effective for borderline patients, who better tolerate interpretations in a group, but their anger and other strong affects are unpredictable; group therapy for narcissistic patients is usually problematic because they have a lack of empathy, a sense of entitlement, and a hunger for admiration, and dropout rates are high; for histrionic patients, group therapy can definitely be helpful since these patients can help energize the group, but scapegoating and dropout rates are high; group therapy is not suitable for antisocial personality disorder patients. For Cluster C patients, avoidant patients can do very well because they are highly motivated; group therapy is regarded as the treatment of choice for dependent personality patients because it provides many opportunities to learn independence and to be expressive; and some obsessive-compulsive patients can benefit, but some tend to act as an additional therapist and to be stubborn and too work oriented (Piper & Ogrodniczuk, 2005). The authors summarized as follows based on the data in the clinical literature: Schizoid, schizotypal, borderline, histrionic, avoidant, and dependent personality disorders are regarded as particularly suitable for group treatment. In contrast, paranoid, narcissistic, and obsessive-compulsive personality disorders are regarded as difficult to treat in group therapy. Most group treatments are contraindicated for patients with antisocial personality disorder (Piper & Ogrodniczuk, 2005).

Verheul and Herbrink (2007) have published a systematic review of the various forms of psychotherapy as treatments for the broad range of personality disorders for the four different treatment settings (outpatient individual, group, day hospital, and inpatient status). They stated that "psychotherapy is the treatment of choice for the personality disorders." They made this statement based on the review of two formal meta-analyses (Leichsenring & Leibing, 2003; Perry, Banon, & Ianni, 1999), a Cochrane review (Binks et al., 2006), two clinical guidelines (APA, 2001; Great Britain, Department of Health, 2003), and six other critical reviews of the literature that help them come to this conclusion. Their systematic review of the literature shows:

> psychotherapeutic techniques have proven to be efficacious with respect to reducing symptomatology and personality pathology, and improving social functioning in patients with Cluster A, B, C, or not-otherwise-specified personality disorders. This is especially true for cognitive-behaviorally or psychodynamically oriented outpatient individual psychotherapies. However, some evidence indicates that this also applies to (1) long-term, psychodynamically oriented group psychotherapy, (2) short-term, psychodynamically oriented psychotherapy in a day hospital setting, and (3) various duration variants of psychodynamically oriented, in-patient psychotherapy programmes. The available evidence mostly applies to borderline, dependent, avoidant and not-otherwise-specified personality disorder, and perhaps also paranoid, obsessive-compulsive, and schizotypal personality disorder. It is unknown whether these conclusions also apply to schizoid, antisocial, narcissistic, and histrionic personality disorder. (Verheul & Herbrink, 2007)

The authors made numerous clinical recommendations and conclusions based on the treatment setting types and the various personality disorder clusters, which are too diverse for the most part to cover here. However, in respect to the added value of pharmacotherapies to psychotherapeutic techniques, they concluded that olanzapine increases the efficacy of psychotherapy for borderline patients, and they cited literature for this conclusion (Soler et al., 2005). They also concluded that fluoxetine does not have added value in addition to psychotherapy for borderline patients, and they cite the literature (Simpson et al., 2004). They stated, "Evidence suggests that pharmacological interventions in general have limited added value in addition to psychotherapy for personality disorders" (Verheul & Herbrink, 2007). They cited two earlier studies to support this conclusion (Teusch, Bohme, Finke, & Gastpar, 2001; Wilberg, Karterud, Urnes, Pedersen, & Friis, 1998). They also stated that effective programs all include a relatively high "dosage," a large amount of structure, and sufficient attention to universally effective factors, and that optimal treatment can take up to many years and large numbers of outpatient sessions, or it can include a day hospital or inpatient phase of several months (Verheul & Herbrink, 2007). They also noted how important it is to use stepped care principles of therapy when starting or stopping therapy, and that stopping therapy usually requires follow-up treatment.

In a review of the different forms of psychotherapy for borderline personality disorder, the most studied variant of the personality disorders, there is an assessment of the similarities and differences with these therapies. This analysis was conducted because there is no single form of psychotherapy that is clearly superior to the others, by the authors' judgment (de Groot, Verheul, & Trijsburg, 2008). They offered an overview of the theory and practice of contemporary psychotherapeutic treatments and their respective similarities and differences. The "results show that similarities concerning (1) the formal characteristics, and (2) the importance of therapeutic techniques in treatments for borderline personality disorder, outnumber the differences."

The remaining conventional approach for treating the personality disorders is under the umbrella called somatic treatments, which includes both the pharmacological approach and electroconvulsive shock treatments. Soloff (2005) reviewed the somatic treatments and stated, "A pharmacological approach to treatment of personality disorders is based on the ability of medication to modify neurotransmitter functions that mediate expression of state symptoms and trait vulnerabilities related to personality disorders." He stated, "Pharmacotherapy in personality disorders is narrowly focused on those few dimensions that command the most clinical attention, such as affective dysregulation (e.g., labile, depressed, angry, or anxious moods), cognitive-perceptual symptoms ('psychoticism'), and impulsive aggression. These symptoms prompt urgent care because they mediate suicidal behavior, self-injury, or assault, and result in emergency department visits or hospitalization. As a result, most drug trials have been conducted in patients with borderline, schizotypal, and antisocial personality disorders." Soloff also described the difficulties in conducting clinical trials with this population and said the "empirical literature, although growing, is still woefully inadequate." He described in some depth the use of the neuroleptics, antidepressants, anxiolytics, and both lithium carbonate and anticonvulsant mood stabilizers. Soloff (2005) stated:

> Pharmacotherapy is an important adjunctive treatment in the overall management of the patient with severe personality disorder. Symptoms of cognitive-perceptual disturbance, affective dysregulation, and impulse-behavioral dyscontrol are appropriate targets for medication trials. Problems of character and interpersonal dynamics are the domain of the psychotherapies and will not respond to medication. Because personality disorders are dimensional syndromes, a symptom-specific approach is warranted, potentially involving multiple medications. It is important to study the effects of each medication before adding a second or third agent. Ineffective medications should be discontinued. Expectations of efficacy should be modest and residual symptoms are the rule.

Again, since the vast majority of clinical research has been conducted on borderline personality disorder, to the exclusion of the other personality disorders, we may assume that the clinical trial results using pharmacotherapies with borderline patients will be informative about the potential use of medications for the other personality disorders. The conclusion to date is not promising. The American Psychiatric Association practice guidelines for the treatment of borderline personality disorder conclude that no pharmacologic or psychosocial treatment has demonstrated efficacy for all aspects of borderline personality disorder, such as affective, identity, and interpersonal disturbances (APA, 2001). A *Cochrane Review* comes to a similar conclusion: "Although several medications have shown efficacy for various symptoms in controlled trials, there is no convincing evidence that any medication is a treatment for borderline personality disorder as a whole" (Stoffers et al., in press). Thus, psychotherapy continues to be the necessary and primary conventional treatment modality for borderline personality disorder (Webber & Farrell, 2008).

Many psychiatrists that specialize in the treatment of the personality disorders combine both therapy and medications. Relief of some symptoms such as depression, phobia, or even panic attacks is the goal here with medications, but it is well understood that these medications cannot cure the underlying disorder. Thus medication is seen as a supportive therapy by some during psychotherapy. Again, it is worth noting, "Evidence suggests that pharmacological interventions in general have limited added value in addition to psychotherapy for personality disorders" (Verheul & Herbrink, 2007).

The medications that are commonly prescribed are in the following categories, with examples for each category: the antidepressants fluoxetine (Prozac, Sarafem), sertraline (Zoloft), citalopram (Celexa), paroxetine (Paxil), nefazodone, escitalopram (Lexapro), and venlafaxine (Effexor); the anticonvulsants that are sometimes prescribed to help suppress impulsive and aggressive behavior are carbamazepine (Carbatrol, Tegretol), valproic acid (Depakote), or topiramate (Topamax); the antipsychotics that are used when people are at risk of losing touch with reality are risperidone (Risperdal), olanzapine (Zyprexa), and haloperidol (Haldol); the anxiolytics as antianxiety drugs are alprazolam (Xanax) and clonazepam (Klonopin); and finally, lithium (Eskalith, Lithobid) is used as a mood stabilizer.

The basic principles, indications, and contraindications of using both pharmacotherapies and psychotherapy for the treatment of patients with personality disorders are discussed at length in a chapter titled "Collaborative Treatment" (Schlesinger & Silk, 2005). While collaborative treatment is widely used for personality disorder patients, most of the research on the topic of combined therapies has been on the Axis I psychiatric disorders, thus again excluding the personality disorders as an area of major importance. Schlesinger and Silk (2005) concluded:

> Thus, for patients with personality disorders, no clear conclusions can be made concerning the effectiveness of a medication versus psychotherapy; furthermore, no conclusions about effectiveness or efficacy can be made if these treatments are combined and performed by one provider versus being divided between two (or more) providers with one providing psychotherapy and the other prescribing medications. The exception may be the study by Kool, Dekker, Duijsens, de Jonghe, and Puite (2003) which found that patients with personality pathology and depression responded best to a combined approach of both psychopharmacology and psychotherapy, although personality pathology of patients with Cluster C diagnoses responded better than that of patients with Cluster B diagnosis.

The treatment of patients with personality disorders is often complicated because of the extreme care that must be taken with patients that are prone to suicide and with those that have a history of suicidal behavior. The other major complications can be with those patients that are violent, self-mutilate, or have problems with substance abuse or dependency, dissociative and psychotic states, and major ego-defensive functioning. While the personality disorders have no doubt existed since the origins of the human race, efficacy and effectiveness research is still in its infancy when compared to that of the Axis I disorders.

The Yogic View on the Etiology of the Personality Disorders

Yogi Bhajan taught a complex yogic model for the structure of the mind that includes 27 different basic personality types that are differentially expressed and combined with the relative and respective strengths and weaknesses in each individual to form our basic personalities and identities (Bhajan & Khalsa, 1998). The 27 different personalities are, respectively, the soldier, ombudsman, prospector, historian, chameleon, judge, runner, integrator, apostle, actor, doer, originator, gourmet, architect, entrepreneur, devotee, enthusiast, creator, scout, coach, guide, protector, commander, pathfinder, educator, expert, and master. Each of these 27 personalities also has a negative, positive, or neutral attribute for how it can be expressed, which then leads to what Yogi Bhajan called "the 81 different facets of the mind" (Bhajan & Khalsa, 1998). I have presented this model of the 81 facets in a condensed format (Shannahoff-Khalsa, 2006). The negative, positive, or neutral way in which each of the 27 personalities is then expressed determines whether a personality is pathological. Yogi Bhajan also taught 27 different meditation techniques that are specific for correcting each of the respective personality types and for helping to develop and refine their talents and skills (Bhajan & Khalsa, 1998).

However, here our interest is with the 10 specific personality disorders as defined by the APA, and how they are grouped into the three respective clusters, A, B, and C, and their unique and aberrant features that characterize each personality disorder, and then how best to help heal these personalities using Kundalini yoga meditation techniques. In the yogic view, these aberrant features and pathological deficiencies emerge as a result of poor and inadequate nurturing, deficient education, and the detrimental influence of the social environment. The yogic view on the development of a personality disorder is not based on the results of mutant genes or neurogenetic anomalies that exaggerate our behaviors and skew our perceptions and personalities. Instead, the origins of pathological personalities are the result of learning, or, more important, a lack of essential learning during the critical developmental stages when it is most important to develop a sound and humane character. We learn virtues. We do not develop them instinctively. There are five core virtues from the yogic point of view that must be learned: the ability to be kind, the ability to be fair, the ability to be organized, the ability to be courageous, and last, the highest of all the human virtues, the ability to be graceful in any and all situations. Learning kindness is the first and most basic of the human virtues. This is the first marker of a humane personality, and all five virtues lead toward the perfection of a healthy and humane personality. If we are not taught these virtues directly and by example from our parents and other primary teachers, there is a strong tendency to develop insecurities, fears, neuroses, and ultimately the extremes of the psychoses. The effects and pressures that are also imposed by a threatening environment on a poorly nourished psyche all too often lead to the development of one or more of the 10 different personality disorders.

There are indeed other human virtues that are each related to these five basic virtues and that certainly deserve mention. Some of these virtues are the ability to be sensitive, sensible, compassionate, loving, patient, tolerant, fearless, bold, self-confident, trusting, stable, disciplined, and devoted. These virtues are like languages. We must learn them from our personal interactions with others. We also require models of expression taught either directly or indirectly by others in our early stages of development. In the best of all circumstances, a parent has the explicit intention to raise a child with these qualities. Many of these qualities and virtues can also be learned at a later stage of life, but frequently the opportunities are not available and people have no conscious concept that they are missing these virtues. Individuals are rarely aware of the voids or deficiencies in their own personality structure. In the yogic view, the basic or prototype model is the personality of a saint. Be kind to all, be fair to all, be organized in all situations, be courageous, be graceful when challenged under any and all circumstances, and excel in the service of humanity. Therefore, there is a broad continuum between the diseased or disordered personality and the personality of the saint. There are ingredients that make for a healthy personality, and these ingredients must be learned as we develop. In many respects, this life is a test of our personalities. We require these five basic core virtues to develop the character so that we can have a healthy, happy, humane, fulfilling, loving, and respectful life. Therefore, the 10 APA definitions of the personality disorders help to set a good foundation for understanding the aberrant side of deficient character. In time, we may see a broader concept evolve on the nature of the personality and the fundamentals of character.

While the above virtues are by definition all positive personality traits, and the ultimate yogic goal for development is their inclusion in the root structure of the personality, there is also work in the academic literature that partly mirrors some of this perspective by focusing on the negative personality traits. First, according to the *DSM-IV* definitions, there are 79 distinct and descriptive criteria that can be included that must be assessed when doing a full differential diagnosis for the 10 respective personality disorders (see the definitions in the first section). This full and comprehensive diagnosis takes considerable time and is usually considered a burden in clinical care. Therefore, others have devised a more focused approach that also gives a fine-grained structure for pathology with a smaller number of elements or facets for detecting an aberrant personality (Krueger, Skodol, Livesley, Shrout, & Huang, 2007). This is the work by Livesley and colleagues that has led to the development of the Dimensional Assessment of Personality Pathology (DAPP), which consists of 30 facets that are closely related to the traits and behavior of the *DSM* criteria. This model contains four broad subgroups that they call emotional dysregulation, dissocial behavior, inhibitedness, and compulsivity, and each has a different number of primary facet traits (Krueger et al., 2007). The 12 primary facet traits that are characteristic of emotional dysregulation are anxiousness, emotional reactivity, emotional intensity, pessimistic anhedonia, submissiveness, insecure attachment, social apprehensiveness, need for approval, cognitive dysregulation, oppositional, self-harming acts, and self-harming ideas. The nine primary facet traits that are characteristic of dissocial behavior are narcissism, exploitativeness, sadism, conduct problems, hostile-dominance, sensation seeking, impulsivity, suspiciousness, and egocentrism. The seven primary facet traits that are characteristic of inhibitedness are low affiliation, avoidant attachment, attachment need, inhibited sexuality, self-containment, inhibited emotional expression, and lack of empathy. The two primary facet traits that are characteristic of compulsivity are orderliness and conscientiousness. In the use of these traits, the person is then further analyzed by how each dimensionally applies to the patient. They have a scale that ranks the patient with a 1 to 4 rating: "(1) Highly uncharacteristic: the facet describes thoughts, feelings and behaviors that are rarely if ever seen in the person; (2) Somewhat uncharacteristic: the facet describes the thoughts, feelings and behaviors of the person on a few occasions, but less than half of the time the person was observed; (3) Somewhat characteristic: the facet describes the thoughts, feelings and behaviors of the person more than half of the time the person was observed; and (4) Highly characteristic: the facet exemplifies the typical thoughts, feelings and behaviors of the person and is a pervasive part of the person's personality" (Krueger et al., 2007). These authors have advanced this model as an effort to improve on the criteria-specific model defined in the *DSM-IV* with an effort to add a dimensional perspective to the description and definition for personality disorders. However, it would be equally possible to construct a dimensional model based on the positive yogic and perennial virtues to help characterize a healthy personality. The positive virtues and negative criteria are two sides of the same coin here, albeit with a different focus for each. Modern mainstream academic psychiatry is very skilled at defining what traits we do not want to develop, but it does little to emphasize what traits we can and should develop. Why this is the case is an interesting topic for discussion by itself.

The Yogic Protocols for Treatment

There are 10 yogic protocols for treating the personality disorders, and each protocol will include a technique that is specifically related to a concrete symbol in nature that is itself characteristic of one of the 10 variants of this group of disorders. These symbols each represent a state of being that is inherent and representative of the nature of the respective personality disorder. These 10 symbol-related techniques will then be included in a larger protocol that is also specific for one of the three APA-defined clusters, A (odd and eccentric disorders), B (dramatic and emotional disorders), or C (anxious or fearful disorders). The 10 symbols as they relate to the respective personality disorders are as follows.

Cluster A Personality Disorders
1. Paranoid: a *cave* where the patient dwells in an effort to escape other people due to his or her "pervasive distrust and suspiciousness of others such that their motives are interpreted as malevolent" (APA, 2000).
2. Schizoid: a *tall tree* that represents the aloof, singular, and isolated nature that patients must overcome due to their characteristic "detachment from social relationships and a restricted range of expression of emotions in interpersonal settings" (APA, 2000).
3. Schizotypal: a *low tree* that symbolizes patients' separateness and nearly singular and exclusive focus on their own weakly rooted belief systems that represent their source for life, that inadvertently stifles their growth and leads to the "social and

interpersonal deficits marked by acute discomfort with, and reduced capacity for, close relationships as well as by cognitive or perceptual distortions and eccentricities of behavior" (APA, 2000).

Cluster B Personality Disorders
1. Antisocial: a *spiral shell* that symbolizes a twisted and self-contained state that needs to become untwisted and opened to the world of others. The spiral shell needs to open up and overcome the failure to conform to social norms, deceitfulness as indicated by repeated lying, use of aliases, conning others for personal gain; impulsive, irritable, and aggressive behavior, reckless disregard for others, consistent irresponsibility, and lack of remorse (APA, 2000).
2. Borderline: a *stick* or *branch* that easily bends or snaps under pressure in an effort to overcome the "frantic efforts to avoid real or imagined abandonment (APA, 2000)." The bending and snapping also leads to unstable relationships, unstable self-images that cause impulsivity, which leads to self-damaging, suicidal, and self-mutilating behavior, affective instability (intense episodic dysphoria, irritability, and anxiety), chronic feelings of emptiness and worthlessness, difficulty controlling anger, and transient paranoid ideation, delusions, or dissociative symptoms (APA, 2000).
3. Histrionic: a *waterfall* that symbolizes the continuous overflow and flooding of everything in their environment with excessive emotionality and attention-seeking behavior (APA, 2000).
4. Narcissistic: a *snake* that symbolizes the low, slick, and sneaky movements of these individuals in the world and their persona of a grandiose sense of self-importance; preoccupation with fantasies; special, unique, and high status that requires excessive admiration; and sense of entitlement. They are interpersonally exploitative, lack empathy, and are envious of others or believe others are envious of them, with arrogant, haughty behaviors or attitudes (APA, 2000).

Cluster C Personality Disorders

1. Avoidant: a *stone* that symbolizes how these people can become solidly and rigidly fixed in place and set in their ways because they avoid significant interpersonal contact and are "unwilling to get involved with people unless certain of being liked," show restraint initiating intimate relationships because of the fear of being shamed and rejected, view themselves as socially inept, and are unwilling to take personal risks (APA, 2000). This stone needs to be turned around in therapy to face the therapist and reality.

2. Dependent: a *claw* that attaches to others with the "pervasive and excessive need to be taken care of that leads to submissive and clinging behavior and fears of separation" (APA, 2000). In their attachment, they have difficulty in making everyday decisions, need others to assume responsibility, have difficulty expressing disagreement and initiating projects on their own, go to obsessive lengths to obtain nurturance and support from others, and are helpless when alone because of exaggerated fears of inadequacy.

3. Obsessive-compulsive personality disorder: a *bird* that symbolizes the state where patients are always up in the air with their wings flapping, flying around and unable to land and find a position to rest. These patients are "preoccupied with details, rules, lists, order, or schedules to the point that the major point of the activity is lost"; they show "perfectionism that interferes with task completion"; they are "excessively devoted to work and productivity to the exclusion of leisure activities and friendships"; they are "over conscientious, scrupulous, and inflexible about matters of morality, ethics, or values"; and they are unable to discard worn-out or worthless objects, reluctant to delegate tasks, miserly, and show rigidity and stubbornness (APA, 2000).

The approach to therapy using the symbols and the techniques described below is an interactive relationship of the therapist and the patient. The two engage in therapy using a disorder-specific symbol-related yogic technique that is to be included in the cluster-specific protocol. One very important key here for understanding this patient population is that they are wholly or largely not accepting of their own condition. They are rarely aware of their behavior or personality deficits. They do not present in the office or clinic and say, "I have a schizoid personality," or "I have a narcissistic personality disorder," or "I have an antisocial personality disorder." They say, "I have come for treatment. Can you help me?" They present for some other reason, which is often the result of a dysfunctional relationship or an Axis I disorder that they perceive as causing their suffering. Therefore, the philosophy here is to modify patients so that they can express themselves using the symbol as a part of nature instead of trying to get them to directly identify with the disorder by name. They have to see how their behavior can affect their life and others around them and the use of the symbol as descriptive of their condition can be more useful and less threatening. The idea is to help them shift their mood or thought processes when they cannot otherwise diagnose their own negative or troublesome behaviors and how they think. Eight of the ten symbols are fairly neutral and easily conceived without stirring much of a negative reaction. However, the snake in most societies is symbolic of evil, and care must be used here with the narcissistic personality disorder patients. The claw may also have a negative connotation with some patients, but less so than the snake. But they also usually understand that clingy and clawlike attachments have been part of how they operate that have led to their suffering.

Therefore, this work proceeds somewhat differently than the Axis I yoga protocols to treat the anxiety, depressive, addictive impulse control and eating disorders, sleep disorders, chronic fatigue syndrome, ADHD, and PTSD, where patients can more readily identify with their respective conditions and symptoms, and where they can also then easily learn to self-administer the respective protocols independently of the therapist if they choose (Shannahoff-Khalsa, 2006). While the yogic approach to treatment for schizophrenia, autism, and the autism spectrum disorders also includes a unique one-to-one therapeutic relationship, the approach here with personality disorder patients will involve a uniquely different interactive therapeutic style. While schizophrenic patients can be told directly of their diagnosis, you will see in Chapter 4 that autistic or Asperger's patients are not told about their diagnosis and, in fact, the approach to therapy is one that only involves play. Other differences will also be apparent when the approaches to treatment are compared.

The treatment of each personality disorder will include a unique personality disorder–specific technique that is related to the symbol, and this technique will then be included in a cluster-specific protocol along with what are called "water" exercises. There are three different water exercises that each relate to one of the three natural symbols of the ocean, river, and rain. The ocean exercise will help the patient "meet the shore in life" using a waveform-like exercise that is symbolic of the curling and uncurling process of the waves breaking on the shore. This exercise helps the patient push himself or herself forward to meet a new shore. The river exercise represents the process of flowing and stretching out in life, and this exercise helps the patient feel a greater flow in life. The rain exercise represents an opening up, blessing, and saturation where these aspects are brought into the psyche of the patient. Each cluster-specific protocol includes an ocean exercise near the start, a river exercise during, and a rain exercise near the end of each protocol. Therefore, there are 10 discrete protocols where each is specific for one personality disorder, where they all include the same water exercises, but each cluster group will also have a disorder-specific nature, and each cluster and its three (A and C) or four (B) variants will then have one of the 10 symbol-based exercises or meditations. These clusters can also include substitutions for some of the core meditation techniques. While the patients can be shown all of the techniques, they must be presented in a manageable sequence that is dependent on multiple factors that vary with the patient. These factors include patients' openness and enthusiasm, physical and mental condition, and why they are presenting in the first place. Here we are going to ignore the various possibilities for why the patients present, and therefore the protocols are presented as if the patient was a "pure" personality disorder patient seeking therapy for their respective condition. However, the various cluster-specific, symbol-specific, and water exercises all have multiple virtues, and some of these are described with each of these unique meditation techniques. Therefore, the overall benefits will also be useful for treating many of the Axis I disorder symptoms. It goes without saying that some conditions, like the addictive and substance abuse disorders, will be better treated by also including the meditation technique specific for addiction that is described in the chapter called "Treating the Addictive, Impulse Control, and Eating Disorders" in Shannahoff-Khalsa (2006). Clearly, the yogic approach to treating complicated psychiatric disorders is also an art where the administration of the formulas requires a patient-based use of discretion.

The 10 Symbol-Related Techniques*

1. **The Cave.** In the cave the patient feels contained, closed off, and withdrawn, and the treatment here includes both an exercise that is symbolic of the contained state and the complement that helps strengthen and open the patient to the world. This is achieved by teaching the patient the classic movements that include the two exercises called camel pose and baby pose, which are also in Chapter 2 as exercise 5 in the series called True Glue. The therapist explains the need to the patient to emerge from the cave (baby pose) and to extend oneself up and out into the world in camel pose. This practice starts with the patient facing the therapist. The patient starts by inhaling through the nose and then coming up into camel pose with the head hanging back and the arms extended down and back with the hands holding the ankles (see Figure 2.8); then the patient exhales and lowers the body into baby pose (see

*Copyright © David Shannahoff-Khalsa, 2008. No portion of this list may be reproduced without the express written permission of the author.

Figure 2.9). This dynamic movement is continued for 2 minutes. In time, once the patient understands how the basic cavelike condition is symbolized by baby pose and how the end goal is the perfected posture in camel pose, the patient can then choose to practice only the camel pose exercise and slowly extend the practice time up to a maximum of 15 minutes. However, even 3 to 5 minutes of camel pose with Breath of Fire will yield a most satisfactory result. But in the beginning, a maximum practice time of 2 minutes of going back and forth from baby pose to camel pose is sufficient.

2. The Tall Tree. As a tall tree, the patient feels aloof, singular, and isolated, and is detached from any meaningful social relationships. In addition, this patient has a restricted range of emotions in any interpersonal settings. The remedy here must help patients to increase their awareness of their inflexible and "planted" condition, their limited desire for reaching out to form new social connections, and their stifled emotional sensitivity, which also reduces their opportunity for any healthy emotional contacts. In part, this can be accomplished by including exercise 6 of True Glue (Chapter 2). This technique helps patients reach around in life and extend themselves in all directions. The therapist explains this symbolism and how this exercise is a good start at healing the condition. The patient starts by facing the therapist and then stands up straight and inhales through the nose while twisting to the left with the left arm extended out and swinging toward the back as far as possible with the right arm then crossing in front of the chest (see Figure 2.10). Then the patient exhales through the nose while reversing the posture and twisting around to the right with the right arm then extended towards the back as far as possible, with the left arm then coming across the chest. The head will also turn with the torso. Keep the hands in lightly closed fists and continue the movement for 2 minutes.

3. The Low Tree. This little tree, which is too attached and grounded in its own root system without additional growth and expansion, needs to reenergize, emerge, and reach up into the fresh air, which provides a new realm for its nourishment, that is, the more kindly realms of the heavens that are far beyond the superficial and surface-only root system that has led to an inadequate nourishment by itself, that is, patients' faulty, limited, and stifling belief systems. The therapist explains the virtues of this technique and patients experience the virtues of the two postures, where they clearly feel a greater comfort in the standing position. The patient faces the therapist. The starting position is with the patient standing up straight with the arms extended above the head and the hands interlocked with the index fingers extended straight up. This is the inhalation posture. The patient exhales while maintaining the arms and hands up as straight as possible and then squats into a low position where the buttocks come close to the floor in what is called crow pose. The feet are shoulder width apart to help provide stability, and the eyes are kept open throughout the movement. Once in the squat position, the patient then inhales through the nose and straightens up with the arms and hands extended up to the heavens. The feet are kept flat in this exercise without the heels coming off the ground. The exercise should begin slowly and 2 minutes is a good practice time here. One great virtue of this exercise is that it will increase the vital energy of the body through the use of the lower body and it will also help change the thought processes of the patient once it has been completed. These patients need a renewed energy and will so that they can reach up and extend toward a higher and more inclusive goal and realm in life.

4. The Spiral Shell. Antisocial patients live in a twisted relationship with almost all of the individuals that they encounter in their lives, and this leads to substantial pain for everyone. They require the experience of the pain of the twisted state compared to the straightforward, open, honest, and untwisted state. This can be taught by having patients first sit in a twisted posture in one direction and then return to the untwisted state, and then twist in the opposite direction, and then again twist to the straightforward posture. Patients first sit facing the therapist. They close their eyes and place their hands on their respective shoulders with the fingers in the front and the thumbs placed toward the back. Then they inhale and twist toward the left with the head, shoulders, and torso all twisted toward the left. This exercise is similar to the exercise in the True Glue portrayed in Figure 2.4, except that the hands are on the shoulders instead of up straight. Patients hold this posture and then exhale as they return to the forward-facing posture. Then they repeat this motion while inhaling and twisting to the right. The first 2 minutes should be done slowly while holding the twisted positions for as long as possible. Then in the final minute, the movement should be rapid, inhaling to the left and exhaling to the right. The therapist times the 2 phases of the exercise. At the end the patient sits facing forward and takes several slow deep breaths. The first phase of the exercise gives the patient the painful experience of the twisted conditions and how the forward-facing posture is so much more pleasant, and the final minute also helps to rapidly change the thought patterns of the patient to a new and more positive state of mind.

5. The Stick or Branch. The marked instability of the stick or branch and the impulsive nature of the borderline patient are both taught through example here. The condition is also corrected in part by the following exercise, which is exercise 7 in Chapter 2 in the series called True Glue. Patients face the therapist while the therapist explains the virtues and symbolism of this exercise. The patient gets down on the hands and knees and starts by extending the left arm directly out in front of the body. The right leg is then also extended straight back like a rigid stick behind the body (see Figure 2.11). The patient makes a right angle with the extended left hand so that it looks like the patient may be pushing against the wall, and the patient also maintains a right angle at the ankle with the extended right foot. The head is raised up, the eyes are open, and the patient visually focuses on a point directly out in front of the body off in an infinite horizon. The patient can hold this position while either doing Breath of Fire (also called Kapalabhati) only through the nose, or by doing long slow deep breathing only through the nose. The patient must maintain this posture perfectly without bending either limb or losing balance, and this is continued with the breathing for 2 minutes. Then the patient comes down and balances on both hands and knees and rests briefly (1 minute or less) and then reverses sides and continues everything for 2 additional minutes. Note that the opposite arms and legs are extended in the first part and then they are reversed for the second part. The difficulty of this exercise will help explain to patients how unstable the "stick" is and in time they learn through experience the virtues of not bending, how rewarding this can be, and how much it helps lead to an inner strength and inner balance that helps them overcome their impulsive nature.

6. The Waterfall. Histrionic patients have to learn the virtues of not overflowing, flooding, or making waves in their environments by the constant release and sharing of their emotions. They have to understand how disturbing this can be for others, and how it can damage their own life when they are always making the effort to become the center of attention. They can begin to learn the negative repercussions of this disturbing hand-waving-like behavior and how much better they can feel by remaining still and silent and the positive experience that comes from this uninterrupted silence. The patient sits facing the therapist. The following technique is a shortened version of a technique that Yogi Bhajan taught in Los Angeles on October 11, 1996, called a meditation for developing and strengthening the subtle body. This technique is invaluable for those who want to become healers as it also helps build and strengthen the subtle body, the immortal body, the working body of the healer and saint. This technique also helps build an incredible aura and arc line that is ultimately what histrionic patients desire in their efforts to attract attention, and the immediate results can produce marvelous benefits when practiced longer or for the maximum times. Things come to us from the universe through the subtle body. The effects of this technique therefore help bring prosperity in all of the positive ways, but they must be earned through the virtues of this practice. It is claimed that the radiance of the practitioner can be increased so much that people really no longer focus on the physical features of their face. They only see the brightness, the glow. While the eyes can be open or closed, here it is best to keep the eyes open so that patients are more easily aware of their own arms and hands in this dramatic motion. The patient inhales and exhales only through the mouth shaped like an O, and the lips are slightly pursed and the sound of the breath is like a hiss. The hands are held with the fingers loose and down by the sides (see Figure 3.1), and then the patient inhales and both hands move rapidly up to the top of the top of head, forming an arclike structure where the left hand comes over the top of the right hand and the right hand is closer to the top of the head (see Figure 3.2). At this point, both palms are over the crown but do not touch each other or the top of the head. On the exhale, both hands come down in a reverse arclike movement all the way to-ward the legs but do not touch the legs or the body on the way down. When the hands are down the backs of the hands are near, but not touching, the floor. The key here is to have the hands and arms making an arclike shape as they ascend and descend. The

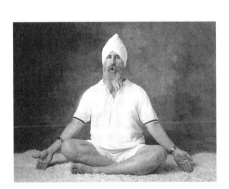
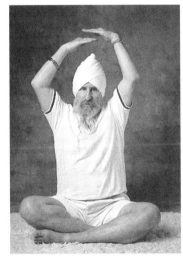

Figures 3.1 and 3.2
Meditation for Developing and Strengthening the Subtle Body

hands and fingers remain relaxed, but the movement is rapid as they are moving up and down with the powerful breath approaching one cycle every 1 to 2 seconds. The technique here ends by interlocking the hands straight over the head while inhaling, holding the breath, and then tightening all of the muscles in the body. Then the patient exhales and relaxes but maintains the posture, and then the inhalation, breath holding, and muscle tightening is repeated two more times. The patient then sits quietly and enjoys the benefits of stillness and the incredible joy that comes from within. A good practice time here is 2 to 5 minutes. This is enough time to help patients understand that the rapid and disruptive movement of their emotional "arms" in life are not only disruptive to others but will ultimately bring them pain. But they also learn that a correct practice of this technique can quickly lead to a much improved state of mind and the true radiance and attractive qualities that they are looking for in life. However, a normal and healthy starting time for this technique, when it is practiced as a single therapy for developing the remarkable healing qualities of the subtle body, would be 11 minutes, building slowly up to 20 or 22 minutes, and finally with a maximum practice time of 33 minutes. When 33 minutes are reached and the technique is finished correctly, the immediate benefits are indescribably magnificent. This may appeal to the histrionic patient, at least in theory.

7. **The Snake.** The slithering and low behavior of the narcissist can be mimicked by the patient facing the therapist in cobra pose (see Figure 3.3). Patients start by lying prone with their legs stretched back with the tops of their feet flat on the floor, keeping the heels together. The hands are spread on the floor near their shoulders as if they were going to do a push-up. The pelvis remains flat on the ground. Then patients begin to inhale and straighten their arms while lifting the chest off the floor until the head is held up as high as possible with the eyes open and focused toward a point on the ceiling. In this posture the spine is stretched as much as possible while working to distribute the effort equally throughout the spine. The entire body is kept as relaxed as possible and the

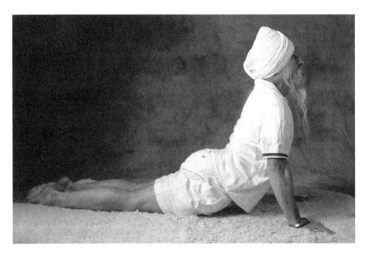

Figure 3.3
Cobra Pose

posture is held for up to 2 minutes as patients do Breath of Fire or slow long deep breathing. When they finish, they relax back down with their head turned toward the side and the arms relaxed along the sides of the body. While holding cobra pose, patients realize the pain of maintaining a snakelike posture and how snakes look to the world when their chest is protruding in the face of others and how they look to others as their head is held too high. But the patient also gains the benefits of having changed their own mental patterns and thought processes through a productive and healthy practice where they stretch themselves out instead of stretching others out in the world. They learn in time that working on themselves, rather than manifesting their grandiose importance, leads to a better internal and more meaningful result.

8. **The Stone.** The stone symbolizes the avoidant personality, which manifests with a "pervasive pattern of social inhibition, feelings of inadequacy, and hypersensitivity to negative evaluation" (APA, 2000). The stone does not like to change or to be moved from its safe space, or to be confronted by anything that represents a potential challenge, difficulty, or threat. Its tendency is to not move. Stones do not move by themselves. Here, patients start by

sitting facing away from the therapist. Then while practicing the breathing technique described below, they slowly rotate counter-clockwise to their left, step by step, to face the therapist. This can be accomplished by using the hands to reposition the body on the ground a few inches at a time, or if they are in a swivel chair or stool the feet can be used to help move themselves. Then they return to the original position facing away from the therapist and continue with the breathing meditation and slowly rotate clock-wise toward their right, step by step. This step-by-step movement slowly forces patients to face the therapist, who encourages and guides the process as needed if patients are reluctant to turn. The therapist also becomes a mirror to patients and their advocate for change. The eyes can be either open or closed in the beginning, depending on the choice of the patient. However, in time patients can also practice the technique with their eyes open so that they are acutely aware of what they are doing and how they look to the world, and how they are not harmed by the slow process of change. There will also be significant and pleasant rewards on a mental and physical level when the following breath technique is practiced. The eight-part breath helps patients experience their expansion, increased awareness, and the integration of their mental processes. Patients sit either on the floor or in a swivel chair (the easier of the two) and maintain a straight spine throughout the practice. If the eyes are closed, they are focused on the third eye, where the root of the nose meets the eyebrows. If patients choose to keep the eyes open, they should be encouraged to focus straight ahead on a fixed point on the horizon that will slowly change as they rotate. The hands are relaxed in the lap. The breathing starts by first inhaling through the mouth using a curled tongue that is slightly extended out of the mouth. The sides of the tongue are curled up and the tongue then has a U-shaped appearance. The inhale is broken into eight equal parts. Then the tongue is brought back into the mouth, which is closed, and the exhale is broken into eight equal parts out through the nose. There is no pause after completing the full inhale or full exhale phases of the breath cycle. The pattern is continued with the cycle of eight parts in through the curled tongue and eight parts out through the nose. This cycle takes about 10 seconds for one complete round. The benefits of this technique can be magnified by using the mantra Sa Ta Na Ma with two silent repetitions of the complete mantra on the inhale and two repetitions on the exhale. Here each of the four syllables is sequentially paired with one step of the inhalation or exhalation, and therefore the mantra is mentally repeated twice through on the inhalation and twice through on the exhalation. This is preferable to counting 1 through 8 for each part of the breath cycle. Patients who are unwilling to use the mantra can mentally focus only on the sounds of the breath. Patients who cannot curl their tongue into the U shape must inhale only through the nose in eight parts, keeping the mouth closed, and exhale only out the nose in eight parts. The ability to curl the tongue is a genetic trait. If the patient can curl the tongue in the U shape, it will help stimulate the thyroid and parathyroid glands. The patient can start with 3 to 5 minutes while slowly rotating first to the left, and then 3 to 5 minutes while slowly rotating to the right. The final end position is facing the therapist. Equal times should be practiced in both directions. Upon finally completing this technique, the patient should take at least three long, slow, deep breaths (unbroken) through the nose and then relax. This is a relatively easy technique and can bring considerable comfort to the patient when practiced correctly. There is no need to make an effort to completely fill the lungs on the inhalation or to completely empty the lungs on the exhalation. This is not a pattern that should strain the patient. This eight-part breath technique can also be practiced while sitting straight for 11 to 31 minutes. But here as a technique for helping the avoidant personality, the slow turning is critical to the patient's benefit.

9. The Claw. The claw symbolizes the approach to life of patients with dependent personality disorder. They latch onto people in their life and are rarely willing to disengage. Other people tend to experience them as thorns or like a cat with claws that insistently tear and scratch at them. Patients have to have a direct experience with the therapist where they attach, but also let go, and where there is a give and take that is balanced and by mutual consent. Their clawlike attachment and how this must change to become a give-and-take relationship is magnified in the following practice of a Venus Kriya. In this practice, patients learn the positive benefits of how a relationship can be with a fair, balanced, and mutual give and take. This Venus Kriya has been previously published and is also called Pushing Palms (Shannahoff-Khalsa, 2006). There are two standard versions of this technique, and the difference is with the mantra employed. The patient and therapist sit facing each other in a cross-legged position on the floor with a straight spine. The right knee touches the left knee of the partner. Sitting in chairs is acceptable, but the knees must still touch. The eyes are open looking directly into the partner's eyes. This technique is practiced with the hands facing forward and up at shoulder level with the palms held flat as if they are going to push something away from themselves. The left palm of each partner touches the right palm of the other. Here, the patient and therapist touch hands palm to palm. Start with the hands at an equal distance from each other (the line just over where the knees meet). Then the right hands push forward and the left hands come back toward the shoulder. With this movement, the woman, who can be either the patient or the therapist if they are of opposite gender, chants the word "Gobinday." Then the left hands push forward and the right hands come back toward the shoulder. During this movement the man chants "Mukanday" (sounds like "mookunday"). The next movement is again with the right hands moving forward and left hands moving back as the woman chants "Udaray" (sounds like "oohdaray"). Again the left hand is pushed forward and the man chants "Aparay" (the A sounds like "ah"). These alternating pushing movements continue as the woman chants "Harying" (sounds like "hareeing"), the man chants "Karying" (sounds like "kareeing"), the woman chants "Nirnamay" (sounds like "nearnamay"), and the man chants "Akamay" (sounds like "aahkamay"). Then the entire mantra is repeated, again with the woman only chanting "Gobinday" and the man only chanting "Mukanday," and so on. Note that the woman chants when the right hands go forward, and the man chants when the left hands go forward, and the respective mantra is chanted only once with each push. The patient and the therapist do not chant together, but alternate the use of the eight sounds. Only the woman chants Gobinday, Udaray, Harying, and Nirnamay, and only the man chants Mukanday, Aparay, Karying, and Akamay. The respective meanings of the eight sounds are the following: "sustainer," "liberator," "enlightener," "infinite," "destroyer," "creator," "nameless," "desireless." The rate of chanting and moving the arms in the pushing movement is about one sound per movement per second. The total time limit for practice is 3 minutes and must not go beyond 3 minutes. When finished, the patient and therapist sit for a moment with their hands separated and relaxed in their laps, and the patient reflects on the need for a mutual give-and-take interaction that must occur if there is a "clawed" interlock. If the therapist and patient are both males, or both females, the therapist should take the role of the male in this meditation technique. Then the patient proceeds to employ the remainder of the protocol. This eight-part mantra is the first version of Pushing Palms. There is also another version that is easier for beginners using the mantra Sa Ta Na Ma. The woman chants "Sa" (the "a" sound as in "father" for each word) as the right hands are pushed forward, and the man chants "Ta" as the left hands are pushed forward. The woman chants "Na" as the right hands are pushed forward and the man chants "Ma" as the left hands are pushed forward. This four-part mantra is repeated with the same sequence for a maximum time of 3 minutes. All other aspects of the practice are the same as the first version with the eight-part mantra. Note also that this is chanting out loud; it is not a silent chant. The sound Sa gives the mind the ability to expand to the infinite; Ta gives the mind the ability to experience the totality of life; Na gives the mind the ability to conquer death; and Ma gives the mind the ability to resurrect and also means "rebirth." In short, the mantra can translate to mean "infinity, life, death, and rebirth." This is a very powerful mantra for cleansing and restructuring the subconscious mind and helping to set a mental framework in the conscious mind to experience higher states of consciousness (Shannahoff-Khalsa & Bhajan, 1988; Shannahoff-Khalsa & Bhajan, 1991). Both mantras here help awaken the individual beyond a finite identity to live in higher states of consciousness. The first version has been my favorite Venus Kriya.

10. The Bird. A bird is best symbolized by the constant flapping of its wings to keep afloat in the air. This is how we see a bird in action. But there is a need for the bird to come back down to earth, to keep things in perspective, and to finish a task. This is an ability that is lost by patients with an obsessive-compulsive personality disorder. The patient will sit facing the therapist and practice a shortened version of a meditation technique called Hast Kriya. This technique helps patients understand how they look to the world (with the constant flapping of the wings) and also helps them achieve a balance between their earth activities and the heavens (Bhajan, 2002). The patient sits in an easy, cross-legged pose or in a chair, maintaining a straight spine with a light neck lock, where the chin is pulled in slightly toward the chest to help straighten the cervical vertebrae. When this lock is pulled, the practitioner immediately feels how straight the neck can become. The lock is also called Jalandhar Bandh. The eyes are kept closed and focused on the third eye point. There is no specific breath pattern and in time it will come naturally. However, the inhale can also be taken when the arms go up over the head and the exhale can be taken when the arms come down with the fingers touching the floor. The patient extends the index fingers on both hands and the other fingers are locked down into a fist with the thumbs coming across the middle and ring fingers. The timing of the movements here is best practiced by listening to a tape with the mantra Sat Nam Wahe Guru (Singh, 1996). Patients touch the index fingers to the floor on both sides near the body (see Figure 3.4) when the musician chants "Sat." Then they touch their index fingers together over the top of their head when the musician chants "Nam" (see Figure 3.5).

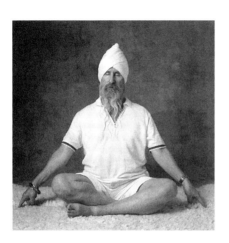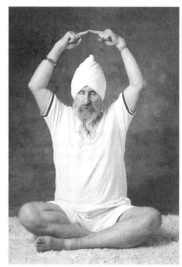

Figures 3.4 and 3.5
Meditation Called Hast Kriya

Then they touch their index fingers to the floor again on both sides when the musician chants "Sat." Then they touch their index fingers again together over the top of their head when the musician chants "Nam." Then the index fingers are touched to the floor on both sides when the musician chants "Wha-hay." Then they touch their index fingers together again over the top of their head when the musician chants "Guroo." Then they touch their index fingers together on both sides when the musician chants "Wha-hay." Then they touch their index fingers together over the top of their head when the musician chants "Guroo." This practice, resembling wings flapping up and down, can continue for 3 to 5 minutes or longer, and the maximum and preferred time is 22 minutes when Hast Kriya is practiced perfectly as an independent technique. To end the technique patients inhale deeply, hold the breath for 10 seconds, then exhale and relax for a few minutes before going on to the next part of the protocol for obsessive-compulsive personality disorder. This procedure will help patients understand how they look in life to others, and it will also help them heal and gain a new perspective and balance that is so profoundly missing in their lives. When Yogi Bhajan taught this technique as a method to help develop a balance of the earth and the heavens, he also commented: "This kriya renews the nervous system and can heal nerve pain and sciatica. It is so powerful it can hold the Hand of God; so powerful, it can hold the hand of death. 'Sat Nam Wahe Guru' is a Jupiter mantra" (Bhajan, 2002). The term Jupiter here also refers to the effects that this technique has via the use of the index finger, which is also called the Jupiter finger. In addition, Yogi Bhajan said, "The most graceful power and knowledge comes from Jupiter. Jupiter controls the medulla oblongata, the neurological center of the brain and the three rings of the brain stem. If you do this kriya for 22 minutes a day, you will totally change your personality. Power will descend from above and clean you out. Anger and obnoxiousness will disappear from your personality."

The Three Water-Related Exercises*

1. The Ocean exercise helps the patient "meet the shore in life." The choice here for an exercise that contains the wavelike actions that help propel the patient forward to meet the shore is called "spine flexing for vitality." This technique is one of the most elementary exercises in Kundalini yoga and when it is practiced sitting on the ground, it is also called camel ride. This technique is the first technique after tuning in for each of the three cluster-specific protocols for the three unique groups of the respective personality disorders. Frequently, even when patients have the right formula, they hesitate to go forward, and the consequence is that they sit in a doldrumlike state. This simple spine-flexing exercise is an easy way to help patients propel themselves forward and overcome their inertia and resistance to engaging in the full protocol. The complete details for practice are provided in the Cluster A protocol as technique 2 in the Three Cluster-Specific Protocols.

*Copyright © David Shannahoff-Khalsa, 2008. No portion of this list may be reproduced without the express written permission of the author.

2. The River exercise helps the patient flow and stretch out in life. When the flow of energy in the body is blocked through the major meridians that are related to the spine, the patient will not easily progress. This technique will help expedite the entire growth process and it is also healing for the sex meridians, sciatic nerves, and lower back. This is the life nerve-stretching exercise with the legs spread wide. See the complete description of the technique in The Eight-Part Kundalini Yoga Meditation Protocol Specific for Treating the Cluster A Personality Disorders.

3. The Rain exercise helps the patient experience an opening up, blessing, and saturation of the psyche. This technique is called "the Meditation with the Magic Mantra." See the description of technique 8 below in the Cluster A eight-part protocol. This technique is always the last exercise for the specific protocols for clusters A, B, and C.

The Three Cluster-Specific Protocols for the Personality Disorders

Three yoga treatment protocols are described here for the personality disorders, and each protocol is specific for one of the three APA-defined clusters, A, B, and C.

The Eight-Part Kundalini Yoga Meditation Protocol Specific for Treating the Cluster A Personality Disorders: Paranoid, Schizoid, and Schizotypal*

1. Technique to Induce a Meditative State: Tuning In

Description of technique (see Figure 2.1): Sit with a straight spine and with the feet flat on the floor if sitting in a chair. Put the hands together at the center of the chest in prayer pose—the palms are pressed together with 10–15 pounds of pressure between the hands (a mild to medium pressure, nothing too intense). The area where

*Copyright © David Shannahoff-Khalsa, 2008. No portion of this protocol may be reproduced without the express written permission of the author.

the sides of the thumbs touch rests on the sternum with the thumbs pointing up (along the sternum), and the fingers are together and point up and out with a 60-degree angle to the ground. The eyes are closed and focused at the third eye (imagine a sun rising on the horizon or the equivalent of the point between the eyebrows at the origin of the nose). A mantra is chanted out loud in a 1½ breath cycle. Inhale first through the nose and chant "Ong Namo" with an equal emphasis on each word. Then immediately follow with a half-breath inhalation through the mouth and chant "Guru Dev Namo" with approximately equal emphasis on each word. (The *o* in Ong and Namo are both long *o* sounds; Dev sounds like *Dave*, with a long *a* sound. The practitioner should focus on the experience of the vibrations these sounds create on the upper palate and throughout the cranium while letting the mind be carried by the sounds into a new and pleasant mental space. This should be repeated a minimum of three times. This technique helps to create a protected meditative state of mind and is always used as a precursor to the other techniques.

2. The Ocean Exercise: The Spine-Flexing Technique for Vitality

See the comments under The Three Water-Related Exercises. This technique can be practiced while sitting either in a chair or on the floor in a cross-legged position. If you are in a chair, hold the knees with both hands for support and leverage. If you are sitting cross-legged, grasp the ankles in front with both hands. Begin by pulling the chest up and slightly forward, inhaling deeply through the nose at the same time. Then exhale through the nose as you relax the spine down into a slouching position. Keep the head up straight, as if you were looking forward, without allowing it to move much with the flexing action of the spine. This will help prevent a whip effect in the cervical vertebrae. Make sure that all of the breathing is only through the nose for both the inhalation and exhalation. The eyes are closed as if you were looking at a central point on the horizon, the third eye. Your mental focus is kept on the sound of the breath while listening to the fluid movement of the inhalation and exhalation. Begin the technique slowly while loosening up the spine. Eventually, a very rapid movement can be achieved with practice, reaching a rate of 1 to 2 times per second for the entire movement. A few minutes are adequate in the beginning. Later, there is no time limit. Food should be avoided just prior to this exercise. Be careful and flex the spine slowly in the beginning. Relax for 1 minute when finished.

3. Ganesha Meditation for Focus and Clarity

Sit with a straight spine with the eyes closed. The left thumb and little finger are sticking out from the palm. The other fingers are curled into a fist with fingertips on the moon mound (the root of the thumb area that extends down to the wrist, see Figure 3.6).

The left hand and elbow are parallel to the floor, with the pad of the tip of the left thumb pressing squarely on the front surface (not on the sides) of the curved notch of the nose between the eyes. The little finger is sticking out. With the right hand and elbow

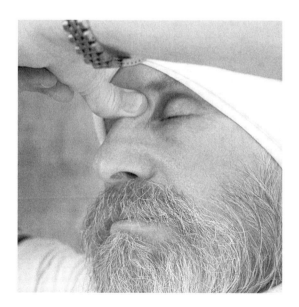

Figure 3.6
Ganesha Meditation

parallel to the floor, grasp the left little finger with the right hand and close the right hand into a fist around it, so that both hands now extend straight out from your head. Push the notch with the padded tip of the left thumb to the extent that you feel some soreness as you breathe long and deep. After continued practice, this soreness reduces. Do this for 3 minutes and no longer. To finish, keeping the posture with eyes closed, inhale and hold the breath, and then push a little more and pull the navel point in by tightening the abdominal muscles for 10 seconds, then exhale powerfully out through the mouth. Repeat the inhale, hold, press, tighten, and exhale one more time for 10 seconds.

4. The River Exercise

See the comments under The Three Water-Related Exercises. Here the choice is to sit on the ground and spread the legs out to the sides as far as possible. The patient grabs around the back of the big toe of each foot with the index and middle fingers of the respective hand and the thumbs hold against the front of the big toes to help secure the grip. Patients who cannot stretch out this far should attempt to grab the ankles or as close as possible to the ends of the lower legs around the calf muscle area. With this stretched position, patients keep the head in line with the spine and on the exhale they pull themselves down slowly, first stretching out toward the right foot. Then they inhale back up while maintaining the grips on the toes and follow by exhaling down toward the center between both legs, followed by inhaling back up straight, and then exhaling as they pull themselves back down to the left leg, and inhale back up. The exhale down and inhale up routine is continued, always following the pattern of right, center, left, right, center, left. This stretching routine will help energize patients further to add to the flow in their life, and it helps to change the mental patterns that are blocking them. With practice, moving through the right, center, and left positions takes about 2 seconds. A good practice time is 1 to 2 minutes.

5. *The Respective Exercise From the 10 Symbol-Related Techniques*

See the detailed description for each disorder-specific exercise in the section The 10 Symbol-Related Techniques. The techniques for the cave, tall tree, and low tree are all described in complete detail.

6. *Gan Puttee Kriya: A Technique to Help Eliminate Negativity From the Past, Present, and Future*

Sit with a straight spine, either on the floor in an easy, cross-legged posture or in a chair. The backs of your hands are resting on your knees with the palms facing upward. The eyes are nine-tenths closed (one-tenth open, but looking straight ahead into the darkness at the third eye point, not the light below). Chant from your heart in a natural, relaxed manner, or chant in a steady relaxed monotone. Chant out loud the sound "Sa" (the *a* sounds like "ah"), and touch your thumb tips and index finger tips together quickly and simultaneously with about 2 pounds of pressure. Then chant "Ta" and touch the thumb tips to the middle finger tips. Chant "Na" and touch the thumb tips to the ring finger tips. Then chant "Ma" and touch the thumb tips to the little finger tips. Chant "Ra" and touch your thumb tips and index finger tips. Chant "Ma" and touch the thumb tips to the middle finger tips. Chant "Da" and touch the thumb tips to the ring finger tips. Chant "Sa" and touch the thumb tips to the little finger tips. Chant "Sa" and touch your thumb tips and index finger tips. Chant "Say" (sounds like the word *say* with a long *a*) and touch the thumb tips to the middle finger tips. Chant "So" and touch the thumb tips to the ring finger tips. Chant "Hung" and touch the thumb tips to the little finger tips.

Chant at a rate of one sound per second. The thumb tip and fingertips touch with a very light 2 to 3 pounds of pressure with each connection. This helps to consolidate the circuit created by each thumb-finger link. Start with 11 minutes, which will be adequate for this protocol. However, patients can also build up the time for Gan Puttee Kriya to 31 minutes of practice if they want additional benefits. To finish, remain in the sitting posture and inhale, holding the breath for 20 to 30 seconds while you shake and move every part of your body with the hands and arms extended over your head. Exhale and repeat this two more times to circulate the energy and to break the pattern of tapping, which affects the brain. Then immediately proceed with focusing the eyes on the tip of the nose (the end you cannot see) and breathe slowly and deeply for 1 minute.

The sounds used in this meditation are each unique, and they have a powerful effect on both the conscious and subconscious mind. The sound "Sa" gives the mind the ability to expand to the infinite. "Ta" gives the mind the ability to experience the totality of life. "Na" gives the mind the ability to conquer death. "Ma" gives the mind the ability to resurrect. "Ra" gives the mind the ability to expand in radiance (this sound purifies and energizes). "Da" gives the mind the ability to establish security on the earth plane, providing a ground for action. "Say" gives the totality of experience. "So" is the personal sense of identity, and "Hung" is the infinite as a vibrating and real force. Together, So Hung means "I am Thou." The unique qualities of this 12-syllable mantra help cleanse and restructure the subconscious mind and help heal the conscious mind to ultimately experience the superconscious mind. Thus, all the blocks that result from an extreme traumatic event are eliminated over time with the practice of Gan Puttee Kriya.

7. Multipart Meditation to Release Pressure From the Subconscious Mind and Overcome Compulsive Behavior Patterns

This technique was first taught by Yogi Bhajan in Los Angeles, California, on March 11, 1997. Sit with a straight spine, either in a chair with both feet flat on the ground or on the floor with the legs crossed. There are five parts to this meditation, with a total practice time of about 26 minutes. This meditation is useful for people that are being tortured by their compulsive behavior and compulsive reactions that result from the intense pressures coming from the subconscious mind.

Part 1

The elbows and upper arms are against the front of the chest with the elbows against the ribcage (see Figure 3.7). The palms are flat and face up toward the heavens, and they are kept flat with the ability to hold something that may fall into the hands. The fingers are together and the thumbs are next to the fingers. The fingers of the right hand are facing out to the right side and the fingers of the left hand are facing out to the left side. The fingers are thus facing in opposite directions. This posture produces a slight pressure on the back of the forearms and forces a stretch on the hands. While

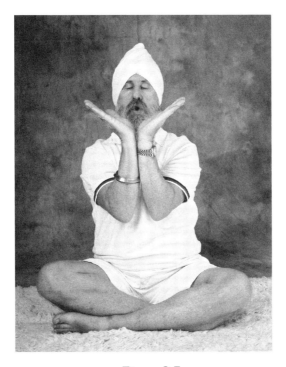

Figure 3.7
Meditation to Release Pressure From the Subconscious Mind and
Overcome Compulsive Behavior Patterns, Part 1

maintaining this posture, keep the eyes open and focused on the tip of the nose. This eye focus point is called "ajna band," which means "mind lock," and this eye posture helps to normalize the activity of the frontal lobes. The mouth is made into a tight O shape, which stimulates the vagus nerves. The breath pattern is slow and deep only through the O-shaped mouth for 13 minutes.

Part 2
Keep the same hand-arm-eye-mouth posture as in Part 1. Now for 6 minutes chant out loud through the O-shaped mouth the mantra Har with a rate of about one Har per second. Each time that you chant "Har," pump/push the navel point out in phase with the mantra. The navel relaxes on its own after it is pumped out. You can either listen to the *Tantric Har* recording while chanting the mantra or not if you know the rhythm of the mantra (Khalsa, 2000).

Part 3
Maintain the same hand-arm-eye posture as in parts 1 and 2. But now whistle out loud to the *Ardas Bhaee* recording for 3 minutes (Anahata, 2001). It is also permissible not to use the recording if you know the beat and rhythm of the mantra.

Part 4
Now close the eyes and focus at the third eye, extend the arms out straight in front of the body parallel to each other with the palms facing up, and do slow deep breathing through the nose for 3 minutes without moving any muscles (see Figure 3.8).

To end Part 4, maintain the arm-hand-eye postures of Part 4 and inhale, hold the breath, and tighten all the muscles in the arms and shoulders. Also tighten the muscles in the back as if to lift the spine up from its base, hold for 10 seconds, and then exhale powerfully. Repeat the entire inhalation and muscle-tightening routine two more times for a total of three times.

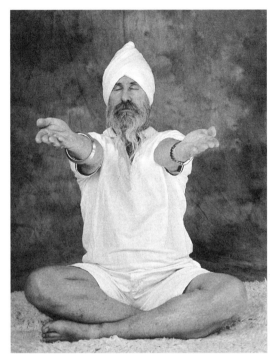

Figure 3.8
Meditation to Release Pressure From the Subconscious Mind and Overcome
Compulsive Behavior Patterns, Part 4

*8. The Rain Exercise to Open Up, Bless, and Saturate the Psyche
With Divine Healing Energy*

The mantra for this technique was taught as the Technique to Turn
Negative Thoughts into Positive Thoughts as part of the 11-part
Kundalini yoga protocol for treating OCD (Shannahoff-Khalsa,
2006). This is the most powerful mantra in the system of Kundalini yoga as taught by Yogi Bhajan. Here this mantra will be taught
as part of a full meditation exercise called the Meditation with the
Magic Mantra that Yogi Bhajan taught on April 26, 1976 (Khalsa,
2006). Patients who can work hard enough to go through the seven
previous exercises deserve to be blessed and saturated with this
glorious healing energy. This technique should be employed while

sitting with a straight spine. The hands are lifted to the level of the heart center with the palms facing up and with the elbows relaxed at the sides. The patient forms a shallow cup with the hands by placing the sides of the hands together along the sides of the little fingers up to where the wrists start (see Figure 3.9). The fingers are kept together as if the patient is forming a bowl. But the thumbs are spread out to the sides away from the hands without holding tension in the thumbs. The edges of the bowl are about a 30-degree angle up from the parallel plane. The important factor here is to keep the line along the sides of the little (Mercury) fingers touching all the way up to where the wrists begin. Normally, there will be no opening whatsoever. However, some people will have a gap between their little fingers, and this gap should be kept to a minimum. During the practice the eyes are closed, but the visual focus

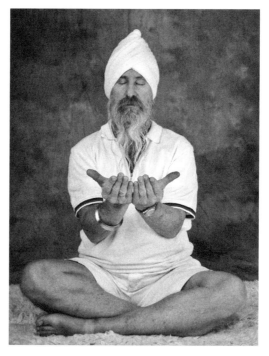

Figure 3.9
The Meditation With the Magic Mantra

is looking into the center of the bowl formed by the hands. This technique must be practiced in a peaceful and serene environment, the more sacred the better. The meditation is practiced by chanting the mantra "Ek Ong Kar Sat Gurprasad Sat Gurprasad Ek Ong Kar" one time per breath with a rate of 4 to 5 seconds per cycle of the mantra. When the mantra is chanted as a single practice in the Technique to Turn Negative Thoughts into Positive Thoughts, it is to be chanted through rapidly up to five full repetitions of the entire mantra per breath. However, that is not the case here and it must be chanted only one time per breath cycle at the rate of 4 to 5 seconds per cycle. The way to chant the mantra is the following: The Ek sound is the same as the "eck" in *neck*. Ong has a long *o* (not "ung"). Kar sounds like *car* but with an emphasis on the *k* sound. Sat has a short *a* sound as in "ah." For Gurprasad, *u* and *a* are short vowel sounds; the *a* sounds like "ah." Eventually, one no longer thinks about the order of the sounds. They come automatically. The mental focus should be on the vibration created against the upper palate and throughout the cranium. If performed correctly, a very peaceful and healed state of mind is achieved that can lead to a blisslike state of being. The maximum practice time for this meditation is 31 minutes. However, even 5 to 11 minutes can produce very powerful effects when it is practiced correctly. That is usually more than adequate to gain the experience of the opening, blessing, and saturation effect that is desired here.

Here are the comments on the Meditation with the Magic Mantra that were given by Yogi Bhajan when he first taught the technique:

Thirty-one minutes of this can keep you very high. A couple of days of practice can give you certain stimulation which is beyond explanation. It is very rare that the Mercury fingers are joined in this way, but that is what makes the difference. Remember to keep the gap between the Mercury fingers as small as possible. Ek Ong Kar Sat Gurprasad Sat Gurprasad Ek Ong Kar is the most powerful of all mantras. The entire Siri Guru Granth Sahib is nothing but an explanation of this mantra. It is so strong that it elevates the self beyond duality and establishes the flow of the spirit. This mantra will make the mind so powerful that it will remove all obstacles. We call it the magic mantra because its positive effect happens quickly and lasts a long time. But it has to be chanted with reverence in a place of reverence. You can mock any mantra you like except this one, because this mantra is known to have a backlash. Normally mantras have no backlash. When you chant them well, they give you the benefit, but when you chant them wrong they don't have an ill effect. If they don't do any good, at least they won't hurt you. But, if you chant Ek Ong Kar Sat Gurprasad Sat Gurprasad Ek Ong Kar wrong, it can finish you. I must give you this basic warning. This mantra is not secret, but it is very sacred. So chant it with reverence; write it with reverence and use it with reverence. Normally we chant to God before practicing this mantra. Either chant the Mul Mantra (Ek Ong Kar Sat Nam Karta Purkh Nirbhao Nirvair Akal Moort Ajuni Sai Bhung Gurprasad Jap Ad Sach Jugad Sach Haibhee Sach Nanak Hosee Bhee Sach) or the Mangala Charan Mantra (Ad Gureh Nameh Jugad Gurey Nameh Sat Gurey Nameh Siri Guru Devay Nameh).

If patients practice all of the techniques in their respective cluster protocol, the chanting of the Mul Mantra or Mangala Charan Mantra is unnecessary. However, all of the other cautions must be respected.

Optional Substitutions for Meditation 7 in the Eight-Part Kundalini Yoga Meditation Protocol Specific for Treating the Cluster A Personality Disorders

1. The Ardas Bhaee Mantra

For those individuals who are less inclined to perform the fourth meditation technique in the part series in the seventh step of the protocol, because of the initially physically challenging arm and hand posture, the easiest substitute is a mantra called Ardas Bhaee. This mantra can be substituted and chanted for 11 to 31 minutes with the eyes closed and focused at the third eye point with the hands in gyan mudra (the thumb tip and index finger tip touch) with the palms facing up resting on the knees. An alternative and slightly more powerful posture is to relax the upper arms at the sides, but to interlock the hands and hold them in front of the heart center and grip them a little tighter than usual if they were only held loosely (see Figure 3.10). With this posture the eyes are focused on the tip of the nose, and this technique can be practiced for 11 to 31 minutes. The full mantra is "Ardas Bhaee, Amardas Guru, Amardas Guru, Ardas Bhaee, Ram Das Guru, Ram Das Guru, Ram Das Guru, Sachee Sahee." Yogi Bhajan described the effects of this mantra, which he taught on January 29, 1986, as follows: "Normally there is no power in the human but the power of prayer. And to do prayer, you have to put your mind and body together and then pray from the soul. Ardas Bhaee is a mantra prayer. If you sing

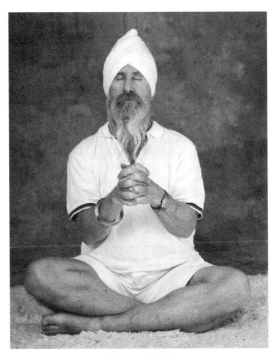

Figure 3.10
Meditation With the Mantra Ardas Bhaee

it, your mind, body, and soul automatically combine and without saying what you want, the need of the life is adjusted. That is the beauty of this prayer" (Bhajan, 2000).

2. A Meditation Technique to Help Overcome
All Psychological Weaknesses

This meditation was taught by Yogi Bhajan in Los Angeles, California, on October 30, 1978. Regarding the effects of this technique, he commented: "This meditation directs your fear toward motivating you to infinity. It will bring a simple polarity of your own magnetic field, and anything which has been neutralized, and is weak with you, it will make strong." Sit in a chair with the feet flat on the floor or in an easy cross-legged pose and maintain a straight spine. Bend the neck and lock the chin down against the chest. Relax the arms down with the elbows bent and raise the forearms up and in toward the chest until the hands meet in front of the chest at the level of the heart. Extend and join all fingers and the thumb of each hand and place the right hand immediately above the left hand. Point the palm of the left hand down at the ground and the palm of the right hand up at the sky. The hands should be parallel to each other and to the ground. This is not an easy hand posture, but it is done most easily by keeping the forearms parallel to the ground (see Figure 3.11). The eyes are open and focused on the tip of the nose (the end you cannot see). Begin the meditation by deeply inhaling and completely exhaling three times. Then inhale and chant out loud the following mantra three times with each breath as the breath is exhaled: Aad Sach, Jugaad Sach, Haibhee Sach, Nanak Hosee Bhee Sach. Begin with 11 minutes and slowly build the time to 31 minutes. Upon completion of the meditation, deeply inhale, hold the breath for an extended period of time, and completely exhale. Repeat the deep inhaling and holding process two more times. The mantra translates as follows: "He was true in the beginning, true through all the ages, true even now. Nanak shall ever be true." This mantra helps protect against the darkest fate and to rewrite the destiny. This mantra helps to institute a new in-

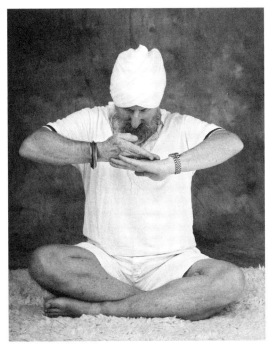

Figure 3.11
Meditation Technique to Help Overcome All Psychological Weaknesses

ternal guidance system that will help to overcome the pitfalls of a defective personality that results from the limiting effects of fears, insecurities, and neuroses. This meditation technique helps elevate the human to new heights.

The Nine-Part Kundalini Yoga Meditation Protocol Specific for Treating the Cluster B Personality Disorders: Antisocial, Borderline, Histrionic, and Narcissistic*

1. Technique to Induce a Meditative State: Tuning In

See Figure 2.1 and the description of this technique as Technique 1 in the Cluster A protocol.

2. The Ocean Exercise: The Spine-Flexing Technique for Vitality

See the description of Technique 2 in the Cluster A protocol.

3. Ganesha Meditation for Focus and Clarity

See Figure 3.6 and the description of Technique 3 in the Cluster A protocol.

4. The River Exercise

See the comments under The Three Water-Related Exercises and the description of Technique 4 in the Cluster A protocol.

5. The Respective Exercise From the 10 Symbol-Related Techniques

See the detailed description for the four disorder-specific exercises in the section The 10 Symbol-Related Techniques. The techniques for the spiral shell, stick/branch, waterfall, and snake are all described in complete detail.

6. Gan Puttee Kriya: A Technique to Help Eliminate Negativity From the Past, Present, and Future

See the description of Technique 4 in the Cluster A protocol.

7. Meditation to Release Pressure From the Subconscious Mind and Overcome Compulsive Behaviors

See Figures 3.7 and 3.8 and the description of Technique 7 in the Cluster A protocol.

8. A Brain-Balancing Technique for Reducing Silliness, Focusing the Mind, and Controlling the Ego

Sit straight with the arms out to the sides. The hands face forward and there is a 90-degree angle at the forearm and upper arm. The hands open completely and close completely, where the thumbs are enclosed by the fingers when the hands form a closed fist. Then the hands open again with all of the fingers sticking up straight and the thumbs are out to the sides, loosely extended, and then alternately the hands close and the thumbs are not enclosed in the fists. Every effort is made to have the fingers extend straight up. This is a rapid open and closing movement, and every effort is made so that both hands open and close together in synchrony. When the technique is practiced appropriately, the opening and closing of the hands can occur two to three times per second. The best practice times are between 2 and 5 minutes. The eyes are closed during the exercise and focused at the third eye point.

9. The Rain Exercise to Open Up, Bless, and Saturate the Psyche With Divine Healing Energy

See Figure 3.9 and the description of Technique 8 in the Cluster A protocol.

Optional Substitutions for Meditation 7 in the Nine-Part Kundalini Yoga Meditation Protocol for Cluster B Personality Disorders

1. Homeh Bandana Kriya for Self-Pride and Vanity

This meditation technique is very suited for those diagnosed with a narcissistic personality disorder. Yogi Bhajan taught this technique in Los Angeles, California, on September 1, 1978. He commented, "This is a very sacred, very simple, but very powerful meditation. It takes away a person's self-pride and vanity. If the number of repetitions of the mantra is increased to the maximum another person should be present with the meditator. The meditator may be rocketed so far into the ethers that he may find it hard to come back down."

Sit either in a chair with both feet flat on the ground or in an easy cross-legged position while maintaining a straight spine. The arms are relaxed down with the elbows bent. Make fists of both hands with the thumbs extended out from the fists. Raise the forearms up and in toward each other until the thumb pads touch each other. Hold the hand position in front of the chest at the heart center level. No fingers of the opposite hands touch each other at any

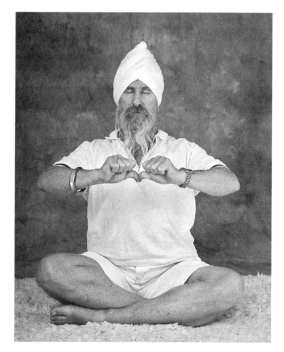

Figure 3.12
Homeh Bandana Kriya for Self-Pride and Vanity

time. Apply 25 pounds of pressure per square inch on the thumbs (see Figure 3.12). The eyes are closed and focused at the third eye point. Deeply inhale and completely exhale as the following mantra is chanted in a monotone voice four times: "Whahay Whahay Whahay Guroo." Four times is the starting number of repetitions of the mantra. It may be increased up to eight repetitions per breath. The mental focus is on the sound and vibrations created by the mantra. Upon completion of the meditation, deeply inhale and completely exhale for about 1 minute. The maximum time for this meditation is 31 minutes, but 11 minutes is a good starting time. Then slowly build up the time to 31 minutes.

2. A Meditation for Ego Problems and Mental Disease

This meditation technique is also very suited for use for those diagnosed with a narcissistic personality disorder, and of course it will also be especially useful for those diagnosed with borderline per-sonality disorder. Yogi Bhajan taught this technique in Los Angeles, California, on September 18, 1978. He commented, "The hand po-sition is known as Shiva mudra. It is a very heavy mudra. The more pressure applied on the hands, the stronger will be the reaction in the brain. The mantra is also very heavy. There must be 5 repeti-tions of the first line per breath. If it is pronounced properly and completely chanted in one breath, on the 5th repetition all the or-gans in the solar chakra or solar plexus area, the pancreas, gall blad-der, spleen, etc. are stimulated and activated to bring about the heavy changes. If a person dedicates himself to this mantra 31 min-utes a day for 90 days, all ego problems and mental diseases are cured."

Sit either in a chair with both feet flat on the ground or in an easy cross-legged position while maintaining a straight spine. The arms are relaxed down with the elbows bent. Raise the forearms up and in toward the chest until the hands meet at the level of the heart. Then make a very weak fist of the left hand with the thumb pointing up. Wrap the right hand around the outside of the fingers of the left hand (they are not to be extended past the larger knuck-les where the fingers meet the hands) with the thumb pointing up. Drop the left thumb down over the two hands on top where it will touch both the index fingers from both hands. Then place the right thumb on top of the left thumb. Then apply pressure to the double fists (see Figure 3.13). Continue to hold the hand position at the level of the heart. Either leave the eyes one-tenth open or close them completely. If the eyes are left one-tenth open, focus on the tip of the nose or on the third eye point. If the eyes are completely closed, attempt to focus on the spot that is the very top and center of the head. The latter posture is the more difficult eye position to hold. Deeply inhale and completely exhale as the mantra is chanted five times in one breath cycle, "Whahay Guru Whahay Guru Wha-hay Guru Whahay Jeeo." The maximum time that this meditation should be practiced is 31 minutes. Starting at 11 minutes and build-ing up to 31 minutes is a good way to start.

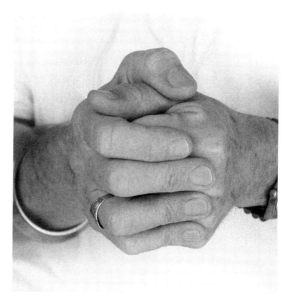

Figure 3.13
Meditation for Ego Problems and Mental Disease

The following simple meditation is especially useful for the Cluster B personality disorders, but it can be useful for anyone, including individuals without any diagnosis.

An Optional Meditation (for Use as Needed) Technique for Tranquilizing an Angry Mind

Sit with a straight spine and close the eyes. Simply chant out loud "Jeeo, Jeeo, Jeeo, Jeeo" continuously and rapidly for 11 minutes without stopping (pronounced like the names for the letters *g* and *o*). Rapid chanting is about 8 to 10 repetitions per 5 seconds. During continuous chanting, you do not stop to take long breaths, but continue with just enough short breaths to keep the sound going. Eleven minutes is all that is needed, no more and no less. The effect can last for up to 3 days. If necessary, it can be chanted for 11 minutes twice a day. This technique is most suitable for treating a "red hot" angry mind.

The Eight-Part Kundalini Yoga Meditation Protocol Specific for Treating the Cluster C Personality Disorders: Avoidant, Dependent, and Obsessive-Compulsive Personality Disorder*

1. Technique to Induce a Meditative State: Tuning In

See Figure 2.1 and the description of Technique 1 in the Cluster A protocol.

2. The Ocean Exercise: The Spine-Flexing Technique for Vitality

See the description of Technique 2 in the Cluster A protocol.

3. Ganesha Meditation for Focus and Clarity

See Figure 3.6 and the description of Technique 3 in the Cluster A protocol.

4. The River Exercise

See the comments under The Three Water-Related Exercises and see the description of Technique 4 in the Cluster A protocol.

5. The Respective Exercise From the 10 Symbol-Related Techniques

See the detailed description for the three respective Cluster C personality disorder exercises in the section The 10 Symbol-Related Techniques. The techniques for the stone, claw, and bird are each described in complete detail.

6. Gan Puttee Kriya: A Technique to Help Eliminate Negativity From the Past, Present, and Future

See the description of Technique 6 in the Cluster A protocol.

7. Meditation to Release Pressure From the Subconscious Mind and Overcome Compulsive Behaviors

See Figures 3.7 and 3.8 and the description of Technique 7 in the Cluster A protocol.

8. The Rain Exercise to Open Up, Bless, and Saturate the Psyche With Divine Healing Energy

See Figure 3.9 and the description of Technique 8 in the Cluster A protocol.

Two Optional Substitutes for Meditation 7 in the Eight-Part Kundalini Yoga Meditation Protocol for Cluster C Personality Disorders

1. Meditation for Overcoming Blocks in the Subconscious and Conscious Mind and Achieving a Deep Meditative State

Yogi Bhajan taught this technique in Los Angeles, California, on September 28, 1978. He commented, "This is a very spacey meditation. It is highly recommended that it only be practiced when there is nothing scheduled for 3–4 hours after the meditation. It is a very powerful meditation whose listing of the effects covers several pages in the holy scriptures. It can totally take you to a different frequency of your meditative capacity."

Sit either in a chair with both feet flat on the ground or in an easy cross-legged position while maintaining a straight spine. The upper arms are relaxed down with the elbows bent. The forearms are raised up and in toward each other until the hands meet in front of the chest at the level of the solar plexus (the region just under where the ribs meet). Press the entire length of the fingers of the opposite hands together, from the mounds where we normally form calluses, to the fingertips but leave the palms spread far apart. Cross the thumbs with the right thumb over the left thumb (see Figure 3.14). There are two positions that the patient can choose for the fingers. The fingers can point up, and this is the position that is traditionally taught. However, the second position, as pre-

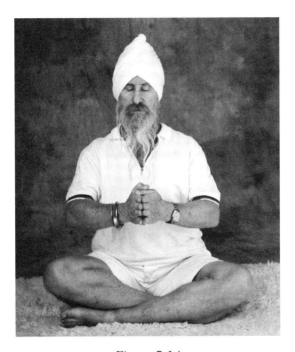

Figure 3.14
Meditation for Overcoming Blocks in the Subconscious and Conscious
Mind and Achieving a Deep Meditative State

sented in the figure, which is much easier and my preference, is to
point the fingers straight forward. The eyes are one-tenth open
with a little light coming in at the bottom, but the focus is maintained at the third eye point. The eye focus is not on the light. To
start this meditation, take several powerful deep breaths to help
open up the lungs before beginning to chant the mantra. This mantra must be chanted for a minimum of two repetitions per breath.
The maximum number of repetitions per breath is five. The mantra is the following: "Aad Sach Jugad Sach Habhay Sach Nanak
Hosee Bhay Sach." This mantra is similar to the second alternate
technique for the Cluster A protocol. However, there are subtle
differences, for the words "Habhay" and "Hosee Bhay" are used here
rather than "Haibhee" and "Hosee Bhee." The maximum time for
practicing this meditation is 31 minutes, although a great starting

time is 11 minutes. When completed, it is best to relax without any other demanding responsibilities for several hours.

2. A Meditation to Block Any Negative Approach to Life: Praan Adhaar Kriya

Yogi Bhajan taught this technique in Los Angeles, California, on August 27, 1979. He commented, "This kriya is very ancient, very sacred, and very secretly given to people. Anyone who can practice it for one hour can intuitively block any negative approach to his life."

Sit either in a chair with both feet flat on the ground or in an easy cross-legged position while maintaining a straight spine. The arms are relaxed down with the elbows bent. Raise the forearms up and in toward each other until they meet in front of the chest at the level of the heart. Interlace the fingers with the palms facing toward the body, and press the pads of the thumbs together (see Figure 3.15). Keep the eyes one-tenth open. Deeply inhale and exhale completely as the following mantra is chanted in a monotone with four complete repetitions per breath cycle: "Whahay Guru Whahay Guru Whahay Guru Whahay Jeeo." Start by practicing this meditation technique for 11 minutes and increase gradually week by week to 31 minutes. Stay there for a long time, and then gradually work up to 1 hour. Yogi Bhajan commented on the times for practice: "Don't be a fanatic."

Since personality disorder NOS is the most common diagnosis for the personality disorders, the therapist must decide which cluster-specific personality disorder protocol and which of the 10 symbol-based techniques is most appropriate for use here. The decision is then made by the array of symptoms. While the symptoms are usually scattered throughout the three clusters, it is probably also the case that they are not randomly distributed, and there may be one cluster and one of the 10 personality disorders where there are more symptoms than the others. The rule of thumb then is to use that cluster-specific protocol and then decide which of the 10 personality disorders is the closest to the patient's condition and then

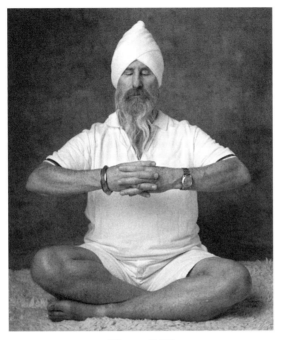

Figure 3.15
Meditation to Block Any Negative Approach to Life: Praan Adhaar Kriya

choose the most appropriate symbol-related technique from the 10 different symbol-based techniques.

Case Histories of Treatment

Case History 1. A Multimorbid Female With Personality Disorder NOS, PTSD, Social Anxiety Disorder, ADHD, and Anorexia Nervosa

Camile is a 42-year-old biracial (African American/Anglo) female. She was born in Dallas, Texas, in the late 1960s when interracial marriages were illegal. Her childhood was complicated by the social stigma of being biracial. Her mother had borderline personality disorder and perhaps other psychiatric disorders including Munchausen syndrome by proxy, now also called fabricated or induced illness. Her father was physically violent with both Camile and her mother, and he may have had intermittent explosive disorder. Camile was diagnosed with personality disorder NOS, PTSD, social anxiety disorder, ADHD, and anorexia nervosa. Below is a long case history that includes the many anomalies and details of her life and her progress using Kundalini yoga. This valuable description was written in her own words.

My earliest memories are of my sobbing mother breaking plates on the floor one by one. Each plate shattered as it hit the kitchen floor. I was, perhaps, 3 years old. This memory is a metaphor for my internal state because inside I have felt like I have been broken into a million pieces. I have suffered from anxiety, depression, and insecurity most of my life. Until recently, I have been secretly suicidal. It wasn't until I started the Kundalini yoga meditation protocol for PTSD that these suicidal thoughts subsided. I have tried many healing modalities, and by far I have had the best results with my most severe symptoms through implementing the Kundalini yoga meditations.

My mother was a brilliant, passionate, and exciting person. She loved nature, animals, art, and food. She had a knack for reviving dying animals and our home was a haven for many rescued animals. Some were odd animals such as the possum and owl that we rehabilitated. Others were more typical such as the abandoned kitten or the bird with a broken wing. In a neighborhood infested with poverty, crime, and violence, my life was filled with unheard-of privileges such as ballet lessons, art lessons, and trips to the local library. I was the only child in my entire grade with a homemade lunch. While other children in my class wore oversized or torn clothing, I was dressed in starched dresses with matching ribbons, and patent leather shoes. Without a doubt, my life was comparatively privileged, and I was the only child in the entire school with a white mother. Like most children I adored my mother, and even now it is difficult to allow myself to feel any anger toward her. Although my childhood was filled with blatant difficulties such as social persecution because I was biracial, regular beatings from my father, and multiple attempted molestations, nothing was more impacting and damaging than the relationship that I had with my mother. Emotional abuse is very hard to explain because it is often subtle, unacknowledged, and invisible.

The best way I can explain my relationship with my mother is through imagery. Imagine someone shoving you into a burning building and then immediately grabbing you, pulling you out while frantically calling an ambulance. Then imagine this same person with great self-sacrifice, devotion, and loyalty nursing you back to health night after night with undying tenderness. This is a metaphor for the maddening vicious cycle of behavior that I had with my mother. My mother was so disassociated that she never saw any of these abuses. When questioned or reminded of them, her face would immediately go blank and then she would become irritated at my ungratefulness for all of her wonderful deeds. Furthermore, no one else saw this dark side of her. To the outside world, she appeared to be a loving and devoted mother. I was nearly 30 years old before I began to uncover the mystery of my mother's changeable behavior. It was through isolated hints and comments that I began to piece together the story of my mom's incest. My mother was molested by her father before the age of 5 and she witnessed her grandfather molesting her best friend through a keyhole at age 12. The events of her childhood were so traumatic that she developed severe disassociation. Before my puberty, my mother was smothering and controlling. I was treated as an extension of her without any identity of my own. My job was to listen to her problems and console her, and this is the role I played in her life until she died 4 years ago. Once I entered puberty, her behavior became much more overtly abusive and provoking, and occasionally with mild sexual abuse. She would accuse me of imagined transgressions and then beat me with straightened coat hangers. She became voyeuristic when my body began to mature. She would constantly barge into the bathroom and make embarrassing comments about my body. She was obsessed with my underpants and would check them to reprimand me for any discharges. She counted how many pads I used during my menses and would punish me for being wasteful. At the age of 12, she told me that I had to make my own money for my clothes and food. I began working by collecting cans from dumpsters. She stopped buying me nice clothes. I was forced to wear one article of clothing until it became full of holes. Between the ages of 11 and 12, five men tried to molest me, and one was a family friend and another was an uncle. I told my mother about it, and she told me it was my own fault for being friendly. By the time that I was 13, I was so emotionally exhausted with my mother that I stopped talking altogether. I didn't speak a word for 6 months. During this time, she took me to a psychologist who also tried to molest me, and later my mom told me, he also tried to molest her. I was so distrustful of this psychologist that I refused to talk to him, so I spent a year in silence with him while he opened his mail and did his paperwork. My teen years are blurry memories of house confinement and an overcontrolling mother who did not allow me the freedom of a teenager. I stayed home and accompanied her on all her errands just as I had at a much younger age of 10. Later, at age 15, I developed anorexia by refusing to eat until I was about 90 pounds (I am 5'7"). Although I never vomited during the 6 months that I refused to eat, I developed severe abdominal pain after recovering from anorexia. It is only in the last few years that the pain has subsided. During the anorexia period, my mother tried to have me admitted to a children's psychiatric ward. They did a full evaluation and determined we needed outpatient family therapy. My mother refused family therapy but agreed to individual therapy for me. This saved my life because the therapist advocated for me. She convinced my mom to allow me to attend a university. Until this period, my mom had insisted that I would never leave home but live with her indefinitely. The opportunity to leave home offered me an escape from an enmeshed relationship that was slowly driving me beyond the edge of normal behavior. Finally, I had a way out.

My mother's behavior was the result of a horrendous childhood and a traumatic adulthood. She had me at the age of 18 and in her naïveté she never foresaw the outcome. At the time, a child out of wedlock was bad enough but a black child was unforgivable in Texas. Her family was quick to reject her, and my father, in the midst of the Vietnam War, was drafted. Left to her own resources, she moved into a housing project where she was the only white woman. The experience was a cruel adventure in a foreign world. She had many experiences that would shape her later erratic and destructive behavior. After a man tried to slash her throat with me watching, she moved back to her mother's house where she was only tolerated. After 2 years in Vietnam, my father returned and she managed to convince him to marry her. She realized her only hopes of surviving with a half-black child were to marry him. Mixed marriages had just become legalized, but they still had a difficult time finding a pastor who would marry them. Our lives, in those years, were barely bearable because we were subjected to constant public humiliation. People stared, pointed, whispered, insulted, and cursed our mixed family. Police officers harassed us by pulling us over and smashing our food beneath their boots. Bricks were thrown through our window. My parents' families refused to invite us to Christmas dinner, reunions, and all family events. At school, as a "zebra," I was taunted, kicked, and teased. Life was hell and I became very self-conscious. I stopped calling my mother "Mom" in public to avoid the disbelieving stares. My dad handled the stress of being a young father and husband by being absent. He and my mother fought incessantly.

As a child, I had no idea why my mother and father fought so much. Their fights were physical and violent. Eventually my mother received a broken nose, and the fights became less physical. Now I know that they fought over my dad's frequent infidelities. Only recently did I discover that he led a double life with an outside woman for over 20 years. My dad was normally a quiet, even-tempered man who showed no emotion or personality. However, when my mother ordered a whipping for me, the beast in him would appear. His routine whippings involved the branches from our rosebushes because the thorns ripped the skin. I was terrified of these whippings that lasted 15–20 minutes. As soon as I knew they were coming, I would run for cover under the bed. He would grab my ankle or any appendage he could reach and swat me anywhere he could. Then our "mad monkey" struggle began. I would run and he would grab. By the time the whippings were over, the room would look like a tornado passed through. The whippings always ended with him telling me to stop crying as he hit me. He would hit and hit and hit until I managed to stifle the cry into a stuttering hiccup. Occasionally, if he didn't feel like chasing me, he would hold me by my ankles for the whippings. I would flop like a fish until he lost his grip. Whippings were a daily routine for minor infractions. I thought they were normal because everyone I knew got whippings. It wasn't until I was much older that I discovered that everyone else only got hit a few times. My dad was a phantom occupant in our house. Except for the whippings, I never saw him. In his absence, my mother was lonely and isolated, so I became her only ally. She relied on me for comfort and unconditional love.

As I started to develop around 11 years old, men started to notice me. I found myself the object of attention more than my immature mind could handle. I was considered exotic and pretty. At the time, I did not actually know what sex was, but intuitively I was able to sense sexuality. None of the men who pursued me were rapists. They were seducers. I knew they were trying to trick and manipulate me so I simply maneuvered to evade their advances. I was always successful, but it still affected my self-esteem. I became very uncomfortable with my developing body and the attention I was receiving. I had my mom cut my long hair to only an inch long. I wore clothes that would conceal my body. My uncle was the only man who attempted to molest me that was overtly mean.

My parents moved to a house next to my maternal grandmother's house when I was about 12 years old. My alcoholic uncle lived with my grandmother. One day he phoned me and asked me to come over when my parents and grandparents weren't home. I walked to the doorway of his room where he was lying in bed. He asked me to come to his bed and I turned and ran as fast I could out of the house. He yelled "nigger bitch" several times as I started running back into my house and locked the door. During this time, we were living in an all-white neighborhood and I was constantly insulted and abused by other children. At school, a few boys who rode my bus decided to make me into a human jump rope. One boy grabbed my wrists and another grabbed my ankles and they twirled me around. The also hit me with their fists in the halls when no one was looking. In machine shop, one of them rammed a grill into my stomach. Those years were really tough because I had no one to protect me. I had to be adaptable and resilient as I moved from one culture to another and as I moved from childhood into adolescence. I left home at 18 and never returned.

I left home 24 years ago. The journey has been long and difficult. In my 20s, I was finishing school and starting a career. At the age of 20, I got involved with a man who was extremely abusive (he put knives to my throat, guns to my head, and he tried to suffocate me). He was sexually violent with me and this resulted in a pregnancy. I realized very quickly that I was in no condition to parent a child and that I could not separate him from his father. So my son was eventually adopted by a family member at the age of 6 months. Because we never bonded and he lived in another state, I rarely saw him, maybe only eight times in 20 years. More recently, I have discovered that he has been diagnosed with borderline personality disorder, bipolar disorder, possible Asperger's disorder, and major drug abuse. When I do see him, I see his father. He looks exactly like his father, he acts exactly like his father, he sounds exactly like his father, etc. Obviously, the dynamics between us are an entangled mess.

Dealing with my sexual identity was the biggest challenge in my 20s. I inherited my mom's psychological problems around sexuality, so I had many psychosomatic symptoms. Whenever I had sexual intercourse, I suffered severe contractions like I was having a baby. At the time, I had no idea what my body was doing or why it was doing this. I went to the doctor and she couldn't find anything wrong with me. At some point, I realized that I had absorbed all my mother's issues around sexuality, and it took me 10 years to finally have sex without pain. Additionally, I had many fears, some reasonable and some unreasonable. I was determined to confront my fears, so I was constantly pushing myself outside my comfort zone. I was afraid of water, so I took swimming lessons. I had developed a type of learned helplessness from my father's frequent childhood beatings and during this time I believe I developed the capacity to dissociate. I would freeze and become immobilized anytime someone was aggressive. For example, I had a job working at a fast-food restaurant where the boss was sexually abusive. He would slap my rear and I would become completely unable to move, so I put myself on a boxing team to learn how to fight back. I had severe social anxiety, so I made myself work as a community youth activist. I created a program to get inner city girls into college-preparatory private schools. Looking back on those years I realize I kept myself very busy, so I didn't have to feel or think. On the outside, I appeared to be an energetic, creative, visionary, but on the inside I was terrified.

As I moved into my 30s I began to have dissociative experiences in my hatha yoga classes. I later discovered that they may have been spiritual experiences. These experiences were varied and unusual. I experienced different states of consciousness where I lost sensation in my body. I was not a spiritual person and I would never have believed this was possible, had it not happened to me. At that time, I participated in yoga for preventive health and not as a spiritual pursuit. At the time, I had no frame of reference for these experiences and when I sought to understand them I became progressively more confused. These experiences were a double-edged sword because they convinced me that it was possible to experience abiding peace and joy, but they also caused me so much confusion that my psychological symptoms worsened. I developed insomnia that impaired my ability to function. I don't think I slept through the night for at least 10 years. I was exhausted all the time and would often fall asleep during the day at work. I also developed panic attacks that felt like a heart attack. Due to my increasing dysfunctions, I became socially withdrawn and my social anxiety increased. I would find myself terrified in groups of three or more. As a result of my spiritual experiences in my 30s, I became more self-aware and thus more aware of my underlying symptoms that had been masked by pure adrenaline and energy in my 20s. Things came to the surface and I was a total mess. In the midst of these occurrences, my mom was diagnosed with an aggressive form of breast cancer when I was 28 years old. She had an agonizing and protracted battle with cancer for 10 years until her death. Her death released me to focus on my own healing in my late 30s when I started to search for a solution to my own trauma.

I was willing to try any healing modality that seemed sensible and likely to produce results. I tried traditional therapy with several psychologists for a period of time. I have never found talk therapy to be of much use because I am so self-aware that there is nothing new to gain from talking. I tried Prozac for a 2-week period. I became very cool and calculating about my depression on Prozac. I emptied all my bank accounts and turned off my electricity, and I began to methodically and secretively plan my own suicide. However, I fell asleep for several hours at the designated time of my planned suicide. When I awoke, I no longer felt suicidal and I called my doctor. She took me off Prozac and told me that the drug has this effect on a small percentage of people. After that, I tried acupuncture and neural therapy for trauma. I also tried several forms of healing methods that involve the whole body such as Rolfing, energy work, muscle-meridian based kinesiology, etc. During this same time period, I practiced hatha yoga and Vipassana meditation for 3 years. Overall, I received some positive benefits from all of these treatment models. However, nothing was bringing lasting changes with my most severe and persistent symptoms of insomnia, anxiety, social anxiety, and depression. Furthermore, for most of my life I have suffered from a peculiar habit of crying for hours on Sundays (sometimes for as long as 8 hours), and nothing was helping with that. Next I tried a 2-week Vipassana meditation retreat that involved 12 consecutive days of silent meditation. During the retreat my panic attacks were more severe, my depression was more severe, and my insomnia was much more severe. Vipassana means to see things as they are, and I certainly saw just how bad things could get. On my return I was determined to find a healing method that would actually produce relief. So, the day after my return, I discovered David's book, *Kundalini Yoga Meditation: Techniques Specific for Psychiatric Disorders, Couples Therapy, and Personal Growth*. I bought the book and began doing a protocol that same day. At first, I practiced each meditation for only a few seconds or minutes. After about a week, I e-mailed David and he suggested I do the PTSD protocol. I noticed an improvement almost immediately. My friends also noticed an improvement in my anxiety levels. I stopped crying on Sundays and I became less reactive to daily life experiences. When I did become upset, I was able to reset very quickly. My panic attacks ceased very quickly. I started to feel less internally fragmented and more integrated. My social anxiety improved as I felt more open, receptive, and less defensive toward others. I also became increasingly less overwhelmed and more in control of my life. With the few phone encounters that I have had with my son in this last year I have also been far less emotionally distraught over the catastrophic problems in his life.

I committed to the PTSD protocol almost exclusively for a year every day, which required about 1 hour. Also, during my lunch break at work, I would occasionally do the left nostril breathing technique for ADD that is in David's protocol for ADHD. In the beginning, I did this technique only a few times a week or randomly. However, during the last month, I have managed to do it for 31 minutes every day. During this year I have had many personal challenges. I lost my job of 8 years and my car stopped running. My dad was diagnosed with Alzheimer's disease and my 20-year-old son was diagnosed with HIV. Furthermore, I thought I was engaged to this guy who I later discovered was a liar and that he had narcissistic personality disorder. I met him through yoga and meditation and he is a family and marriage therapist. He told me he was divorced, but I discovered he was married. I never suspected ill will from him because of his avid spiritual practices. In hindsight, I realize that he used his training in hypnosis and other techniques to manipulate and control my mind. He knew my history and he exploited my weaknesses and insecurities. He presented himself as the ideal lover, father, brother, friend, and ally that I had never had in my life. Once I discovered the extent of his lies, I told him I never wanted to speak to or see him again or I would tell his wife. He then had a restraining order filed against me and he began to taunt me (he called 13 times) and attempted to goad me into reacting so that he could have me arrested. I did not want to jeopardize my career by having this on my record so I had to stay in hiding at a friend's house because he broke into my house. Through all of this I kept my composure and focus. I put together my own defense and represented myself in court. In the end, I was victorious. The restraining order on me was lifted, but he received a 120-day restraining order and a year of domestic violence classes, which I thought was very ironic since he was contracted as a psychotherapist for the victim's board in my city. Throughout my legal preparation, I did my PTSD protocol every day and I also worked on my navel point by doing Nabhi Kriya [see techniques, Chapter 5]. This legal victory was the most empowering moment of my life. For the first time I realized that I can defend myself, that I have a voice, and that I have my own power. I no longer have debilitating symptoms that impair my ability to function or handle life's challenges. The PTSD protocol gave me an anchor and it grounded me. I can now handle all of my problems with balance, fortitude, and clarity. For the first time in my life, I also feel like a whole person. My feet are planted and my head is held high. I am proud.

Before I started the PTSD protocol, I was at the end of my rope in my life. I felt that my coping skills were no longer sustaining me. I could no longer handle my high-stress job working with inner city children as a schoolteacher. Each second and minute of the day was a struggle because I felt so depleted and fragmented inside. I was considering moving to a developing country and living in a hut because I was so tired of my life. I wanted to rest. After starting the protocol, I bought a house and a car. I moved to a great job working with students in a diverse university community with like-minded people. The school curriculum supports wellness, yoga, and creativity. I reconnected with my son and our relationship has improved. I find myself connecting with others and being successful in my communication. I have also been asked to teach the protocol to soldiers with PTSD. My life has completely turned around.

Recently I participated in a women's study on domestic violence. They contacted me through public records. The interview, which consisted of IQ tests and trauma questions, was set for 3 hours. It took me 2 hours and the graduate student administering the test told me I did very well on the IQ test. She said I was the only person out of over 200 people to get the last question correct. Life has been so hard for me and I have made so many mistakes that I have always felt stupid. I couldn't believe that I am smart. It made me feel so much better about myself. She also told me that the university pays for all students who pursue a doctorate in clinical psychology. I have secretly always wanted to pursue a doctorate in psychology. I have always wanted to find a way out of my misery so I could help others. I left there with a dream. Maybe I can get a PhD and help victims of trauma. In the end it all came full circle. Maybe, just maybe there is a light at the end of this very long tunnel.

Camile first contacted me by e-mail on June 25, 2007. She contacted me approximately 70 times by e-mail up until the end of June 2008, at the time that this case history was written. I have never seen her in person, although in November 2007 she sent me a picture of herself. We have had only one phone conversation that she initiated at the time of her legal battles with her ex-boyfriend, and this call lasted for approximately 1 hour. Her self-described case history verges on the conservative side when I compare it with the e-mail exchanges. Her progress is striking and it is a testimony both to her own determination to eliminate her suffering and to the potency of the PTSD protocol and the occasional use of the ADD meditation technique and Nabhi Kriya. She no longer has PTSD, social anxiety disorder, ADHD, or anorexia nervosa, and she no longer fits the inclusion criteria for a personality disorder NOS. If I had the opportunity to learn more about her condition in the beginning, my approach to treatment with her would have included the Cluster B protocol and symbol-specific technique for borderline personality disorder. However, she only slowly revealed the facts about her life and her multimorbid condition through e-mail over many months. Fortunately, she was able to benefit without using a cluster-specific protocol.

Case History 2. A Case of Histrionic Personality Disorder, Depression, Anxiety, and Insomnia

Alessandra is a very attractive 44-year-old Italian female. She comes from a very wealthy family in Milan, Italy, and she has two older brothers, one aged 54 and the other 56, who both remain living in Italy. Her father died in an auto accident when she was 5 years of age and her mother never remarried. However, there were always different lovers in her mother's life that were frequently brought into the home. Her mother never had to work and had a life of considerable leisure due to the husband's fortune. Alessandra was very close to her father, and she was devastated by his death. He had been the center of her life. After that, she was primarily raised by the servants who lived in the home, and they were instructed by the mother to meet her needs and wishes. Her mother was often too busy to see to her upbringing. Alessandra felt abandoned as a child, and she remembers that more often than not, the only way that she could get her mother's attention was through tantrums and other hysterical outbursts. Soon after the father's death, her brothers were no longer living at home. They were attending a university in Rome. Alessandra never felt like she had to work to achieve anything in her life, and mostly remembers being an unhappy and lonely child after her father's death. In her later adolescent years, she discovered that her physical beauty and charm could be a means for obtaining what she wanted, especially from men. When she was 19, she met an American man while she was attending the University of Milan. He was 24 years of age and working on a doctorate in the arts. He was struck by her beauty, and they soon started a romantic relationship. Six months later she found that she was pregnant. She insisted on keeping the child, and they got married. They lived in Milan for another 2 years until his education was complete, and then they moved to Los Angeles where his family was living. The marriage faced many difficulties, including her relationship with his parents, who never accepted Alessandra or the idea that their son was married to her. Due to the conflict, the marriage lasted only 2 more years and she remained living in Los Angeles until 2004, when her daughter was admitted to the University of California, San Diego. Alessandra's family wealth met all of her financial needs and afforded her the luxuries of her youth. However, she also was not able to find a man that could "adjust to her emotional needs." Her beauty and wealth made it easy for her to meet men. However, the relationships never seemed to last, and she never felt like she was appreciated. She felt like the men in her life did not understand her and that they "could never be there for her emotionally." They wanted sex, but they did not want to commit to her in a serious way. She later told me that she felt that these were "shallow" men. The loneliness of her youth and the emotional isolation that she later felt when she was married and living in Los Angeles was finding its way back into her life. And she did not understand why this was happening to her.

When Alessandra sought my help at the advice of a female friend, she complained of the loneliness in her life and her depression, anxiety, and difficulties sleeping. When I met her, I could see why men were physically attracted to her. However, I could also see why she was unsuccessful in all of her relationships with men. Her physical attributes were well exposed with her provocative dress style, and it was clear that she wanted me to listen to every complaint about her life without interrupting so that I could learn all that I needed to know about her. She was the quintessential drama queen. Not only was her voice dramatic, but it was annoying, with a whiny tone. I realized that she had a classic "waterfall" personality. She was flooding the session with her emotions and she had a need to be the center of attention. Alessandra was the most classic case of histrionic personality disorder that I have ever met. After she complained about the men in her life, I asked her to tell me about her depression and anxiety, even though I understood why she felt that way. She went on to explain that she did not understand why these relationships were never working, and that she needed a man in her life that would stand by her. She was tired of having short-term relationships that never amounted to anything that was meaningful or lasting. I suggested that perhaps one of the reasons that she was not successful was because she herself required a greater balance emotionally. She agreed and commented that on occasion some men told her that she was too much for them emotionally. I also told her that I thought that she had to refine her value system with men, and she agreed. She knew that she needed to start meeting men who were more stable and sincere. She said, "Why don't men love me? Why don't they respect me?" I said, "Did you ever learn to earn love or respect?" At that moment she stopped cold, became silent, and looked at me like I had hit on something that might help her better understand. I never told her that my diagnosis was that she had a histrionic personality disorder. She, like others with a personality disorder, would find this label and diagnosis too much to accept. They simply cannot compute these deficits. So I agreed to treat her for her depression, anxiety, and insomnia. This is why she came for therapy. She agreed to therapy twice a week and returned to learn techniques for her problems 2 days later.

At our second appointment I taught her the the nine-part protocol for the Cluster B disorders with the substitution at step 5 for the Meditation for Developing and Strengthening the Subtle Body as the appropriate match for her histrionic personality disorder based on the 10 Symbol-Related Techniques. I explained to her that this protocol would meet all of her needs for her depression, anxiety, and sleep problems. I also told her that this protocol would help her flow more easily in life so that she could avoid much of the emotional stress and strain that was the source of her problems. I also told her that the technique for the subtle body would help her attract a man of greater caliber and character. She very much liked this idea. She was athletically inclined and quickly adapted to the protocol. While she never did it on her own at home, the twice weekly sessions soon seemed to meet her needs for her depression, anxiety, and insomnia. She was very disciplined in the sessions, and she commented on how it began to help her have a much improved emotional balance in her life. I saw her twice a week for 2 months. During this time, I could also see that she was far less needy, much less demanding, and much less emotional. She was much more relaxed, and she developed a new inner balance over these 2 months. She no longer dressed in the same provocative style when coming for therapy. She called me after several months and told me that she was grateful for my help and that she had started to attend a local Kundalini yoga class. She also told me that Kundalini yoga had become an important part of her life. She said that she now had less need to have the attention and company of a man, but that she hoped in time to find a healthy and suitable match in the future.

Case History 3. A Case of Depression and Avoidant Personality Disorder

I first saw Ellen in October 2008. Ellen was 53 years old and had never married. She was raised in Texas and is the fourth child of five siblings, with a brother being the oldest, followed by two sisters, herself, and a younger brother. When growing up, she felt like she had been given the least parental and sibling attention. Years later she discovered that her parents were always hoping to have another son. Her father was in the military and his family had a long military history. Ellen did not fit into her father's equation.

She was physically unattractive and never dated during high school. She had very little social life in or outside of the home. She had attempted to play the violin during her middle school years but failed to develop an ear or an affinity for music. However, her brothers and sisters played in the school band. She was often criticized by her siblings for her looks and social inactivity. She often felt rejected by her family. The little self-worth that she did have during her youth came from her scholastic efforts. However, she also failed to achieve scholastically to her parents' satisfaction. After completing her bachelor's degree in biology at the University of Texas at Austin, she failed to be accepted into graduate school. She took employment as a lab technician in a hospital performing routine assays. She later found more gainful employment at a nuclear power plant in south Texas, again performing routine assays. Her work required little social interaction, and her personal life in a small town essentially led to the life of a hermit. She went to work, shopped for food, and came home. After 10 years of social isolation, she moved to north San Diego county and took a similar job sampling radioactive contamination at the San Onofre nuclear power plant. However, again she found herself in the same routine without a social life and with little or no ambition to attempt to develop one. She became depressed and sought help through a psychiatrist. She was diagnosed with major depressive disorder and prescribed 30 mg of paroxetine. After 6 weeks she found little to no improvement in her depression and the dose was increased to 50 mg. She failed to improve. However, she began to suffer with drug-induced side effects, including somnolence, nausea, sweating, insomnia, and headaches. The psychiatrist changed her prescription to citalopram (40 mg). This sudden switch led to a case of "Paxil flu." Without understanding what was going on, she had extreme dizziness, headaches, profuse night sweats, nightmares, severe body pain, and lesions in her mouth. She thought she had contracted a virus. This went on for 10 more days without letting up. She was unable to report to work. When she first reported her new symptoms, her psychiatrist told her that they could be the result of getting off the paroxetine too quickly, which happens in a small percentage of cases, but they would probably dissipate once the citalopram took over. However, the symptoms failed to abate and eventually her psychiatrist realized that he would have to help her restabilize on the paroxetine, and then later slowly lower the dose milligram by milligram using a liquid preparation. After stabilizing her again on 50 mg paroxetine, her physical symptoms subsided, and she was eventually fortunate enough to be successful in using the slow reduction method. But this took 2 months. She was also unable to tolerate two more antidepressants (citalopram, venlafaxine). Her symptoms of depression never remitted. However, she regarded her depressive symptoms as much less problematic than the physical symptoms from her medication. Her depression was now severe. She started seeing a psychologist recommended by her psychiatrist. During this time she was unable to work. She had exhausted her sick days and vacation time, and she was advised to take disability insurance. She mostly slept when she could and avoided leaving her apartment. In fact, she now avoided nearly everything. She stopped cleaning her apartment and frequently went for days without attending to her personal hygiene. Her diet now consisted of frozen foods, ice cream, and well-buttered toast. She did not open her windows and mostly lived in the dark. Her TV was her sole source of stimulation. She made little to no progress in psychotherapy and was unwilling to follow her therapist's advice to get out in the world, to go "walk on the beach, attend a gym for exercise." Her therapist realized that she was recalcitrant to change and diagnosed Ellen with avoidant personality disorder. Ellen had contemplated suicide, but realized it was contrary to her religious beliefs and her upbringing. Her psychotherapist had attended one of my full-day course presentations at the American Psychiatric Association and thought that Ellen might be a candidate for Kundalini yoga meditation. Ellen and the therapist both realized that they had exhausted practically every other avenue. I got a call from her therapist, and Ellen agreed to make an appointment. However, it was 4 more weeks before she called. Ellen was coming to be treated for her depression, and she was hoping that I could help her change her life. She knew she was stuck in her life, but she wanted to have a better life. She was personally disgusted with her present state of affairs. She just did not know how to go about changing her life for the better.

My strategy was to teach Ellen the eight-part Kundalini yoga protocol for the Cluster C disorders, using technique 8 of the 10 Symbol-Related Techniques, for the "stone" persona. I explained to her that she needed to learn the value of changing her own life. She agreed. However, I never told her that she had a diagnosis of avoidant personality disorder, and her psychotherapist also never divulged this possible diagnosis. Her therapist was not sure of the diagnosis because she also knew that Ellen's condition might have been only the result of her severe depression. But she knew, given Ellen's history, that the personality disorder diagnosis was a likely complicating factor in her condition. The first four times that I taught Ellen the protocol, I left out technique 7, the meditation to release pressure from the subconscious mind and overcome compulsive behaviors. I did not want to overly stress her with the physical difficulty of the protocol. I realized that Ellen was not an energetic or athletically inclined individual, and that she was still suffering from depression. Also, I did not want to set her up for failure. In the beginning, we practiced each technique for the minimum time. She understood that the stone-related technique was symbolic of her inability to change in her life or try new things. This eight-part breath not only helps expand the practitioner's awareness but improves energy levels. Ellen liked this idea. Fortunately, her first experience was rewarding. She felt immediate improvements in her mood, anxiety, and energy levels. She also felt much more relaxed, and she agreed to come back once a week. She said that if she could afford to see me more often that she would. While she had some savings, she was also concerned about losing them. However, Ellen had renewed hope in her life. But she also knew that she had a difficult road ahead. She knew the only way to progress was through her own efforts. Ellen had the basic intelligence, but she lacked confidence in herself and had very little self-respect. After the third meeting, she said that she liked the idea that she was able to engage with the protocol and that she could help herself. By this time we were practicing the stone technique without her having any resistance to the turning movement. She understood the symbolism behind it and started to trust in the concept. She also started to practice some of the techniques on her own at home. After 6 weeks, we were practicing the entire protocol. We met for six more sessions, and Ellen decided that she was now able to manage her life and return to work. On occasion she would call me to tell me about her home practice and to ask for additional guidance. I gave her the two optional substitutes for Meditation 7. Several months later, I received another call from Ellen. She thanked me for helping her regain a normal life. She no longer had symptoms of depression, and she said that she had much greater confidence in herself.

FOUR

Treating the Pervasive Developmental Disorders

Autistic Disorder, Asperger's Disorder, and Pervasive Developmental Disorders– Not Otherwise Specified

Wealth is in the health of your communication. And communication is the essence of your commitment. Commitment is the character you project. That projection should penetrate the heart and head of its object.

Yogi Bhajan, date unknown

How can two people live together without quarreling? The arc body and the eyes must connect for someone to feel that you want to communicate. That is where relationship is created—psyche to psyche.

Yogi Bhajan, date unknown

Teach your child to negotiate with his parents. Who brings war? The nonnegotiating child, the egomaniacs who are narrow minded, stupid and mentally retarded but macho in their behavior, they bring war.

Yogi Bhajan, date unknown

Subtypes and Diagnostic Features, Prevalence, Etiology, and Results Using Conventional Treatment Modalities

The pervasive developmental disorders (PDDs) are a group of five disorders that have considerable overlap in symptoms, which may include delays in the development of socialization and communication skills, along with restricted and stereotyped behaviors, interests, and activities. The five PDDs are autistic disorder, Asperger's disorder (or Asperger's syndrome), Rett's disorder, childhood disintegrative disorder, and pervasive developmental disorder not otherwise specified (PDD-NOS). The PDDs are a distinct subgroup of disorders that are included and often confused with the more inclusive group called the specific developmental disorders (SDDs), which also include the communication disorders, learning disorders, and motor skills disorders as defined by the *DSM-IV-TR* (APA, 2000). All of the SDDs are usually first diagnosed in infancy, childhood, or adolescence. Besides the PDDs, the SDD group includes the attention-deficit and disruptive behavior disorders, feeding and eating disorders, tic disorders, elimination disorders, and other disorders like selective mutism, separation anxiety disorder, and reactive attachment disorder (APA, 2000). Autistic disorders are also called the autism spectrum disorders or autism spectrum conditions, with the word *autistic* sometimes replacing *autism* (WHO, 2003). Here I will only cover the PDDs. However, treatment protocols and case histories are not included for either childhood disintegrative disorder or Rett's disorder due to their rarity, and since I have had no direct experience with patients with either condition.

The symptoms of the PDDs are frequently detected in infancy or by the age of 3, and these children differ widely in their abilities, levels of intelligence, and behaviors. While all have problems with age-appropriate social skills, others do not speak at all, or speak only in limited phrases or conversations, while others develop normal language skills. Repetitive, ritualistic, and limited range in play skills are also general features of this broad spectrum of disorders.

Many also have unusual responses to sensory stimuli, such as lights or loud noises, and a substantial inflexibility with changes in their routines and surroundings.

Autistic children share three key traits: (1) they are slow to develop language; (2) they are poor at social interactions; and (3) they repeat stereotypical behaviors that commonly include hand flapping, making sounds, head rolling, and body rocking; compulsive behaviors that appear to follow rules and typically include the arranging of objects; keeping things the same with a resistance to change, whether it is with furniture or resisting interruptions; doing daily activities the same way each day, whether it is eating or dressing rituals; restrictive behavior, whether it is limited to a single television program or a special toy; and last, self-injury, which can include eye poking, skin picking, hand biting, or head banging (Johnson & Myers, 2007). One study found that self-injury affected up to 30% of children with autism and that the "atypical behaviors tended to have a lower nonverbal IQ, lower levels of expressive language, more severe social deficits, and more repetitive behaviors" (Dominick, Davis, Lainhart, Tager-Flusberg, & Folstein, 2007). However, overall some forms of autism are subtle, whereas others devastate every aspect of the individual's capacity to function.

Interestingly enough, about 0.5% to 10% of individuals with PDD also show unusual abilities or an "island of genius," ranging from splinter skills such as obsessive preoccupation with and memorization of music, sports trivia, license plate numbers, maps, historical facts, or obscure items such as vacuum cleaner motor sounds, to the extraordinarily rare talents of prodigious autistic savants that include musical, artistic, or other special abilities (Rimland, 1978b; Treffert, 1989). One study of 583 facilities of those institutionalized with a diagnosis of mental retardation found a prevalence rate of 1.4 per 1,000 for patients with savant skills (Hill, 1977).

Treffert (2006) reviewed the newest findings on savants, which have a relationship to the yogic insight into the PDDs that I address in the section on etiology. Treffert described the literature that supports the insight of a left brain injury and a right brain compensation to explain the nature of the savant condition, and this has a bearing on the PDD condition in general. He stated, "One theory that does provide an increasingly plausible explanation for savant abilities in many cases is left brain injury with right brain compensation. . . . The skills most often seen in savant syndrome are those associated with the right hemisphere (Tanguay, 1973)" (2006) and they usually occur in one of five general categories including music, art, calendar, calculating, mathematics in the absence of other simple arithmetic abilities, and mechanical or spatial skills. Rimland (1978a) also pointed out the selective use of right brain activity in savants with autism, which differs strongly from the sequential nature of left brain activities. Treffert went on to say:

> In autistic disorder itself, left brain dysfunction, compared to right brain activity, has been demonstrated in a number of studies. Even as early as 1975, before CT scans and MRI studies were available, pneumoencephalograms demonstrated left hemisphere abnormalities, particularly in the temporal lobe areas in 15 of 17 patients with autism, four of whom had savant skills. Investigators in this study concluded that motor and language functions were "taken over" by the right hemisphere because of deficits in the left hemisphere (Hauser, DeLong, & Rosman, 1975). A 1999 PET study showed low serotonin synthesis in the left hemisphere of persons with autistic disorder and other studies have confirmed such left hemisphere deficits as well (DeLong, 1999). Boddaert and coworkers demonstrated in five children with autism and eight controls that at rest and listening to speech-like sounds, the volume of activation was greater on the right side and diminished on the left among children with autism; the reverse pattern was found in the control group (Boddaert et al., 2003). Escalante-Mead and colleagues demonstrated an atypical pattern of cerebral dominance among individuals with autism and a history of early language disorder when compared to both healthy participants and individuals with autism and persons with normal acquisition of early language skills (Escalante-Mead, Minshew, & Sweeney, 2003). (Treffert, 2006)

Treffert further elaborated on the savant syndrome and described a number of case histories. One was of a "typically developing 9-year-old boy who was left mute, deaf and paralyzed by a gunshot wound to the left hemisphere" and after the injury the boy developed "unusual savant mechanical skills, presumably from the undamaged right hemisphere (Brink, 1980)" (2006). He reviewed other reports that included left hemisphere injuries, one of a musical savant and another of a mathematical savant (Treffert, 2006). Treffert also noted that "the most powerful confirmation of the left brain dysfunction/right brain compensation theory in savant syndrome, however, comes from a 1998 report by Miller and coworkers who described five previously nondisabled patients with frontotemporal dementia (FTD) who acquired new artistic skills with the onset and progression of FTD (Miller et al., 1998). Several of these individuals had no previous history of particular artistic abilities, yet prodigious art skills emerged as the dementia proceeded. Consistent with characteristics and traits of savants, the modality of skill expression in these five older adults was visual, not verbal; the images were meticulous copies that lacked abstract or symbolic qualities; episodic memory was preserved but semantic memory was devastated; and there was intense, obsessive preoccupation with the artwork. Neuroimaging studies showed dominant (left) hemisphere injury and dysfunction" (2006).

Treffert pointed out some other key findings in an attempt to understand the nature of the savant syndrome and autism. First, he noted that males outnumber females about four to one in both autism and with the savant syndrome (Treffert, 2006). Others are more specific and arrive at a ratio of 4.3 to 1 males to females (Newschaffer et al., 2007). Treffert also pointed out that Geschwind and Galaburda (1987) showed that the left hemisphere develops after the right hemisphere and is thus more highly sensitive to detrimental prenatal influences. Geschwind and Galaburda showed that very high levels of circulating testosterone, especially in the male fetus, can retard growth and impair function in the "more vulnerable exposed left hemisphere, with actual enlargement and shift of dominance favoring skills associated with the right hemisphere" (1987). They postulated a "pathology of superiority" where the right brain then compensates for left brain injury or impaired development.

In keeping with the theory that early injury or trauma plays a causal role in the development of a PDD, a study links autism and very premature births (less than 28 weeks). Researchers tested the hypothesis that children born preterm are more likely to screen positive for a PDD (Kuban et al., 2009). They compared the Modified Checklist for Autism in Toddlers (M-CHAT) in extremely low gestational age newborns. They found a positive increase on the M-CHAT for those with cerebral palsy, cognitive impairment, and vision and hearing impairments when compared to those without these disorders. More specifically, when comparing to children who could walk, the odds for screening positive on the M-CHAT were increased 23-fold for those unable to sit or stand independently, and more than a 7-fold increase for those requiring assistance to walk. Those with quadriparesis were 13 times more likely to screen positive, and those with hemiparesis were four times more likely to screen positive on the M-CHAT. Those with a major vision or hearing impairment were eight times more likely to screen positive than those without. Similar positive results were found for those living with a mental impairment. They concluded, "Major motor, cognitive, visual, and hearing impairments appear to account for more than half of the positive M-CHAT screens in extremely low gestational age newborns. Even after those with such impairments were eliminated, 10% of children—nearly double the expected rate—screened positive" (Kuban et al., 2009). These data show that one in five children born more than 3 months prematurely screen positive for a PDD, and that even after excluding the children with a motor, vision, hearing, or cognitive impairment, 10% still screen positive for PDD symptoms. These results support the theory that a premature birth, which probably results from early gestational trauma, may play a role in the development of a PDD.

Diagnostic Criteria for Autistic Disorder (299.00)

The APA in the *DSM-IV-TR* (2000) lists the following essential diagnostic criteria for autistic disorder:

A. A total of six (or more) items from (1), (2), and (3), with at least two from (1), and one each from (2) and (3):
  (1) qualitative impairment in social interaction, as manifested by at least two of the following:
    (a) marked impairment in the use of multiple nonverbal behaviors such as eye-to-eye gaze, facial expression, body postures, and gestures to regulate social interaction
    (b) failure to develop peer relationships appropriate to developmental level
    (c) a lack of spontaneous seeking to share enjoyment, interests, or achievements with other people (e.g., by a lack of showing, bringing, or pointing out objects of interest)
    (d) lack of social or emotional reciprocity
  (2) qualitative impairments in communication as manifested by at least one of the following:
    (a) delay in, or total lack of, the development of spoken language (not accompanied by an attempt to compensate through alternative modes of communication such as gesture or mime)
    (b) in individuals with adequate speech, marked impairment in the ability to initiate or sustain a conversation with others
    (c) stereotyped and repetitive use of language or idiosyncratic language
    (d) lack of varied, spontaneous make-believe play or social imitative play appropriate to developmental level
  (3) restricted repetitive and stereotyped patterns of behavior, interests, and activities, as manifested by at least one of the following:
    (a) encompassing preoccupation with one or more stereo-

typed and restricted patterns of interest that is abnormal either in intensity or focus
(b) apparently inflexible adherence to specific, nonfunctional routines or rituals
(c) stereotyped and repetitive motor manners (e.g., hand or finger flapping or twisting, or complex whole-body movements)
(d) persistent preoccupation with parts of objects
B. Delays or abnormal functioning in at least one of the following areas, with onset prior to age 3 years: (1) social interaction, (2) language as used in social communication, or (3) symbolic or imaginative play.
C. The disturbance is not better accounted for by Rett's Disorder or Childhood Disintegrative Disorder.

Diagnostic Criteria for Asperger's Disorder (299.80)

In children with Asperger's disorder, language, curiosity, and cognitive development proceed normally while there is a substantial delay in social interaction and "development of restricted, repetitive patterns of behavior, interests, and activities" (APA, 2000). However, there is no clinically significant delay in language as there is with autistic disorder, nor is there a clinically significant delay in cognitive development, or self-help skills, and curiosity about the environment.

The *DSM-IV-TR* lists the following essential diagnostic criteria:

A. Qualitative impairment in social interaction, as manifested by at least two of the following:
(1) marked impairment in the use of multiple nonverbal behaviors such as eye-to-eye gaze, facial expression, body postures, and gestures to regulate social interaction
(2) failure to develop peer relationships appropriate to developmental level
(3) a lack of spontaneous seeking to share enjoyment, interests, or achievements with other people (e.g., by a lack of showing, bringing, or pointing out objects of interest to other people)
(4) lack of social or emotional reciprocity

B. Restricted repetitive and stereotyped patterns of behavior, interests and activities, as manifested by at least one of the following:
    (1) encompassing preoccupation with one or more stereotyped and restricted patterns of interest that is abnormal either in intensity or focus
    (2) apparently inflexible adherence to specific, nonfunctional routines or rituals
    (3) stereotyped and repetitive motor mannerisms (e.g., hand or finger flapping or twisting, or complex whole-body movements)
    (4) persistent preoccupation with parts of objects
C. The disturbance causes clinically significant impairment in social, occupational, or other important areas of functioning.
D. There is no clinically significant general delay in language (e.g., single words used by age 2 years, communicative phrases used by age 3 years).
E. There is no clinically significant delay in cognitive development or in the development of age-appropriate self-help skills, adaptive behavior (other than in social interaction), and curiosity about the environment in childhood.
F. Criteria are not met for another specific Pervasive Developmental Disorder or Schizophrenia. (APA, 2000)

Diagnostic Criteria for Pervasive Developmental Disorder Not Otherwise Specified (Including Atypical Autism; 299.80)

"This category should be used when there is a severe and pervasive impairment in the development of reciprocal social interaction or verbal and nonverbal communication skills, or when stereotyped behavior, interests, and activities are present, but the criteria are not met for a specific Pervasive Developmental Disorder, Schizophrenia, Schizotypal Personality Disorder, or Avoidant Personality Disorder. For example, this category includes 'atypical autism'—presentations that do not meet the criteria for Autistic Disorder because of late age at onset, atypical symptomatology, or subthreshold symptomatology, or all of these" (APA, 2000).

PDD-NOS is frequently and incorrectly referred to as simply PDD. However, the term PDD refers to the entire group that includes all of the autism like disorders, but it is not a diagnosis in itself. PDD-NOS is a diagnosis. PDD-NOS is difficult to describe because of the "not otherwise specified" factor. People with PDD-NOS are close to having full-syndrome autism or Asperger's syndrome, but do not fulfill all conditions.

Diagnostic Criteria for Rett's Disorder (299.80)

The key to the diagnosis of Rett's disorder is a normal development and functioning in every way for the first 5 months of life. After that point there are a number of different and characteristic deficits that develop. The *DSM-IV-TR* criteria are the following:

A. All of the following:
  (1) apparently normal prenatal and perinatal development
  (2) apparently normal psychomotor development through the first 5 months after birth
  (3) normal head circumference at birth
B. Onset of all of the following after the period of normal development:
  (1) deceleration of head growth between ages 5 and 48 months
  (2) loss of previously acquired purposeful hand skills between 5 and 30 months with the subsequent development of stereotyped hand movements (e.g., hand-wringing or hand washing)
  (3) loss of social engagement early in the course (although often social interaction develops later)
  (4) appearance of poorly coordinated gait or trunk movements
  (5) severely impaired expressive and receptive language development with severe psychomotor retardation (APA, 2000)

Diagnostic Criteria for Childhood Disintegrative Disorder (299.10)

The key to the diagnosis of childhood disintegrative disorder "is a marked regression in multiple areas of functioning following a period of two years of apparently normal development" (APA, 2000).

This disorder is usually associated with mental retardation and there are a variety of nonspecific neurological symptoms. It has been suggested that it results from an insult during development, but no specific mechanism has been postulated. The *DSM-IV-TR* criteria are the following:

A. Apparently normal development for at least the first 2 years after birth as manifested by the presence of age-appropriate verbal and nonverbal communication, social relationships, play, and adaptive behavior.
B. Clinically significant loss of previously acquired skills (before age 10 years) in at least two of the following areas:
   (1) expressive or receptive language
   (2) social skills or adaptive behavior
   (3) bowel or bladder control
   (4) play
   (5) motor skills
C. Abnormalities of functioning in at least two of the following areas:
   (1) qualitative impairment in social interaction (e.g., impairment in nonverbal behaviors, failure to develop peer relationships, lack of social or emotional reciprocity)
   (2) qualitative impairments in communication (e.g., delay or lack of spoken language, inability to initiate or sustain a conversation, stereotyped and repetitive use of language, lack of varied make-believe play)
   (3) restricted, repetitive, and stereotyped patterns of behavior, interest, and activities, including motor stereotypes and mannerisms
D. The disturbance is not better accounted for by another specific Pervasive Developmental Disorder or by Schizophrenia. (APA, 2000)

Prevalence and Etiology

Thirty years ago it was believed that one in 2,500 children had autism (Waldman, Nicholson, Adilov, & Williams, 2008). But a study by the Centers for Disease Control in Atlanta now calculates a prevalence rate for autistic spectrum disorders at one in every 150 children (Kuehn, 2007). One survey finds a rate for all PDDs at about 60 per 10,000 or 1 per 166 individuals, with the majority of cases being in the PDD-NOS group, along with an estimated rate for autistic disorder at 13 per 10,000 or 1 per 769 individuals, and for Asperger's disorder at an estimated rate of approximately 3 per 10,000 or 1 per 3,333 individuals, and childhood disintegrative disorder, which is very rare, at about 0.2 per 10,000 or 1 in every 50,000 individuals (Fombonne, 2005). Fombonne also states that the "assessment process, sample size, publication year, and geographic location of studies all have an effect on prevalence estimates" (2005).

While there is no clear indication or agreement on the exact causes of PDDs, in more recent years there has been a very heated debate about whether environmental factors, including vaccines, play a causal role in their onset. This debate has been sparked by the alarming 8-fold rise in new cases reported over the last decade in California. While some researchers believe that this increase can be explained by artifacts that include a broadening of the diagnostic criteria and greatly increased diagnosis at younger ages, Hertz-Picciotto and Delwiche (2009) studied this trend to help explain this phenomenon by investigating the changes in age at diagnosis and the inclusion of milder cases. They looked at the autism cases identified from 1990 through 2006 in the databases from the California Department of Developmental Services, and they calculated "population incident cases younger than age 10 years for each quarter, cumulative incidence by age and birth year, age-specific incidence rates stratified by birth year, and proportions of diagnoses by age across birth years" (Hertz-Picciotto & Delwiche, 2009). Here are their results: "Autism incidence in children rose throughout the period. Cumulative incidence at 5 years of age per 10,000 births rose consistently from 6.2 for 1990 births to 42.5 for 2001 births. Age-specific incidence rates increased most steeply for 2- and 3-year-olds. The proportion diagnosed by age 5 years increased only slightly, from 54% for 1990 births to 61% for 1996 births. Changing age at diagnosis can explain a 12% increase, and inclusion of milder cases, a 56% increase." They concluded, "Autism incidence in California shows no sign yet of plateauing. Younger ages at diagnosis, differential migration, changes in diagnostic criteria, and inclusion of milder cases do not fully explain the observed increases. Other artifacts have yet to be quantified, and as a result, the extent to which the continued rise represents a true increase in the occurrence of autism remains unclear." Another study looked at rain precipitation rates in counties in California, Oregon, and Washington to investigate the possibility of an environmental trigger for autism with children born between 1987 and 1999 (Waldman et al., 2008). They compared the county-level precipitation with county-level autism prevalence rates and counts. This careful study also controlled for time trends, population size, per capita income, and demographic characteristics. They found that the "county-level autism prevalence rates and counts among school-aged children were positively associated with a county's mean annual precipitation" and that "the amount of precipitation a birth cohort was exposed to when younger than 3 years was positively associated with subsequent autism prevalence rates and counts in Oregon counties and California counties" (Waldman et al., 2008). The authors concluded that these results are consistent with the existence of an environmental trigger for autism that is positively associated with rain precipitation. They also suggested that additional studies should be conducted to help establish whether such a trigger exists and to identify the specific trigger.

However, another study assessed the continuing increase in autism in California to study the possible effects of thimerosal (ethylmercury) exposure from vaccines as a primary cause of autism (Schechter & Grether, 2008). The researchers noted that the exclusion of thimerosal from childhood vaccines was accelerated from 1999 to 2001 and they investigated the time trends in the prevalence by age and birth cohort of children with autism who were active status clients of the California Department of Developmental Service (DDS) from January 1, 1995, through March 31, 2007. They found that the "estimated prevalence of autism for children at each year of age from 3 to 12 years increased throughout the study period" and "the estimated prevalence of DDS clients aged 3 to 5 years with autism increased for each quarter from January 1995 through March 2007" (Schechter & Grether, 2008). However, they also found, "Since 2004, the absolute increase and the rate of increase in DDS clients aged 3 to 5 years with autism were higher than those in DDS clients of the same ages with any eligible condition including autism." Therefore, they concluded, "The DDS data do not show any recent decrease in autism in California despite the exclusion of more than trace levels of thimerosal from nearly all childhood vaccines. The DDS data do not support the hypothesis that exposure to thimerosal during childhood is a primary cause of autism." One can interpret this result in one of three ways. There is some evidence that ethylmercury in vaccines does not lead to an increase in autism, or it may be that the large increase in the number of vaccines administered alone plays an important role as a causative agent in the development of autism. The number of diseases that children were vaccinated for in 1985 was 7, and now that number is 16 and children endure about 37 separate vaccination encounters. The final interpretation is that the continued increase in autism is too high due to all factors combined, and thus these multiple factors overshadow any real causative effect of thimerosal. Regardless of the nature of the causative agents, which are likely to be many and multiple, the fact that autism is increasing at an alarming rate tells us that it is highly likely that environmental factors are far more important here than previously expected. Therefore, investigating the role of environmental factors deserves much greater attention and funding. This is further supported by a study that examined mercury exposure from maternal dental amalgams during pregnancy among 100 children born between 1990 and 1999 and diagnosed with autism or the more mild variant of autism spectrum disorder. The authors used logistic regression analysis (age, gender, race, and region of residency adjusted) by quintile of maternal dental amalgams during pregnancy, which revealed that children of subjects that had greater than six amalgams "were 3.2-fold significantly more likely to be diagnosed with autism (severe) in comparison to ASD (mild) than subjects with less or equal to 5 amalgams" (Geier, Kern, & Geier, 2009). They concluded, "Dental amalgam policies should consider mercury exposure in women before and during the child-bearing age and the possibility of subsequent fetal exposure and adverse outcomes." One may conclude that this highly toxic heavy metal has a serious deleterious effect on children in the womb and perhaps with mothers who are also nursing (Daschner & Mutter, 2007; Mutter, Naumann, & Guethlin, 2007), and that mercury, like lead, should be avoided under any and all circumstances, including amalgam fillings, regardless of the age.

There has been a long-standing controversy and interest to know if PDDs are in fact genetically determined. "Two previous epidemiological studies of autistic twins suggested that autism was predominantly genetically determined, although the findings with regard to a broader phenotype of cognitive, and possibly social, abnormalities were contradictory" (Bailey et al., 1995). The same researchers, after increasing their British twin database, now state that there is evidence to support the view that PDDs are heritable (Bailey et al., 1995). More recently, others have added, "autism spectrum disorders are neurodevelopmental disorders of complex etiology with a recognized substantial contribution of heterogeneous genetic factors" and that "specific genetic mechanisms underlying this heritability have not yet been discovered" (Yrigollen et al., 2008). Others noted that "the search for susceptibility genes in autism and autism spectrum disorders has been hindered by the possible small effects of individual genes and by genetic (locus) heterogeneity" (Liu, Paterson, & Szatmari, 2008). The following summary comment on the controversy made by a group of expert geneticists (Yrigollen et al., 2008) is based on the Autism Genome Project Consortium Report: "the dominant hypothesis regarding the etiological factors underlying autism spectrum disorders is oligogenic inheritance with possible epistatic interactions among common risk-predisposing genetic variants and detrimental environments" (Szatmari et al., 2007). However, no clear evidence has conclusively demonstrated any causal role of "risk-predisposing" genes to date in the development of the PDDs. Indeed, if there is a risk factor based on specific genes, it would potentially be with a relatively large array of genes, and therefore, there is very little chance that anything can be done to either prevent or treat these spectrum disorders based on an understanding of the genetics alone. My pessimistic view is further supported by a comment by experts on this complexity: "Recognition of the complexity of the genetic mechanisms of autism explains why its biology remains elusive and molecular mechanisms underlying this biology are mostly speculative or unknown" (Yrigollen et al., 2008).

Results Using Conventional Treatment Modalities

Most recently, King and colleagues commented on the pharmaco-logical approach to treatment of the PDDs: "no medications are approved by the Food and Drug Administration for core symptoms of autism spectrum disorders" (2009). Others have asserted that there is an "absence of clear and present guidelines" for children and adolescents with PDD when using psychopharmacologic agents (Filipek, Steinberg-Epstein, & Book, 2006). However, a more re-cent article based on the "limited clinical and empirical experiences of the author and a few other investigators" presented a psycho-pharmacological treatment plan for a wide range of comorbid psy-chiatric disorders that are potentially responsive to drugs, includ-ing the variants of the anxiety disorders, mood disorders, ADHD, Tourette's syndrome, sleep problems, and psychotic symptoms that frequently accompany Asperger's disorder (Tsai, 2007). This au-thor also stated that while he was successful with children with Asperger's syndrome, the "older adolescents and adults with this disorder and comorbid mental conditions refused to accept the di-agnostic conclusion and would not cooperate with any profession-als' interventions including medications."

One study characterized the widespread use of psychoactive medications among children and youth with PDDs over the course of one calendar year (Oswald & Sonenklar, 2007). These authors found that 83% of their subjects were taking at least one drug during the study year and that the prescribed drugs came from 125 different therapeutic classes. "The seven most frequently prescribed classes of psychoactive drugs were antidepressants, stimulants, tranquilizers and antipsychotics, anticonvulsants, hypotensive agents, anxiolytic/sedative/hypnotics, and benzodiazepines." They pointed out that these children and adolescents are frequently treated with medication due to target symptoms that may be commonly associated with other mental disorders. More specifically, they found "that about 70% of children with autism-spectrum disorders age 8 years and up receive some form of psychoactive medication in a given year." Clearly, a major effort has been made by physicians to treat PDDs with psychoactive medications. This major effort is further supported and inspired by the fact that the global market for autism therapeutics is estimated at $2.2 to $3.5 billion and that the greatest global market share (59%) is accounted for by the antidepressants in the category of the selective serotonin reuptake inhibitors (SSRIs) (King & Bostic, 2006). One of the most problematic symptoms of children and adolescents with PDDs is the repetitive behaviors, which vary widely and persist over time. These behaviors typically include stereotypic movements, inflexible routines, repetitive play, and limited and oddly patterned speech, all of which may cause anxiety, argumentative behavior, self-injurious behavior, and aggression when others attempt to interrupt them. These repetitive behaviors are also the greatest predictors that an early diagnosis of autism will endure (Richler, Bishop, Kleinke, & Lord, 2007). Since researchers have hoped that the SSRIs would reduce or eliminate repetitive behaviors with the autistic disorders, because there is evidence that it helps with these symptoms in obsessive-compulsive disorder, this has been one major reason for attempting to treat PDDs with SSRIs. While one older 10-week study of children and adolescents showed that a serotonin reuptake blocker called clomipramine, with unique antiobsessional properties, was superior to both placebo and desipramine on ratings of autistic symptoms (including stereotypes), anger, and compulsive, ritualized behaviors (Gordon, State, Nelson, Hamburger, & Rapoport, 1993), a later study comparing clomipramine with haloperidol and placebo in adults with autistic spectrum disorders showed no differences between the drug and placebo, with the exception of a high rate of adverse events with the drug (Remington, Sloman, Konstantareas, Parker, & Gow, 2001). Another 12-week study of 30 autistic adults compared the SSRI fluvoxamine with placebo, and this study showed that the SSRI was superior to placebo in reducing repetitive thoughts and behavior, maladaptive behavior, and aggression, and improving some aspects of social relatedness, especially language usage (McDougle et al., 1996). Other than mild sedation and nausea in some patients, the drug was well tolerated. However, in another placebo-controlled study of fluvoxamine in children, only 1 of the 18 subjects demonstrated improvement on the active drug, and 14 of the 18 children treated with fluvoxamine showed adverse events that included hyperactivity, insomnia, agitation, and aggression, which suggests a very high sensitivity of autistic children to this SSRI (Posey & McDougle, 2000). In 2005, one group of researchers noted that there were "no published placebo controlled trials with SSRIs that documented safety and efficacy in children with autism" (Hollander et al., 2005). Therefore, they conducted an 8-week placebo-controlled trial with fluoxetine studying repetitive behaviors and global improvement. Their results showed that with low doses fluoxetine was only slightly, and not significantly, superior to placebo on the Clinical Global Impressions Scale autism score, that fluoxetine was marginally superior to placebo on a composite measure of global effectiveness, and that the drug did not significantly differ from placebo on treatment-emergent side effects. The authors concluded that "fluoxetine in low doses is more effective than placebo in the treatment of repetitive behaviors in childhood autism" (Hollander et al., 2005). Most recently, due to this scant positive evidence and high incidence of prescribing of SSRIs to youth with PDDs, a very large study looked at psychotropic medication use among Medicaid-enrolled children with PDDs to examine the child and health system characteristics associated with psychotropic medication use. This study looked at claims for the calendar year 2001 from all 50 states and Washington, DC, and examined 60,641 children with a PDD (Mandell et al., 2008). They found that 56% of these children used at least one psychotropic medication and that 20% were prescribed three or more medications concurrently. They also found, "Use was common even in children aged 0 to 2 years (18%) and 3 to 5 years (32%). Neuroleptic drugs were the most common psychotropic class (31%), followed by antidepressants (25%) and stimulants (22%)" (Mandell et al., 2008). They also found that those children most likely to be medicated were male, older, and white, in foster care or in the Medicaid disability category; those with additional psychiatric diagnoses; and those who utilized more autism spectrum disorder services. They also found that children who lived in counties with a lower percentage of white residents or greater urban density were less likely to use such medications. They concluded that "psychotropic medication use is common among even very young children with autism spectrum disorders. Factors unrelated to clinical presentation seem highly associated with prescribing practices. Given the limited evidence base, there is an urgent need to assess the risks, benefits, and costs of medication use and understand the local and national policies that affect medication use" (Mandell et al., 2008).

Given the apparent need for much greater therapeutic efficacy in a rapidly emerging, troubled, and costly population, the National Institutes of Health created a network called Studies to Advance Autism Research and Treatment (STAART). This group decided for various reasons to do a placebo-controlled trial of citalopram for repetitive behavior in children with PDD. They believed that citalopram would improve global functioning by reducing repetitive behavior and that the use of a low starting dosage, followed by gradual upward adjustment, would identify an effective well-tolerated dosage range with few adverse events (King et al., 2009). In a multisite trial, they studied 149 children and adolescents between the ages of 5 and 17 who met the criteria for either an autistic disorder, Asperger's disorder, or PDD-NOS. They found "there was no significant difference in the rate of positive response on the Clinical Global Impressions, Improvement subscale between the citalopram-treated group (32.9%) and the placebo group (34.2%)." They also found that there was no difference in score reduction on the Children's Yale-Brown Obsessive Compulsive Scales modified for pervasive developmental disorders. However, they did find that "citalopram use was significantly more likely to be associated with adverse events, particularly increased energy level, impulsiveness, decreased concentration, hyperactivity, stereotypy, diarrhea, insomnia, and dry skin or pruritus" (King et al., 2009). Therefore, citalopram exhibited significant adverse effects without any therapeutic benefits in children. The authors concluded, "Results of this trial do not support the use of citalopram for the treatment of repetitive behavior in children and adolescents with autism spectrum disorders." They also noted that about one third of their placebo-control patients showed a positive response. This was the largest randomized controlled medication clinical trial in children with PDD (Volkmar, 2009). Their careful choice of a psychotropic agent here, along with their careful administration of initial low and slowly titrated doses, and the results of earlier trials with several other and older SSRIs, does not lend much hope for this drug category as an effective agent for the treatment of PDD, despite the widespread and current prescribing habits of physicians in the United States.

While the SSRIs do not appear to be a favorable class of drugs for treating children with PDD, there is one study using the atypical antipsychotic agent called risperidone that has shown promising results for children who have serious behavioral disturbances (McCracken et al., 2002). This group of researchers conducted an 8-week, multisite, randomized, double-blind placebo-controlled trial for 101 children (82 boys and 19 girls) with a mean age of 8.8 years (range 5–17) that had autistic disorder accompanied by severe tantrums, aggression, or self-injurious behavior. They measured outcomes using the score on the Irritability subscale of the Aberrant Behavior Checklist and the rating on the Clinical Global

Impressions–Improvement (CGI-I) scale. Forty-nine children took risperidone and 52 took placebo. There was a 56.9% reduction in the irritability score for the risperidone group and a 14.1% decrease in the placebo group. "The rate of a positive response, defined as at least a 25 percent decrease in the Irritability score and a rating of much improved or very much improved on the CGI-I scale, was 69 percent in the risperidone group (34 of 49 children had a positive response) and 12 percent in the placebo group (6 of 52)" (Mc-Cracken et al., 2002). However, the antipsychotic medication was also associated with an average weight gain of 5.94 pounds compared with 1.76 pounds with placebo, and there was also a significant side effect profile with the medication group that showed increased appetite, fatigue, drowsiness, dizziness, and drooling. They also found that two thirds of the children with a positive response to medication at 8 weeks maintained their benefits at 6 months. The authors concluded, "Risperidone was effective and well tolerated for the treatment of tantrums, aggression, or self-injurious behavior in children with autistic disorder. The short period of this trial limits inferences about adverse effects such as tardive dyskinesia." "Despite strong evidence in its favor, the FDA has not felt that the risk/benefit profile was strong enough to warrant granting risperidone a specific indication for use in autism" (Filipek et al., 2006). No doubt this current ruling is based mostly on the significant and serious negative side effect profiles that are associated with the typical and atypical antipsychotics. Overall, there is insufficient information on the vast majority of medications used in children and the long-term effects of any psychotropic medication on the developing brain are unknown (Blumer, 1999; Steinbrook, 2002). In addition, since there is no known neurochemical basis for PDD, extreme caution must be used when prescribing for this vulnerable population. To date, the primary directives for use in this population are listed as the following four conservative rules (Filipek et al., 2006): (1) rule out all potential medical etiologies that may lead to symptoms of PDD; (2) all behavioral management strategies must be attempted before medication is initiated; (3)

there remains a clear need for pharmacological intervention; and (4) the medication management protocol must proceed in a responsible and conscientious manner.

Behavioral as opposed to pharmacologic treatment is the hallmark of effective intervention for autism, and these approaches include the more traditional language communication therapies, occupational and sensory integration therapies, special education services, and those under the rubric called applied behavioral analysis (Filipek et al., 2006). There have also been considerable advances in the area called educational law and special education recommendations to help protect these vulnerable patients and the rights of their families, and to help ensure that they are receiving the best that standard school systems have to offer toward education. Today this law is called the Individuals With Disability Education Act, and it covers six critical areas: (1) a zero reject policy; (2) nondiscriminatory evaluation; (3) an individualized education plan; (4) providing a least restrictive environment; (5) due process, which is a set of legal procedures to ensure fairness of education procedures; and (6) ensuring parental participation in the development of the individualized education plan and a right of access to educational records.

The scientific evidence provided in the National Research Council report for the effectiveness of early education and intervention with young children with autistic spectrum disorders has been described at length (Mirenda, 2001; NRC, 2001). A summary comment on the report concerning the nature of effective treatments and interventions for young children with autistic spectrum disorders is the following: "The absence of knowledge cannot be used as a reason to withhold appropriate assessments, treatments, or educational programs, for young children with autism. Nevertheless, there is a tremendous need for more knowledge about which interventions are most effective for which children and how they are best integrated into comprehensive treatments for individual children and their families" (Lord et al., 2002). This tells us that there is a huge gap between the treatments that are employed for PDD and the scientific research that is needed to support any therapies that may be truly efficacious. This gap is further reflected by the Autism Society of America, which stated, "Finally, we need boldness. A child with autism needs help right away. There are more and more such children every day. And people with autism need help through the lifespan. We need to help now. We need to overcome the disconnect between treatment and science, and learn from our present treatments so we can have better treatments in the future" (Herbert, 2008).

While psychoanalytic approaches may not appear to be an obvious way to treat autistic children, who by definition have impaired communication skills, they have been discussed using a select case history that showed a marked improvement in a 7-year-old severely troubled autistic male child (Parks, 2007). This young male did not contain the inner representations of "self with mother," "self with father," and "self with mother and father together." However, he developed a representation of "self with analyst" (Parks, 2007). The author commented about parents with children with significant developmental problems that increasingly turn to psychoanalysis for help: "As a result, child analysts today see many more patients who have turned to psychoanalysis as the 'treatment of last resort'" (Parks, 2007). This approach has some bearing on the yogic approach to treatment (see the section Yogic Protocols for Treatment).

The Yogic View of the Etiology of the Pervasive Developmental Disorders

The pervasive developmental disorders are the most difficult-to-treat disorders of the three groups covered in this book. From a yogic point of view, there is no single causal factor that will always lead to the onset of autistic disorder, Asperger's disorder, or PDD-NOS. However, the causal factors or triggers can be singular, multiple, or varied, and of course the respective incidents must occur during the earliest months and years of the life cycle. The trigger must be an insult or trauma that affects the central nervous system during the most vulnerable and critical stages of development. Sometimes the event occurs while in the womb, or during the birthing process, or additive events may occur while in the womb plus the birthing process that result in the development of PDD. Or it may be a singular event that occurs after birth. Regardless of the event, or cascade of events, the trigger acts as a shock that disrupts the highly sensitive process of early normal development. The end result here and the key to understanding PDD is that these patients are lost and must themselves recognize the split part of their being through a unification exercise. Much here also depends on the basic and initial stability of the psyche of the individual taking the affected incarnation. It is worth considering that not all souls who take an incarnation have a well-integrated psyche prior to their entry into the womb and that these individuals are thus more vulnerable to an often subtle but traumatic event or series of events. These individuals are frequently lost prior to their entry into the earthly world, and therefore they may have the fate of attracting a life to live out this experience of being lost in a new incarnation. Here, like attracts like.

Several obvious questions here are what does it mean to be lost, how can this happen, and how can we help these people to become whole again. One unique quality that varies in degree, which is also central to the variants of the psychoses and the personality disorders, is the disconnection and the lack of adaptation that these patients have with their respective cultural or commonly accepted version of reality. By definition, individuals in these three classes of disorders have skewed views of reality that can and do vary in severity. While the idea of a single version of a healthy normal reality is indeed open to much debate, people with PDD, psychosis, or personality disorder all have an experience of reality that does not serve their needs effectively in society because of their respective perceptions of reality. They do not fit in. That is, their perception and behavior are not considered functional or appropriate for members of a healthy society. There is a discordant perception of self in relationship to the world. With the autistic patient, and to a lesser degree the Asperger's patient, the patient is living in a world much to themselves where their practical and daily living skills remain undeveloped. Autistic and Asperger's patients are isolated in their own world and they are not aware of the difference in their perception compared to that of others. Consequently the PDD patient remains disconnected with some varying degree of separation. One mechanism for the autistic patient is that this person lives almost totally in the world as perceived by their right hemisphere, which dominates their waking conscious awareness, intelligence, and personality. As noted in Chapter 2, the schizophrenic patient may only experience hallucinations during the left nostril–right hemisphere dominant state, and of course during this state, their reality is far from being connected to the culturally accepted version of a normal world. We have some scientific evidence to support this case for the autistic individual. Dane and Balci (2007) studied the nasal cycle in children that are autistic and noted that approximately 80% of the time the children were left nostril dominant during the waking state compared to age- and sex-matched healthy controls, who exhibited approximately equal dominance between the left and right nostrils under the same testing conditions. Therefore, according to this study, autistic children are primarily right hemisphere dominant during the waking state. This fits with the findings described in the first section of this chapter, where the case is made for left hemispheric damage or underactivity (to the more vulnerable hemisphere) with the resulting consequence of greater right hemispheric activity in the PDD patient, including the savant. These patients are living in a world of their own. Their perceptions, patterns of behavior, and ability to connect to those in the world around them remains inadequate and they are not aware of this difference. From the yogic perspective, the left hemisphere is the primary home of our daily languages, basic living and working skills, and mental tools that we use to make our way in or conquer the world, and tools that are used for everyday survival. Our hunting skills are lateralized to the left brain. In a nutshell, the right brain gives us a look at the bigger picture, and it can support modes of intelligence that are beyond time and space. When people are living in this realm almost exclusively, they are unaware of the other realm, and often they do not develop the other skills that better serve their daily functions, like language. Normal, healthy individuals will have a balance of both brains, although they too are usually not consciously aware of the shift back and forth since it is usually gradual and slow. They do not notice the physical markers of this shift in state. This is one reason why the nasal cycle is an important parameter. It clearly marks both states. Once individuals are aware of the nasal cycle, they can more easily compare and contrast variations in moods, emotions, energy levels, and cognitive performance efficiencies.

Parents of PDD children intuitively recognize that their child is in another world. But it does not mean that the child's world is not a real world. Simply put, the child's world is not in sync with the more outwardly productive and earthly world. The question is how to bridge the gap, how to get these children to connect, adapt to, and experience a richer and fuller life, a life that fits better with the world around them where they can excel and be totally independent. How can we best help them to achieve a state of wholeness and unity?

The Yogic Protocols for Treatment

The intention and direction for treatment here is to help patients develop a lasting experience of wholeness and unity in their conscious awareness. This is a slow process, and it involves different ministages that are often dependent on the age and status of the patient, and the talent and charisma of the individual that helps to coordinate this process.

This protocol is called the Dance of the Heart.* The first step in this protocol is to reach out to the individual in the form of a dance

*Copyright © David Shannahoff-Khalsa, 2008. No portion of this protocol may be reproduced without the express written permission of the author.

that is perceived as playful for the subject. This must be done in such a way that the subject does not understand the therapeutic motive for the activity. It must appear to be a playful game. This process does not have to be carried out by a psychiatrist, psychotherapist, or parent. Therefore, we can call this person a coordinator. The coordinator can be an older brother or sister, or even a younger brother or sister if the patient is older and the coordinator has the skills. The coordinator can also be a neighbor or a family friend with whom the patient already has a natural affinity. In principle, this process is not that different from what a therapist or yogi does with anyone who has been traumatized and is seeking help. But the outward steps here are very different. At the start, the coordinator can be either in a standing or sitting posture. A standing posture is much preferred, but not all patients may be able or willing to join in a standing posture. The coordinator must first touch hands without leaning forward, but the patient is coaxed to lean forward and reach out and touch hands with the coordinator. The fingers can be interlaced to form a comfortable secure link and interlock. At this point, if standing, the coordinator then leads the individual in an unstructured playful dance where the patient is being guided while in a receptive mode. It is imperative that the coordinator leads, but the dance can take any playful form. The second critical part of the protocol includes a breathing technique where the coordinator first begins to practice a breathing pattern that is recognized by the patient. Three patterns with increasing complexity are suggested below. This can happen while the two are still moving or while the two are standing still for a moment. Once the patient recognizes the pattern as part of the game, the coordinator then asks the patient to make the same breathing pattern. The next step after the patient makes the same breathing pattern is that the coordinator asks the patient to join in by making and holding eye-to-eye contact with the coordinator. It is not always necessary to ask the patient to hold the eye-to-eye contact out loud. This can also happen spontaneously without the verbal input, but it is rare. At first the patient may not want to join in with the breathing pattern or to initiate or maintain eye contact. The most critical component here is that patients have fun so that they will continue again on another day. The next stage of the process is where the coordinator begins to chant a mantra out loud, but in phase with the breath pattern. At this stage the coordinator then asks the patient to join in with the chanting while maintaining the breathing pattern and eye contact. However, the chanting with breathing can be started either before or after the eye contact is made. But eventually, the eye-to-eye contact, the regulated breathing, and the chanting must all occur together. This is in fact a meditation practice, but one that is perceived as play, a game. This process of the dance, where the patient is being led and is breathing and chanting, continues until a connection is perceived, which is ultimately critical to the final step of the process. The next step of the process is a balance in the standing position without the patient leaning on the coordinator and while the breathing, eye-to-eye contact, and chanting continue, where both feel centered and stable and where the patient feels like he or she is drawing in a measure of love from the coordinator. This final step then includes the subject consciously identifying and experiencing the heartfelt connection and the flow of love. This final step is why this process is called the Dance of the Heart. This multipart description is the ideal sequence and it includes all of the essentials. However, the coordinator cannot expect the subject to follow through the first time, or even the second, third, or fourth time. It can take months of play and practice to arrive at the final stage of this sequence. Much is dependent on the frequency of the play. It is very important that the coordinator must not go into this process with any expectations and intentions other than to enjoy it and to help the patient have immediate fun, and ultimately to help the patient have the experience of creating a personal and loving connection. This healing process is different with each individual, and much depends on the extremes of the subject's condition, and the magnetism and playful nature of the coordinator, and his or her ability to help create a loving heartfelt connection that touches the soul of the patient.

A variety of options are listed below that can be used for the specific breathing patterns and for the choice of mantra. The choices here will vary depending on the comfort, familiarity, and ability of the coordinator, but mostly they should be determined by the condition, cooperative nature, and age of the patient. The positions and forms of the dance too can vary. Both the patient and coordinator have to enjoy this playful process. Sometimes the process is best initiated by the coordinator, who first begins to dance alone and then starts chanting along with the dance, where it is obvious to the patient that the coordinator is having a great deal of fun. This is a process that has to be repeated over and over and over again. This is play that comes from the heart, not from the head. This is not an intellectual process. The head has to bow to the heart in this game. In reality, we all seek love, but none of us want to be told that we are not already normal, united, or whole, or that our world is unreal and that we are not adequate. We all want to live in love and union. But rarely are we willing to reach out for it, or acknowledge that our lives are missing this divine quality. The PDD patient is certainly no different in this regard. The initial position, breathing patterns, chants, and the final balance position are all somewhat variable. The key here is to make it fun and to make the experience of the techniques playful, healing, and rewarding for the PDD patient. For this to happen, the experience must also be fun for the coordinator. There is a sequence and an end point. But there are no minimum times for each of the respective stages of play. The chanting, breathing, and eye-to-eye contact should not be practiced longer than 11 minutes. Three minutes is usually an adequate time for the chanting, eye-to-eye contact and breathing part of the protocol. If the child (or adult) can reach 3 minutes in this phase, this is a great achievement.

Patients who make substantial progress may be willing to forgo the earlier stages of the dance and leaning. At this point, the procedure can start by locking the hands and looking eye to eye while the breathing and chanting occur in synchrony with the coordinator. The coordinator and patient can also practice a variety of techniques at this stage called Venus Kriyas, which are published elsewhere (Shannahoff-Khalsa, 2006). However, the best results with any of the Venus Kriyas for the PDD patient will be achieved by practicing the techniques where the eyes are open, eye looking into eye, and the mantra is chanted out loud. For this purpose, I recommend the one called Pushing Palms. But the intent must still be one that is playful and loving, a play of the heart and soul. The final and fine-tuning stages of healing and growth can be achieved by the PDD patient learning to practice a variety of Kundalini yoga meditation techniques that are described below in the sections for Additional and Elementary Brain-Balancing Techniques for the PDD Patient and the Advanced Techniques for the Accomplished PDD Patient. The latter techniques will help the patient overcome any final symptoms and "residue."

This procedure must begin with the coordinator tuning in with the mantra "Ong Namo Guru Dev Namo." This is the standard and an essential practice for any of the protocols or individual techniques that are taught in this book or for any of the techniques in general that are part of the system of Kundalini yoga as taught by Yogi Bhajan. The coordinator can chant the mantra out loud or silently, but it must be practiced before entering into the dance relationship with the patient. If the coordinator chooses, he or she can do it silently while in the same room with the patient before starting. Or the coordinator can chant it out loud prior to entering the room. This decision is based solely on what is most convenient and comfortable for the patient and the coordinator. The coordinator can also start by doing a meditation in the same room, with the patient only observing, or not observing. Some of my clients use this as a key to help interest the patient in the activity. Most PDD patients enjoy the mental state of the coordinator once they tune in and begin to practice. They may not show this openly, but on one level they may begin to connect. The world of meditation is more familiar to them than the ordinary world of daily life. They too are living in another world.

Technique to Induce a Meditative State: Tuning In

Sit with a straight spine and with the feet flat on the floor if sitting in a chair (see Figure 2.1). Put the hands together at the center of the chest in prayer pose—the palms are pressed together with 10–15 pounds of pressure between the hands (a mild to medium pressure, nothing too intense). The area where the sides of the thumbs touch rests on the sternum with the thumbs pointing up (along the sternum), and the fingers are together and point up and out with a 60-degree angle to the ground. The eyes are closed and focused at the third eye. A mantra is chanted out loud in a 1½ breath cycle. Inhale first through the nose and chant "Ong Namo" with an equal emphasis on each word. Then immediately follow with a half-breath inhalation through the mouth and chant "Guru Dev Namo" with approximately equal emphasis on each word. (The *o* in Ong and Namo are each a long *o* sound; Dev sounds like *Dave*, with a long *a* sound. The practitioner should focus on the experience of the vibrations these sounds create on the upper palate and throughout the cranium while letting the mind be carried by the sounds into a new and pleasant mental space. This should be repeated a minimum of three times. This technique helps to create a protected meditative state of mind and is always used as a precursor to the other techniques.

Suggested Breathing Patterns

1. The first and most basic pattern is to simply and consciously inhale and exhale through the nose, with a slow and distinguishable breath rate, where it is apparent to the patient that the breathing is being consciously controlled. When it is used with any of the following mantras, the mantra is only chanted on the exhalation phase of the breath cycle. However, remember that the mantra does not have to be added right away. (Note that the inhalation is not taken through the mouth, only through the nose.)

2. The second breath pattern can be a four-part breath cycle through the nose where the inhalation phase of the breath cycle is broken into four equal parts. This is also called a four-part broken breath, where there are four distinct and approximately equal steps for the inhalation phase. After the inhalation phase the breath is exhaled through the nose in a single breath without breaking the exhalation into parts. After the patient learns to comply and match the pattern, the coordinator then continues with the four-part inhalation but then chants one of the mantras on the exhalation phase. It is natural to chant out loud only during the exhalation phase.

3. The third permissible pattern here is the eight-part broken breath, which is similar to the four-part broken breath, except that it includes eight steps (stages/parts) on the inhalation through the nose. The exhalation is again only through the nose in a continuous unbroken slow expiration of the breath, or later when a mantra is chanted out loud.

Suggested Mantras

These mantras must all be chanted out loud. They are listed with increasing complexity, but the practice can include any of the following. The choice here depends on the age, skill, appeal, and willingness of the patient. However, it is obviously much preferred to attempt the simplest mantras first, using either Ma, Ra, Um, Ee, or Oooh. The patient is likely to have a greater affinity to one sound than to the others.

1. Ma should be chanted as one long word on the exhale. The sound means mother, rebirth, resurrection, and renewal. This sound helps to awaken the primary feminine principle and essence of the psyche. This is a good starting place and may have a high appeal.

2. Ra should be chanted as one long word. The sound relates to the primary male principle and essence of the psyche. It is simple and may have a high appeal.

3. Um, Ee, and Oooh are three individual sounds that must be chanted as single long words. They can be chanted individually in a

practice session, or with approximately equal times for all three in the order of Um, Ee, and Oooh. It is also permissible to only chant Um for a few minutes followed by Ee for a few minutes. But the order should not be altered if they are combined with a few minutes for each (Shannahoff-Khalsa & Bhajan, 1988). I recommend starting with Um for a short time. These are simple sounds that are very easy to reproduce and very basic to the psyche, and they may already be sounds that are practiced by some children in their repetitive behaviors. They give a very pleasurable sensation when they are vibrated correctly. Patients may find that they like one of these three sounds better than another. Or they may show no preference. If they have a preference, they should use that sound until they are willing to have fun chanting any of the other two sounds.

4. Sat Nam is a seed or bij mantra, and it is one of the most basic mantras in the system of Kundalini yoga. Sat translates as truth and Nam is the manifestation of that truth. It is a very simple mantra that helps to merge the infinity and finite identities of the practitioner. When it is used in practice here, it is best chanted in the long version, called long Sat Nam, where there is a quick and punchy sound to Sat followed immediately by a long extended Nam. Here it is meant to be chanted completely through in one breath cycle, all chanted on the exhale.

5. Sat Nam Sat Nam Sat Nam Sat Nam Sat Nam Sat Nam Whahay Guru is a powerful healing mantra that helps to awaken and elevate the psyche. Sat Nams is repeated six times, followed by Whahay Guru once. Eventually the practitioner can learn to chant the entire mantra through quickly on one breath cycle or even to chant it through twice on a single breath cycle. Here Sat and Nam are of approximately equal length and there is no extension of the sound Nam or the sounds Whahay or Guru.

6. Sa Ta Na Ma is called the Panj Shabad and is the combination of the five primal sounds of the universe. Sa is the vibration that gives the mind the experience of the Infinite. Ta gives the mind the experience of the totality of life. Na gives the mind the ability to conquer death. And Ma gives the mind the power of rebirth and

resurrection. (The fifth sound is Ah, which is common to all four basic sounds, and this is why it is called the Panj Shabad, where the word Panj means five.) Here the four syllables can be repeated all in one breath with approximately equal emphasis on each sound on the exhale, or it can be practiced where Sa is chanted on the first breath, then Ta on the second breath, Na on the third breath, and Ma on the fourth breath, and the cycle is repeated in exactly the same sequence using all four syllables. This is one of the most powerful and frequently used mantras in Kundalini yoga. While it is not likely that the coordinator and patient would ever reach 11 minutes, this time is technically the longest time that this mantra should ever be chanted out loud as a single mantra, unless specified otherwise with another meditation technique.

7. Whahay Guru is called the Guru Mantra, or the mantra of ecstasy. It is not readily translatable, but chanting it elevates the spirit and gives the practitioner a natural high and the experience of the Infinite in its totality. There is equal emphasis on both words.

8. Whahay Guru, Whahay Guru, Whahay Guru, Whahay Jeeo: The meaning essentially translates to "the ecstasy of consciousness is my beloved." All four segments of the mantra are to be practiced with equal times and emphasis. With extended practice and capacity, it can be repeated through more than once per breath cycle.

9. Hum Dum Har Har. This mantra opens the heart chakra and means, "We the universe, God, God." The sound Dum sounds like the word *dumb*, and Hum rhymes with the sound *dumb*. The four sounds should be chanted with equal times and emphasis, and the entire mantra can be repeated more than once per breath cycle.

10. Ong Namo Guru Dev Namo is the Adi Mantra that precedes any Kundalini yoga practice. This mantra tunes us into our higher self. Ong means, "Infinite creative energy in manifestation and activity." (Om or Aum is God absolute and unmanifested and is not used here.) Namo means "reverent greetings," implying humility; Guru means "teacher or wisdom"; Dev means "divine or of God"; and Namo reaffirms the state of humility and reverence that

242

is experienced when this mantra is mastered. In all it means, "I bow to the infinite creative energy, and I bow to the divine wisdom as it is awakened within me."

11. Ang Sung Whahay Guru means, "Every cell of my body vibrates with the divine wisdom, indescribable happiness that carries me from darkness to light." This mantra eliminates haunting thoughts and gives the experience of the divine within each fiber of the being. Here it should be chanted through in a monotone with equal emphasis on each sound. It can also be chanted through more than once if the lung capacity can support it.

12. Guru Guru Whahay Guru Guru Ram Das Guru—the word *guru* means the technique, teacher, or guide that brings one out from the darkness into the light; the sound Whahay gives the experience of divine ecstasy; the words Ram Das translate as "servant of God," the name of the guru who is the royal yogi and father of the lineage of Kundalini yogi as taught by Yogi Bhajan. This mantra is very healing and it gives a feeling of balance, elevation, guidance, and protection. The earth and ether qualities of human existence come into balance. The first four words relate to the etheric realm and the last four words cover the earthly realm of existence.

13. Ra Ra Ra Ra Ma Ma Ma Ma Rama Rama Rama Rama Sa Ta Na Ma is a healing mantra that helps balance the sun and moon qualities, or left and right brain hemispheres, respectively. This mantra also helps to eliminate the pain from earlier experiences that are left as residues in the psyche and subconscious mind and it is a unique aid in the process of development. While this mantra includes 16 parts, the 16 parts should be chanted with approximately equal emphasis. It can be chanted quickly enough to be completed in one breath cycle.

14. Sa Ray Sa Sa, Sa Ray Sa Sa, Sa Ray Sa Sa, Sa Rung, Har Ray Har Har, Har Ray Har Har, Har Ray Har Har, Har Rung. This is obviously the most complex and most difficult mantra in this group. The meaning is, "That infinite totality is here, everywhere. That creativity of God is here, everywhere." The syllable Sa sounds like *sah* or *saw*; Ray sounds like *ray*; and when Har is chanted the

tongue tip flicks the upper palate to induce the correct impact on the brain. The *r* in Har is a slightly rolled *r*. The power and effect of this mantra can help set a perfect foundation for the developing psyche and ultimately take the practitioner into the realm of the infinite. The whole mantra is meant to be chanted in one breath cycle. However, it can also be chanted halfway through (ending at Sa Rung) on one breath for those with a lesser lung capacity, and completed on the next breath cycle. In a lecture in Los Angeles, on July 3, 1989, Yogi Bhajan said about the effects of this mantra, "It takes away the ugliness of life. It will bring peace to those on whose forehead it is not written. It will bring prosperity to those who do not know how to spell it. It will bring you good luck when you have done nothing good, ever. Because this is the lotus, this is the opening of the lotus and turning the Mother Divine power back to the navel point. It is a path."

Additional and Elementary Brain-Balancing Techniques for the PDD Patient

These simple techniques can be used once the patient is willing to practice Kundalini yoga meditation techniques in addition to the essential core practice using the Dance of the Heart protocol. These techniques will further accelerate the patient's healing. However, they are not essential to recovery. But they can help patients develop the excellence and neurodevelopmental capacity that is their birthright. However, practice with these individual techniques must also include the tuning in technique.

1. A Brain-Balancing Technique for Reducing Silliness, Focusing the Mind, and Controlling the Ego

Sit straight with the arms out to the sides, the hands facing forward, and a 90-degree angle at the forearm and upper arm. The hands open completely and close completely, so that the thumbs are enclosed by the fingers when the hands form a closed fist. Then the hands open again with all of the fingers sticking up straight and the thumbs are out to the sides but not extended stiffly (they are extended loosely), and then alternately the hands close and the thumbs are not enclosed in the fists. But every effort is made to have the fingers extend straight up. This is a rapid opening and closing movement and every effort is made for both hands to open and close together in synchrony where the thumbs are enclosed when the hands close and then the thumbs are closed outside of the fists when the hands close again. This is a rapid alternating of thumbs in and thumbs out as the hands close into fists. When the technique is practiced appropriately, the opening and closing of the hands can occur two to three times per second. The best practice times are from 2 to 5 minutes. The eyes are closed during the exercise and focused at the third eye point.

2. A Brain Exercise to Enhance Communication Skills and Activate the Frontal Lobes

Sit straight and raise the hands to the shoulder level with the hands facing forward and the elbows are by the sides. The first three fingers (index, middle, and ring finger) are kept straight and point up. The thumb tip and the tip of the little finger continuously touch and let go at a very rapid pace at about two to five times per second, the faster the pace the better. The eyes are kept closed. Continue the rapid contact and release of the thumb and little finger for a maximum time of 3 minutes. Effort should be made to move both the thumb and little finger in the movement, not just the thumbs. After 2 minutes the individual can begin to create the desired effect of helping to normalize and balance the frontal lobes, but 3 minutes is ideal. The immediate effects can last up to a maximum of 4 hours. Over time this technique will enhance the development and cooperative nature of the frontal lobes. Once practitioners develop the ability to do this technique, they will begin to excel in their communication skills and gain the confidence and focus of a real leader.

3. For Mental Development and Mental Coordination

Sit straight with the hands facing forward near and at shoulder level with the elbows relaxed by the sides. Use both hands, and follow the sequence of thumb tip touching to the respective fingers: Touch your thumb to (1) the little finger tip, (2) the index finger tip, (3) the tip of the ring finger, (4) the tip of the index finger, (5) the tip of the ring finger again, and (6) the tip of the middle finger. Then repeat the entire cycle 1–6, building up the pace until the cycle takes 2–3 seconds and it becomes a learned exercise that does not require any conscious focus on the pattern. This is when the real benefits are achieved. The eyes are closed once the pattern is learned. Build up the time to 11 minutes with a rapid pace. This is an excellent technique for mental development and mental excellence. There is a similar pattern with a slightly different finger tapping order that also includes additional elements that has been published and is specific for treating dyslexia and the other learning disorders (Shannahoff-Khalsa, 2004, 2006).

4. A Technique for Brain Balancing and Mental Development

Sit with a straight spine and, if seated in a chair, keep both feet flat on the floor. Place the arms straight up and over the head and with the upper arms against the ears. Enclose the thumbs with the fingers, then slowly extend and straighten only the index fingers keeping the other fingers in a fist and then close the index finger down, then extend only the middle fingers and then close the middle fingers down, then extend the ring fingers (usually the most difficult finger) and close ring fingers down, then finally extend only the little fingers. Then start the full cycle again with index, middle, ring, and little, all the time trying to keep the other fingers down in place. The eyes remain closed throughout. Try to build up the pace with a maximum time of 3 minutes.

Advanced Techniques for the Accomplished PDD Patient

1. Meditation to Balance and Synchronize the Cerebral Hemispheres

This technique was first published in the multipart protocol for treating ADHD and comorbid disorders (Shannahoff-Khalsa, 2006).

Sit with a straight spine. The eyes are open and focused on the tip of the nose (the very end, which is not visible to the patient). Both hands are at the shoulder level with palms facing up and forward with the hands loosely open, the fingers are spread wide as if holding a heavy ball in each hand (see Figure 4.1). Chant out loud "Har Har Gur Gur," and with each sound (Har or Gur) rotate the hands to where the palms face toward the back and as if still holding a heavy ball (see Figure 4.2) and then quickly return them to the face forward position. The left palm rotates in the clockwise direction and the right hand rotates in the counterclockwise direction (the only natural direction for rotation of each hand when starting with the palms facing forward). Make sure that the tongue quickly touches (flicks) the upper palate on Har and the lower palate on Gur. Also pump the navel point lightly with each Har or Gur. The rate of chanting for the entire mantra and rotating the hands reaches 2 seconds per round of the mantra. The time for practice is 11 minutes. The effects are that the frontal lobes and other paired regions of the hemispheres are synchronized to bring clarity, peace, vitality, and intuition.

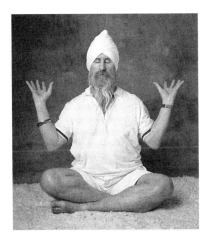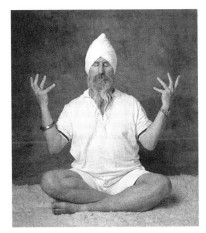

Figures 4.1 and 4.2
Meditation for Balancing and Synchronizing the Cerebral Hemispheres

2. Gan Puttee Kriya: A Technique to Help Eliminate Negativity From the Past, Present, and Future

Sit with a straight spine, either on the floor or in a chair. The backs of your hands are resting on your knees with the palms facing upward. The eyes are nine-tenths closed (one-tenth open, but looking straight ahead into the darkness at the third eye point, not the light below). Chant from your heart in a natural, relaxed manner, or chant in a steady relaxed monotone. Chant out loud the sound "Sa" (the *a* sounds like "ah"), and touch your thumb tips and index finger tips together quickly and simultaneously with about 2 pounds of pressure. Then chant "Ta" and touch the thumb tips to the middle finger tips. Chant "Na" and touch the thumb tips to the ring finger tips. Then chant "Ma" and touch the thumb tips to the little finger tips. Chant "Ra" and touch your thumb tips and index finger tips. Chant "Ma" and touch the thumb tips to the middle finger tips. Chant "Da" and touch the thumb tips to the ring finger tips. Chant "Sa" and touch the thumb tips to the little finger tips. Chant "Sa" and touch your thumb tips and index finger tips. Chant "Say" (sounds like the word *say* with a long *a*) and touch the thumb tips to the middle finger tips. Chant "So" and touch the thumb tips to the ring finger tips. Chant "Hung" and touch the thumb tips to the little finger tips.

Chant at a rate of one sound per second. The thumb tip and finger tips touch with a very light 2 to 3 pounds of pressure with each connection. This helps to consolidate the circuit created by each thumb-finger link. Start with 11 minutes and slowly work up to 31 minutes of practice. To finish, remain in the sitting posture and inhale, holding the breath for 20 to 30 seconds while you shake and move every part of your body with the hands and arms extended over your head. Exhale and repeat this two more times to circulate the energy and to break the pattern of tapping, which affects the brain. Then immediately proceed with focusing the eyes on the tip of the nose (the end you cannot see) and breathe slowly and deeply for 1 minute.

The sounds used in this meditation are each unique, and they have a powerful effect on the mind, both the conscious and subconscious mind. The sound "Sa" gives the mind the ability to expand to the infinite. "Ta" gives the mind the ability to experience the totality of life. "Na" gives the mind the ability to conquer death. "Ma" gives the mind the ability to resurrect. "Ra" gives the mind the ability to expand in radiance (this sound purifies and energizes). "Da" gives the mind the ability to establish security on the earth plane, providing a ground for action. "Say" gives the totality of experience. "So" is the personal sense of identity, and "Hung" is the infinite as a vibrating and real force. Together, "So Hung" means "I am Thou." The unique qualities of this 12-syllable mantra help cleanse and restructure the subconscious mind and help heal the conscious mind to ultimately experience the superconscious mind. Thus, all the blocks that result from an extreme traumatic event are eliminated over time with the practice of Gan Puttee Kriya.

3. Meditation for Balancing the Brain Hemispheres

This meditation will correct and adjust the impulses of the brain hemispheres, and it is a very powerful meditation that will greatly benefit the PDD patient or anyone else. There are no limits on who can benefit from this technique. This technique was originally taught by Yogi Bhajan in Salem, Oregon, May 24, 1984, and this technique has not been published elsewhere to date. Yogi Bhajan said that this technique will "clean out the karma, and create a very sharp mind, and that it will bring health, wealth, and happiness."

Sit with a straight spine, and if sitting in a chair, keep both feet flat on the ground. The forearms are up in front of the chest and parallel to the ground at the heart center level with the elbows pointing out toward the sides and the hands about 4 to 5 inches in front of the chest. The hands do not touch, and the palms are face down. The first movement is touching the respective thumb tips and little finger tips (see Figure 4.3), then they release. Then touch the thumb tips to the ring finger tips, and release. Then touch the thumb tips to the middle finger tips, and release. Then touch the

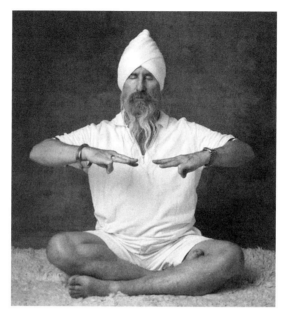

Figure 4.3
Meditation for Balancing the Brain Hemispheres

thumb tips to the index finger tips, and release. The thumb tips and finger tips touch with a light 2–3 pound pressure, not intense. This pressure helps to stimulate a circuit in the brain. The tapping sequence continues at a rate of once per second. Note that the finger tapping pattern is the opposite of Gan Puttee Kriya. With each tap, the mantra "Har" is chanted as a whisper. It is not chanted out loud as is done with Gan Puttee Kriya. When chanting, the mouth is open wide enough so that the upper and lower teeth show, and the lips never touch. The tip of the tongue is flicking the upper palate on the sound Har. The eyes are kept closed and focused at the point where the eyebrows meet with the root of the nose—the third eye point. To end the meditation, inhale deeply and hold the breath for about 15 to 20 seconds, then let it go. A good starting time is 11 minutes. It can also be done twice a day for 11 minutes, first in the morning and then in the evening. The patient can progress to practicing the technique once a day for 31 minutes. Once this level is reached, a significant achievement is to practice it for

40 consecutive days and it will have a powerful and transformative effect. It can also be practiced daily for years and years.

4. A Meditation to Balance the Western Hemisphere of the Brain
With the Base of the Eastern Hemisphere

This meditation balances the left or western hemisphere of the brain with the base of the right or eastern hemisphere of the brain. This technique enables the brain to maintain its equilibrium under stress or the weight of a sudden shock. It also keeps the nerves from being shattered under those circumstances. This technique will also help PDD patients to further recover from their chronic condition. Yogi Bhajan taught this meditation on October 24, 1978, in Los Angeles, California.

The patient sits in a chair with both feet flat on the ground or in easy pose on the floor while maintaining a straight spine. The right upper arm is extended straight out to the right parallel to the ground with the elbow bent and the forearm drawn in toward the body until the hand is in front of the chest near the level of the throat. Extend and join the fingers of the right hand together without allowing them to spread apart, with the palm facing the ground and the fingers pointing to the left. Draw the thumb back and point it at the body. Relax the left arm down with the elbow bent. Draw the left forearm straight up until it is directly in front of the upper arm with the left hand at the same height as the right hand. Extend and join the fingers together. Bend the hand back to a 90-degree angle and face the palm up with the fingers also pointing to the left. Pull the thumb to the rear and point it back in the direction of the body. Do not move an inch once you are in the position (see Figure 4.4). The eyes are open and focused on the tip of the nose, the end you cannot see. This employs the eye posture called Ajna band. Deeply inhale and completely exhale as the mantra is chanted. Upon completion of the meditation, deeply inhale and completely exhale five times. Then deeply inhale and hold the breath while the arms are stretched over the head. Exhale as they are relaxed down. Repeat twice more with the inhalation, hold, and

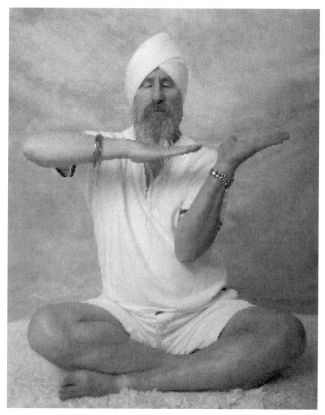

Figure 4.4
A Meditation to Balance the Western Hemisphere of the Brain
With the Base of the Eastern Hemisphere

stretch. The following mantra is chanted out loud in a monotone, repeated three times with one breath as the breath is completely exhaled: "Sat Nam Sat Nam Sat Nam Sat Nam Sat Nam Sat Nam Whahay Guru." There are essentially eight parts to this mantra with equal beats and equal efforts for all eight parts. The words "Sat Nam" are each one part, making six parts all together, and the words "Whahay" and "Guru" also each make one part, totaling eight parts. This meditation is to be practiced for 11 to 33 minutes. Eleven minutes is a great starting time if the patient has the ability. If not, then start with 3 to 5 minutes and slowly build up the time.

5. A Meditation to Balance the Two Brain Hemispheres and to Correct Any Spiritual, Mental, and Physical Imbalance

Yogi Bhajan taught this meditation technique on March 20, 1979, in Los Angeles, California. Yogi Bhajan commented on this technique: "It affects the two brain hemispheres to bring you into balance. Breathing through the mouth stimulates meridian points on a ring around the throat, which affects the parasympathetic nervous system. Breathing in strokes affects the pituitary gland." The patient sits in a chair with both feet flat on the ground or in easy pose on the floor while maintaining a straight spine. The patient raises the arms with the elbows bent until the hands meet at the level of the heart in front of the chest (see Figure 4.5). The fore-

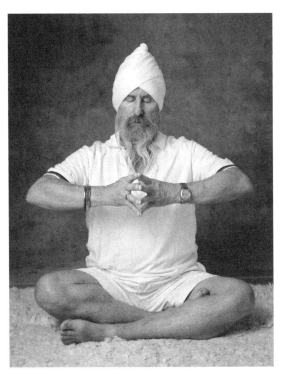

Figure 4.5
Meditation to Balance the Two Brain Hemispheres and to Correct Any Spiritual, Mental, and Physical Imbalance

arms make a straight line parallel to the ground with the fingers kept straight. Press the fingers and thumbs of both hands together from the tip to the first joint. The fingers are spread apart and point away from the body. The thumbs are stretched back and point toward the body. The fingers are bent back at the knuckles, but the base of the fingers do not meet because maximum pressure is applied at the fingertips. The breath pattern is the following: Inhale deeply and completely through the nose, and then exhale in eight strokes through the mouth, and continue this pattern. The eyes remain open and are kept focused on the tip of the nose. The pressure on the fingers is the key to this kriya. Be sure it is maintained correctly and strongly. There is no mantra for this meditation. The patient starts by practicing this technique for only 3 minutes, and then can work up to 5, then 11. Eleven minutes is the maximum recommended time.

6. A Meditation to Correct Language and Communication Disorders: Ad Nad Kriya

Yogi Bhajan taught this meditation on April 23, 1978, in Los Angeles, California. He said, "This Nad, this secret language or technique existed with a very powerful sect of yogis, called Ai Panthis. Now very few of them exist. It will clear your language. Even if you mumble words, if you practice this for a long time, you will be clearly heard by another person. It is called Gupt Gian Shakti, secret power of the knowledge. If you perfect this, you need not speak. You can just send a mental thought, and the other person will totally know about it." Therefore, this meditation technique is useful for people who have problems speaking and communicating on any level.

The patient sits in a chair with both feet flat on the ground or in easy pose on the floor while maintaining a straight spine. The patient relaxes the arms down with the elbows bent and the upper arms are resting against the ribs. The forearms are pulled up and in toward the chest until the hands meet between the levels of the solar plexus and the heart. The fingers are interlocked with the right index finger on top of the left index finger and the thumbs joined side by side and stretched back so that they point straight up (see Figure 4.6). The heels of the hands are also joined. The eyes are kept closed and focused on the third eye point. The patient starts the meditation by taking a deep inhalation and chanting the entire mantra as the breath is completely exhaled. The mantra is the following: "Ra Ra Ra Ra, Ma Ma Ma Ma, Sa Sa Sa Sat, Haree Har Haree Har." Each sound has approximately equal emphasis, time, and effort. The mental focus is on the breath and the sound effects of the mantra. There are no time restrictions on this technique. Starting with 3, 5, or 11 minutes is a great beginning.

Case Histories of Treatment

The following three case histories describe children for whom a family member acted as the coordinator. This is a process that can-

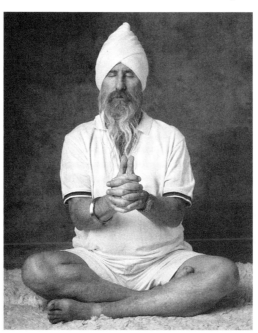

Figure 4.6
Meditation to Correct Language and Communication Disorders:
Ad Nad Kriya

not easily be scheduled like a normal office visit. There usually has to be some spontaneity with the event and a relaxed and receptive child. The more severe the condition, the more need there is for waiting for a spontaneous and appropriate moment, especially with the autistic child. However, Case History 2, a 9-year-old male with Asperger's syndrome, worked best with a fairly rigid schedule. Otherwise, scheduling a child for an office visit would likely be counterproductive and defeat the spirit of the process. Again, a key component of the process is to make this a time for play. This is not a therapy in the more classical sense. Therefore, in the following cases, I trained the individuals who acted as the coordinators. In the first case history, the 18-year-old sister played the role of the coordinator, and in the next two cases, the mothers played this role. Fortunately, all three individuals had prior experience with Kundalini yoga as my students. All three independently asked me if there was a way that Kundalini yoga could help a family member who had either autism or Asperger's disorder. In the following cases, the details and the rate of progress are less well defined compared to most of the other case histories reported in this book. The reason for this is that the coordinators relayed generalities and were less attentive to reporting details.

What will become abundantly clear here is how each of the three cases is really very different, and how each child has to be approached as an individual with his or her own unique qualities and complications. The application here of the Dance of the Heart is an excellent example of how Kundalini yoga meditation is truly both an art and a science, perhaps much more so with the PDD child and adolescent than with any of the other disorders.

Case History 1: An Autistic Male Child, Age 6

William was 6 years old when his sister Whitney requested my help for him. Whitney was an undergraduate at UCSD in 2006 who was taking my Kundalini yoga class and living at home with her family. Whitney had one older brother, Jonathan, age 24. William's conception was not planned and his mother was 44 years of age at the time of conception. William was born 4 weeks prematurely. William's parents are both attorneys with active and stressful careers, and William's mother worked up until near the time of the delivery.

William's development was typical for many autistic children. He failed to smile and showed little facial expression during his first year of life, and he was socially unresponsive with minimal changes for the first 18 months. At this time he began to hum sounds but failed to speak in words. Originally, his mother was concerned that he might be hearing impaired or retarded. At 3 years of age he was diagnosed as autistic. William had rocking movements that were atypical and repetitive. By the time he was 6, he showed some improvement in both his use of words and social interaction. However, he appeared to his parents to be living in a world of his own. He avoided any room where the TV was playing, and much of the music that his sister or his parents listened to. His older brother was not living at home as William grew up. William's closest social bond was with his sister. When Whitney practiced Kundalini yoga at home, William would come into her room and observe. He would sit, usually facing another direction, and occupy himself with one of his toys. He seemed content. Perhaps he was intrigued by her repetitive body movements and chanting, which may have appeared to him to be her way of humming sounds. Whenever she starting playing a CD with a special mantra (*Humee Hum and Peace and Tranquillity*, Kaur, Nirinian), he would appear in a heartbeat. This may have given William some comfort. Perhaps their worlds were now more alike than ever.

After I taught the Dance of the Heart to Whitney, she was optimistic that she could use it as a way to help William. She also thought that at the very least, it might be a good way to help better connect with him. As her brother and as a special needs child, William always had a special place in her heart. I realized that Whitney was an ideal candidate for the role of William's coordinator. Prior to their efforts here, the longest sustained eye-to-eye contact that they would have together was when she would play with him in their swimming pool. William loved the water and Whitney had taught him to swim. Sometimes she would play with him while he was using a float, and this was one of the only events when they would maintain sustained eye contact for any period of time. Whitney quickly learned the protocols and already knew some of the mantras. The ones that she had to learn took only a few minutes. These were the Ma, Ra, Um, Ee, and Oooh mantras. When she told me that he would hum using a sound that was similar to Um, I suggested that she first start by using Um as the mantra.

Whitney invited William to dance with her, and frequently after her yoga practice she would put on music and dance in her room. So one time, she asked him to join her in a dance, but without playing any music. He got up and joined her and she started by pulling him with her as she danced. However, she realized this could not be her usual free-form style of dance that William was used to seeing. She would have to revise her style so that he would be able to hold onto her. She was in the lead, and William seemed to enjoy joining her with interlocked hands. The first time, she decided not to push it, and she played with him only for a few minutes without attempting the later steps. A few days later she went through the same routine. But this time she slowed the dance and tried to get him to notice the simple breath pattern of inhaling and exhaling through the nose. He did not pick it up. However, she then started to chant Um on the exhale. After a few minutes he responded to her invitation to join in, but he used his own "mantra" instead, as the sound was not that much different than Um. She smiled and asked him to try Um. He refused. Perhaps he did not understand why. Apparently, his mantra was working for him. In the following weeks, she continued with her yoga, meditation, and chanting routine and ended by inviting William to join her. They had started to develop a practice together. Finally, William was willing to breathe with her in synchrony. However, he would only sustain it for a minute or two in the beginning. After some weeks Whitney decided to include the Um, Ee, and Oooh sounds for several minutes in her own chanting practice to help give William the insight to using specific but singular sounds. He was soon able to grasp the difference between using his mantra and the Um mantra, and he joined her.

After about 2 months he was able to sustain the dance, the breathing (simple inhalation and exhalation), the chanting of Um, and the eye contact for about 5 minutes. She then decided to spend 2 minutes chanting Um, then 2 minutes chanting Ee, and finally 2 minutes chanting Oooh. After 2 more weeks he was fully engaged with her and maintaining a stable eye contact and breathing pattern. They also ended the practice with a moment of loving silence and standing still looking eye into eye. They would finish by hugging. Rarely was William willing to hug anyone. Now he seemed to enjoy the opportunity with Whitney, and he started to communicate more openly and closely with her. He started making progress with longer and more meaningful communications with his mother. She was working 2 days a week and trying to spend more time with William now that he was more willing and able to communicate with her. He was even willing to hug his parents. Whitney continued her Dance of the Heart sessions with William two to three times per week. She also started using different mantras. After Um, Ee, and Oooh, she tried Whahay Guru, and on some days she would use Hum Dum Har Har. He liked both mantras, and he now seemed open and able to use more complex practices. After several more weeks of both mantras, she progressed to the four-part inhalation and one-part exhalation with the chants. William enjoyed each practice and the variety. Sometimes he would ask her if they could practice one or the other. They now had considerable practice with the triplet (Um, Ee, and Oooh) and Whahay Guru and Hum Dum Har Har. After another 2 weeks they progressed to more complex mantras (Whahay Guru, Whahay Guru, Whahay Guru, Whahay Jeeo, and Aung Sung Whahay Guru), and he began to develop a preference for the breathing pattern. He now chose to use the four-part breath pattern, and he asked if they could now only continue with it instead of the single inhalation and exhalation.

William's bond with his sister grew, and he seemed to be mak-

ing his way out of his old world. He also started to be more responsive to his parents, and on occasion he would initiate a conversation with them, even if it was only about minor things. He was
beginning to emerge from his world. He even started to show progress in his school curriculum, and his special education teachers
noticed the improvement. After another 3 months of practice with
his sister two to three times per week, he was showing marked
changes, and his parents and neighbors commented on how much
he seemed to fit in with the other children in the neighborhood.
After 8 months of doing the Dance of the Heart, William asked
Whitney if he could join her with some of her regular yoga and
meditation practices. She was delighted. He had thought of it, and
he had taken the initiative to ask her. Their play was beginning to
take on a whole new level of practice. She decided that the best
thing to do would be to practice more simple meditation techniques than she had been using and to practice them for relatively
short times. In addition to some of her easier yoga exercise sets, she
decided to teach him the eight-part breathing technique with the
mantra Sa Ta Na Ma (see Chapter 3, technique 8 for the stone in
the 10 Symbol-Related Techniques). She knew that the eight-part
breath was something that he could easily comprehend since he
had already learned the four-part inhale and one-part exhale pattern. She had also learned that technique from me in an earlier
yoga class. She also decided to teach him the first two techniques
in the Additional and Elementary Brain-Balancing Techniques for
the PDD Patient, A Brain-Balancing Technique for Reducing Silliness, Focusing the Mind, and Controlling the Ego, and A Brain Exercise to Enhance Communication Skills and Activate the Frontal
Lobes.

By the time William was 8 years old, he was in many ways a
normal healthy child. His progress at school was continuing to accelerate and he appeared to have near normal social skills, although
he remains a shy child. To date, William is the child that started
with the greatest deficit and made the greatest progress. He has
had the most ideal circumstances for making progress—the rela-

tionship that he now enjoys more than ever with his loving, attentive, and devoted sister. Whitney has chosen to make psychology her major, and she hopes to attend graduate school in clinical psychology. While William still attends special education classes, he has amazed his teachers and his parents.

Case History 2: A Male Child, Age 9, With Asperger's Syndrome

Andy had one sibling, a sister 4 years older. The family lived in an upscale beach neighborhood, and the father was a pioneer in the communications technology industry. Andy's mother, Barbara, had a career in academia. Barbara stayed home for the first 3 months after her daughter's birth, and she had the same plans for Andy after his birth. When she returned to work, she had a nanny attend his needs during her working hours, as she had with her daughter. However, after 2 years, Barbara returned home to help manage Andy's needs. From an early age, Andy was an exceptionally particular eater. He refused most foods, and found cereal, pizza, and coca cola to be his diet of choice. At age 6, Andy was diagnosed with ADHD and was prescribed methylphenidate in an attempt to help manage his reckless and seemingly callous behavior with people at school and with his sister and parents. However, the methylphenidate did not help him improve his behavior, sensitivity, or relationships to others, and his parents noticed that he started having sleep problems. While on the medication his diet also became even more rigid. At this point, the psychiatrist changed the diagnosis to Asperger's syndrome and the medication was stopped because of the side effects and the apparent lack of benefits.

Andy had many classic symptoms of a young child with Asperger's syndrome. He was socially inept, insensitive to others around him, often unwilling to communicate with others, and when he did he failed to make eye contact. When he started a conversation, it was frequently only about himself, often at inappropriate times, and unidirectional. He was a loner and mostly entertained himself. When other children came over, he showed little interest, and when he did, it was for very short periods of time. Soon, other children no longer showed interest in playing with Andy. He showed no interest in his sister and never asked to go out and play with other children in the neighborhood. Andy had several obsessions. His earliest obsession was with his mechanical toys. He started to take them apart, and he tried to figure out how they worked. He had little interest in toys that were not mechanical. He also spent endless hours playing with his building blocks, and he built elaborate structures. His latest obsession was with his computer. He often played computer games for hours at a time. He was above average intelligence in most cognitive areas. To his mother and other family members, he lived with them, but in a world apart. Andy attended special education classes. His parents and teachers made every attempt to help him develop the sensitivity to others and the social graces that he had been lacking. He was performing adequately academically in school, but he also had the social graces of a young male child with Asperger's syndrome.

Barbara starting taking Kundalini yoga classes from me in early 2008 to help better cope with her own stress and anxiety. Although she was an attentive mother, and she loved Andy dearly, she also felt like she often lived too close to the edge of life and that this was starting to impact her other relationships, including the relationships with her husband and daughter. Barbara also wanted to develop a greater capacity to cope with Andy without becoming frustrated, disappointed, and distant. After several months of doing Kundalini yoga in class, Barbara started to develop her own practice at home. Fortunately, Andy had a strong interest in learning how things worked. Andy had noticed his mother's practice, and the structure and sequence of the different activities caught his attention. She practiced several different breathing exercises that all had unique patterns, and she chanted different mantras for long periods of time. Andy became curious about her new practice. He asked her about what she was doing, and he wanted to know how it worked. While she failed to provide him with an adequate answer to how it worked, she did manage to capture his interest, perhaps because the techniques had many different parts, which seemed to be Andy's key interest. He did not question if they worked. He only wanted to how they worked.

After some weeks, Barbara suggested to Andy that he try some of the techniques. She had already learned the Dance of the Heart protocol from me in the interim, hoping for an opportunity to use it with Andy. She asked for suggestions on how to start, and I told her that I did not have a boilerplate solution for her, but that she would have to find a way on her own. Andy was not physically well coordinated, and Barbara thought that this was the angle that she could use to help entice him to make the experience easier for him and where they could engage in the dance protocol. She said, "Let me hold your hands. I want to help you learn to practice these techniques, and we have to start by doing them together." She told him in advance what they would try to do, and this gave him the apparent satisfaction that he needed to become an experimentalist. Andy quickly understood the mechanical elements in the protocol, and he was eager to give it a try. The first time that he did a very simplified version of the protocol, his only difficulty was in holding the eye gaze. He was more focused on the breath patterns and learning to do the mantras correctly. He seemed to resonate with the various sounds. He was obsessed with doing things correctly so he could understand how they worked. In time, it was clear that the more detailed the techniques, the more interest he had and the more he enjoyed the practice. He was fixated on the specifics of the techniques, and he was determined to know how they worked. He told his mother that maybe he could know by observing what effects they would have on him. He was captivated by the details and fascinated by the process.

Barbara had a new partner for her yoga sessions. She practiced at home three times a week and timed it to match Andy's arrival after school. Andy had a new obsession and Barbara was absolutely thrilled. She finally started to develop the bond with Andy that she had always wanted. After about 10 sessions, he had learned to do the dance perfectly. He had a talent for following procedures exactly according to the instructions. After a month, Barbara felt like he was no longer only doing the practice automatically. After 3 more months, they had worked through all 14 mantras and had tried all 3 breath patterns with most of the mantras. Both Barbara and Andy soon found that he was becoming slowly altered by the practice. He now saw that he could focus more clearly on the details of his toys and that he could achieve higher scores with his computer games. He also soon noticed that he could see more around him, and that he felt larger, and that his mind would sometimes slow down. His behavior with others began to change. He was beginning to develop the ability to be receptive and show limited interest in other people. He even started listening to his sister and holding normal conversations, for a 9-year-old male.

After 4 months of practice, Barbara also started to teach Andy different meditations from the list of Additional and Elementary Brain-Balancing Techniques for the PDD Patient after they practiced the dance. Andy wanted to try all of them. First they went through techniques 1 through 4 in sequence, and then Andy started to choose. He wanted to compare them. At first he could only do them for a minute or two, but after several more weeks, he was able to do techniques 2 and 4 for full times, technique 1 for half time, and near maximum time on technique 3. He was definitely intrigued by these techniques. After several more months of practice, he decided he was ready to try some of the more advanced techniques. He was especially intrigued by Gan Puttee Kriya because of its structure. By this time Andy was showing much more normal behavior and sometimes his comments and receptivity amazed his family members and his teachers. He had started interacting normally with the children in his neighborhood and he became a star pupil in class. After that school year was completed, they hoped to enroll Andy in a mainstream education class. A year of at-home play therapy made a major difference in Andy's life and his family's. Andy was unique in that he did not conceive of the dance as play or therapy. For him it was a mechanical process that he wanted to investigate, but he also clearly appeared to enjoy the warmth of the connection that developed with his mother. He even started calling her "Mother." Previously, he had neither called her Mother or Barbara.

Case History 3: An Autistic Male Child, Age 8

Brandon was a first child, and at the age of 34 months he was officially diagnosed with autism. His mother, Merriam (age 38), had an older brother who had a severe case of autism, and she was all too familiar with the classic symptoms. Merriam's brother was eventually institutionalized in a special facility at the age of 15 when his family could no longer care for his needs. Merriam's parents attempted medication and special therapy for him, but he proved too difficult to manage at home. He was also diabetic, and he had self-destructive behaviors of biting himself and banging his head. Merriam had nearly panicked after noticing Brandon's earliest signs. She had fears that Brandon would follow in her brother's footsteps and also require institutionalization. However, while her early suspicions of autism were later confirmed, she also found that Brandon was easier to manage compared to her brother. Merriam became fiercely devoted to Brandon's needs. While she had been reasonably well informed about the approaches to treatment in the earlier years, she started reading whatever she could find to help bridge the gap and study any new advances in treatment. She was acutely aware of what her brother had gone through in his early years at home, with polypharmacy from a young age, and that now he could be managed only by high doses of an antipsychotic, antidepressant, antiepileptic, and a hypnotic for sleep. Her brother also now had other medical needs. He had diabetes and epilepsy. The years of difficulty and torment for her brother and her parents turned out to be an excellent preparation for her current responsibilities.

Instead of engaging in a pharmaceutical approach with Brandon, she decided to try everything else that might help him first. When he was 4, she looked into dietary care and took him to herbalists and acupuncturists. She found that Brandon was lactose intolerant and highly sensitive to wheat. She immediately put him on a gluten-free nondairy diet and he seemed to improve a great deal. His constant mucous problems quickly disappeared and he no longer appeared to have abdominal pains and discomfort. He cried much less often, and she also found that it was much easier to get him to eat. However, he was still clearly autistic. She started massage therapy using special aromatherapy oils, and she also started using the Bach Flower Rescue Remedy for his emotional needs. She experimented with music to see what might help him relax and where he would be more responsive. Merriam's husband was a physician, and fortunately his income afforded her the luxury of time and financial means so that she could devote herself entirely to Brandon's care. She also knew that the earlier she could help him, the more likely that he would make progress. She employed a teacher with special education training to come into their home in an attempt to home school him. She also took Brandon to the beach and the park every day to help him enjoy nature as much as possible and to help develop his tactile and agility skills by playing in the sand and the water.

In early 2007, she ran into me on the beach in Del Mar just after purchasing my first book on Kundalini yoga. After getting the book, she realized that she had often crossed my path on the beach. This time, she introduced herself and Brandon and asked me if there were any techniques for helping autistic children. Brandon also showed a strong interest in my golden retriever, Bubba, and she said he always showed a lot of affection to animals. I told Merriam about the Dance of the Heart protocol and she said that she wanted to learn it because she had heard that Kundalini yoga was a powerful therapy, but that she did not know if it could be practiced by autistic children, and especially at such a young age. We met on three occasions over the next 2 weeks. She was new to Kundalini yoga, and she also wanted to learn techniques that she had seen in the book so that she could better manage her own stress levels. She knew that her ability to relax was not her strong suit.

When she started meditating at home, she noticed that Brandon was more peaceful and that her practice seemed to have a calming effect on him too. He also showed more interest in her during her practice. Brandon spoke, but he had limited vocabulary. She decided to practice her meditation routine and then follow by giving him his massage. After his massage, he was always the most peaceful and receptive. She invited him to play with her, with the intention to teach him the Dance of the Heart. At first he did not respond, and as usual he appeared to be in his own world. She knew she would have to be patient if he was going to join her by choice. She began to practice her meditation routine and follow with his massage three times a week. Each time, she invited Brandon to play and dance with her. On the fourth invitation, he showed more receptivity and without explaining the details of what they were going to do, she simply extended her hands to him in an effort to reach out to him. While the ideal approach is to get the child to lean forward, with the will and intention to reach out to the coordinator, she realized this might not happen soon. So she amended the protocol and interlocked her hands with Brandon's. She began to slowly pull him around the room and their arms moved in a slow artistic dance. She then began to chant while looking him in the eyes. While he wondered what she was doing, he did not seem to be averse to this new game. At the age of 8, he was mostly hesitant to do anything new and change his routine, which is a classic symptom for the autistic child. However, occasionally he was also inquisitive and more open. These events were few, but at least they did occur. Fortunately, he was not intellectually judgmental or skeptical, as is often the case with adults. His autism was mild to moderate, not severe. While he mostly appeared to live in another world, it was one that appeared to have portals to the world around him. He had no siblings and he was clearly the center of the universe for Merriam and her husband. However, his father played little role in his life because of his long working hours as a surgeon.

Merriam would always practice a mantra by herself that she

had planned to use with him during the dance. She started with the mantra Ma. On occasion Brandon would call her Ma. Therefore, she thought this mantra might be a good link to him. After a few more times with the playful dance, she made the effort to use a simple inhalation and exhalation pattern before starting the chanting, in following with the preferred approach. She would stand still with him, look into his eyes, and request that he do the same, and she began to use the simple breath pattern. He was aware that she added the new breathing component to the dance, and when she asked him to join her, he was willing. However, it never seemed to last long. He might go for 2 minutes and then quit. So she decided to add the Ma chant to the breathing pattern on the exhalation, and he seemed to join her for longer periods. Now his challenge seemed to be more about holding the eye contact. After about 6 weeks, he could last about 6 minutes with her, and he was also willing to stand still at the end and stare into her eyes and enjoy her smile. He was also appearing to open up more to her, and he was willing to hug her back at the end. For Merriam, this seemed like a new beginning for them. While she always believed that he loved her too, she now had more reason and hope that in time she could have a more normal relationship with him, one where he could have a future. There are always stages or events in therapy that can give one hope for a better future. And the hugs and lasting eye contact and smiles gave her every reason to hope.

Merriam and Brandon continued their dance play, and he seemed more open and interested in the variations that she would occasionally make with the routine. While he enjoyed the routine and knowing what to expect, he also seemed to be progressing with the therapy and experiencing some overall benefits. In time, they progressed to the Ra, Um, Ee, and Oooh mantras, and eventually to the four-part inhalation and one-part exhalation with the mantras. Brandon slowly started to show changes in his behavior with less agitation, and his language skills also started to improve. He also showed more openness to his father when his father was around. When at the park, he also showed some interests in interacting with others. Brandon was starting to come out of his shell and join the world around him. While his language skills were not par for his age, he showed a marked improvement over the previous 6 months, and Merriam had every intention of increasing both his and her Kundalini yoga practice. She was looking forward to the times when the dance could be replaced by a regular meditation practice. Brandon was always insistent on watching her during her practice, and then on following up with their joint practice. After some months he seemed to forget that there was a massage in between her practice and the dance with him. And at this point the massage became less important to him and he was more intent on joining his mother with their dance.

FIVE

Treating Multimorbidity in Psychiatric Disorders

There are three areas where the subconscious can lock your mind and you will not be aware of it. You can be interlocked in your insecurity, your incompetence, or your projection of your personal reality.

Yogi Bhajan, date unknown

The subconscious was not given to you to collect garbage and make you afraid, and go through dramas, and traumas and tantrums. It was given to you to record in you the proofs of life, so that you can live provingly and approvingly.

Yogi Bhajan, date unknown

If you do not have the power to elevate others, you have absolutely no power.

Yogi Bhajan, date unknown

Multiple Morbidities: Principles and Hierarchy in Treating Complex Patients

This chapter briefly addresses the general topic of the broad spectrum of multimorbidities and presents a partial landscape for the problems and consequences in comorbid psychiatric patients and how they may be best approached using Kundalini yoga meditation. This chapter is not limited to the psychoses, personality, and pervasive developmental disorders (PDD). The reason for this is that most psychiatric patients present with the complex problems that result from comorbidities, regardless of their primary diagnoses, and the three disorder categories in this book are often comorbid with the other common psychiatric disorders.

When we look at the evolutionary process of defining discrete psychiatric disorders, it turns out that the number of bona fide psychiatric disorders according to the *DSM* system of diagnosis and categorization has increased from 106 in the first edition (*DSM-I*) to 292 in the third edition (*DSM-III-R*), and to about 400 in the current edition (*DSM-IV-TR*). This large increase in the number of the diagnosable disorders is partly due to the newer *DSM* subtypings within the major categories, and this one reason contributes to diagnoses of multiple disorders. However, it is also well known that "both clinical and community samples have consistently shown that the frequency of subjects with comorbidity is more common than that of single disorders" (Angst et al., 2002). Both clinical studies and epidemiological studies have consistently shown high rates of comorbidity in anxiety and mood disorder patients (Kessler et al., 1994, 1996, 1997; Kessler, Stein, & Berglund, 1998; Regier, Rae, Narrow, Kaelber, & Schatzberg, 1998). More than 50% of primary anxiety disorder patients have at least one additional anxiety or mood disorder (Brown & Barlow, 1992; Goisman, Goldenberg, Vasile, & Keller, 1995; Sanderson, DiNardo, Rapee, & Barlow, 1990). It is also true that rates of comorbidity for certain primary anxiety disorder patients can be even higher (Brawman-Mintzer et al., 1993; Massion, Warshaw, & Keller, 1993). A study by Brawman-Mintzer and colleagues (1993) looked at a population of 109 adults (61 women, 48 men, mean age = 43 years) with primary generalized anxiety disorder, where the researchers first excluded patients who also had a concurrent major depressive episode. In this preselected population, they found that only 26% of their patients had no additional current or lifetime psychiatric diagnosis. They also stated that their results "support the findings of previous studies of high rates (range 45%–91%) of comorbid psychiatric diagnoses in the generalized anxiety disorder population." Therefore, they found a lifetime 74% occurrence rate for another Axis I diagnosis, other than depression, with this generalized anxiety disorder population. A 2002 study from the general community in Zurich, Switzerland, with 591 young adults, found that the average number of lifetime disorders was 2.1 with a range of 0 to 7 (Angst et al., 2002).

With schizophrenia, there has been a long-held interest in "an etiologic overlap between schizophrenia, schizoaffective disorder, and bipolar disorder" (Laursen, Agerbo, & Pedersen, 2009). This overlap was studied over a 35-year period with a Danish population of more than 2.5 million people. Subjects in this study were followed from 1970 to 2006. These researchers also introduced a new index of comorbidity for measuring the magnitude of the overlap between these three disorders. They assessed 12,734 schizophrenic patients, 4,205 bipolar disorder patients, and 1,881 schizoaffective disorder patients. They found that "a female bipolar patient's risk of also being admitted with a schizoaffective disorder by the age of 45 years was approximately 103 times higher than that of a woman at the same age in the general population. Thus, we defined the comorbidity index between schizoaffective disorder and bipolar disorder at age 45 years to be 103. At age 45 years, the index between schizophrenia and schizoaffective disorder was 80, and between schizophrenia and bipolar disorder the index was 20. Similar large comorbidity indexes were found for men" (Laursen et al., 2009). They concluded, "A large comorbidity index between schizophrenia and schizoaffective disorder was found, as well as a large index between bipolar disorder and schizoaffective disorder. But, more surprisingly, it was clear that a substantial comorbidity index between bipolar disorder and schizophrenia was present. This study supports the existence of an overlap between bipolar disorder and schizophrenia and thus challenges the strict categorical approach used in both *DSM-IV* and ICD-10 classification systems." Regardless of the etiological origins of this overlap, it is clear that there is a relatively high psychiatric comorbity among schizophrenia, schizoaffective disorder, and bipolar disorder that exceeds the occurrence rate in the general population. These comorbidities clearly lead to difficulties and complications when treating these patients.

An assessment of psychiatric comorbidities with schizophrenia has been published (Buckley et al., 2009). The authors stated, "Substance abuse comorbidity predominates. Anxiety and depressive symptoms are also very common throughout the course of illness, with an estimated prevalence of 15% for panic disorder, 29% for posttraumatic stress disorder, and 23% for obsessive-compulsive disorder. It is estimated that comorbid depression occurs in 50% of patients, and perhaps (conservatively) 47% of patients also have a lifetime diagnosis of comorbid substance abuse" (Buckley et al., 2009). This article also gives a very thorough and detailed review and summary of the extensive psychiatric comorbidities in the schizophrenic patient population for those interested in more specific details. They commented on the unique complexity of this patient population: "The clinical heterogeneity of schizophrenia is indisputable. Virtually no 2 patients present with the same constellation of symptoms. Moreover, even in the same patient, symptoms can show dramatic change over time, and there is significant interplay between different sets of symptoms: e.g., 'secondary' negative symptoms might be ameliorated with resolution of positive symptoms, while core 'deficit' negative symptoms are more enduring but can worsen over the longitudinal course of illness." They further added to the complexity of this picture by describing examples of how comorbidities can further complicate the patient's condition: "Depression can cause secondary negative symptoms, panic attacks can drive paranoia, and cannabis abuse can worsen positive and disorganization symptoms. Conversely, depressive symptoms seen in the context of a florid psychotic relapse often resolve with treatment of the positive symptoms but may re-emerge in the 'postpsychotic' state and in turn worsen the longitudinal course of the illness." The authors also provided some very important insights into the problems of multimorbidities in this population: "These observations may contribute in part to the high rates of polypharmacy that are observed in the treatment of schizophrenia. At present, the therapeutic implications of this clinical heterogeneity are poorly understood and are largely manifested in 'trial and error' treatment choices. The most parsimonious conclusion at the present time is that these comorbidities are certainly more common than chance in schizophrenia, but their etiopathological significance and treatment implications thereupon are poorly understood at the present time."

Volkow (2009) reported on the substance use disorder (SUD) rates in the schizophrenic population based on a range of published studies and compared these rates to the general adult population that were derived from the 2007 National Survey on Drug Use and Health (SAMSA, 2008). The rates for the schizophrenic population versus the general population are the following: nicotine, 60–90% versus 25.9%; cannabis, 17–80.3% versus 5.8–16.4%; alcohol, 21–86% versus 2.9–17.9%; and cocaine, 23% versus 0.7–1.7% (Volkow, 2009). Volkow stated,

> In summary, addressing comorbidity of SUD in schizophrenia has important clinical implications for both the prevention and treatment of these 2 disorders and also for decreasing morbidity and mortality. Moreover, research shows that treatment of patients with comorbidity should include interventions for both disorders because lack of adequate treatment of one of the disorders interferes with recovery (Goldsmith & Garlapati, 2004). These reasons highlight the urgency of addressing the need for integrated treatment interventions for SUD in patients with schizophrenia and for training psychiatrists in the proper screening and treatment of SUD in patients with schizophrenia and other mental illnesses.

There has been a long-standing interest in the relationship of the schizophrenic and other psychotic patients to the potential for violence. The belief has been that the schizophrenic poses an increased risk of committing violent crime, four to six times the level of the general population of individuals without psychoses (Fazel, Langstrom, Hjern, Grann, & Lichtenstein, 2009). However, a recent meta-analysis of 20 individual studies that included 18,423 individuals with schizophrenia and other psychoses compared against 1,714,904 individuals from the general population showed somewhat different results (Fazel, Gulati, Linsell, Geddes, & Grann, 2009). The meta-analysis was conducted on 20 studies published from 1970 to February 2009 that reported on the risk of interpersonal violence or violent criminality. A key factor in their analysis was also the influence of substance abuse on the effects of crime. These researchers found that the "risk estimates of violence in individuals with substance abuse (but without psychosis) were similar to those in individuals with psychosis with substance abuse comorbidity, and higher than all studies with psychosis irrespective of comorbidity" (Fazel, Gulati, et al., 2009). They also found that the association between violence and substance abuse in the psychotic patient population was even stronger in women and that the risk for homicide was almost 20 times greater in the psychotic population (with and without comorbid substance abuse) compared with the general population. In general, they concluded, "Schizophrenia and other psychoses are associated with violence and violent offending, particularly homicide. However, most of the excess risk appears to be mediated by substance abuse comorbidity. The risk in these patients with comorbidity is similar to that for substance abuse without psychosis. Public health strategies for violence reduction could consider focusing on the primary and secondary prevention of substance abuse" (Fazel, Gulati, et al., 2009). Again, it is clear that there is an imperative to attempt treatment using an integrated approach to care. Treating the SUD schizophrenic without treating SUD makes very little sense.

This association of SUD, violence, and the schizophrenic patient population suggests that there may be an even greater need to attempt to use Kundalini yoga as a therapy for treating the comorbid SUD schizophrenic population. The protocol for treating the addictive, impulse control, and eating disorders (Shannahoff-Khalsa, 2006) would be a most useful adjunctive protocol when treating this comorbid population.

Given the complex nature of many psychiatric disorders, there is also a very serious potential for misdiagnosing the patient due to common features. For example, PDD and infantile schizophrenia were initially thought to be the same disorder. Both share some common features including perceptual abnormalities, thought disorder, catatonia, and deficiencies in reality testing. It was only after much research that distinct differences were described (Starling & Dossetor, 2009). In addition, the process of arriving at a complete and accurate diagnosis is often complicated by how the physician obtains the critical information. Unfortunately, "Most clinicians rely on patients' mention of depression, anxiety, or substance use to identify disorders, without assessing specific criteria" (Alegria et al., 2008). It is unlikely that this error is only specific for depression, anxiety, and substance abuse. These authors also commented, "Differential discussion of symptom areas, depending on patient ethnicity, may lead to differential diagnosis and increased likelihood of diagnostic bias." Given the expediency of care today, we can only imagine how much goes missing with the average diagnostic intake.

Perhaps one of the most important relationships to consider here is the comorbidities of the Axis I and Axis II personality disorders. It has become increasingly clear in more recent decades that many if not most psychiatric disorders start in adolescence and even in early childhood (Crawford et al., 2008; Kim-Cohen et al., 2003; Rutter, Kim-Cohen, & Maughan, 2006). Crawford and colleagues made the point that a worse prognosis and long-term dysfunction are linked to personality disorders, which are now increasingly recognized as clinically significant disturbances in adolescents (Crawford et al., 2008; Kim-Cohen et al., 2003; Rutter et al., 2006). To put the current reality of this problem into the broader clinical picture, Crawford and colleagues made a number of important points here:

Although placement of personality disorders on Axis II was intended to encourage greater attention to their clinical significance, their separation from Axis I disorders may paradoxically cause them to be overlooked at times. Early epidemiological studies, including the Epidemiological Catchment Area Study (Robins & Regier, 1991) and National Comorbidity Survey (Kessler et al., 1994), largely ignored personality disorders, as have most longitudinal epidemiological studies that began in the participants' childhood. Researchers conducting these studies may have ignored personality disorders based on common (but then untested) assumptions that personality disorder symptoms were not stable before late adolescence or early adulthood. Partly for these reasons, diagnostic assessments by structured clinical interviews were developed for personality disorders well after comparable measures existed for Axis I disorders. Current instruments for assessing personality disorders in children or adolescents are limited in number and their coverage of Axis II pathology is often incomplete. (Crawford et al., 2008)

When comparing the comorbid Axis I and Axis II population with patients that were only in Axis I or Axis II groups, the comorbid group had "almost a 9-fold increase in risk of subsequent psychiatric disorders" (Crawford et al., 2008). It is clearly worth restating a quote from Chapter 3 here: "Most psychiatrists ignore axis II pathology" (Gabbard, 2005).

We know that the Axis I and Axis II comorbidity problems, even when not including substance abuse and dependence, increase the problems in a markedly significant way for academic, occupational, interpersonal, and psychiatric functioning. However, when adding the Axis I problems to substance abuse, these problems are only magnified, and there are additional tragic consequences. If we only consider alcohol abuse and dependence, we find substantial increases in car crashes (Chou et al., 2006), domestic violence (Caetano, Nelson, & Cunradi, 2001), fetal alcohol syndrome (Lemoine, Harousseau, Borteyru, & Menuet, 2003), neuropsychological impairment (Bates, Bowden, & Barry, 2002), poor medication adherence (Bazargan-Hejazi, Bazargan, Hardin, & Bing, 2005), and economic costs and lost productivity (Harwood, Fountain, & Livermore, 1998). Hasin, Stinson, Ogburn, and Grant (2007) summarized the results of the National Epidemiologic Survey on Alcohol and Related Conditions: the "Prevalence of lifetime and 12-month alcohol abuse was 17.8% and 4.7%; prevalence of lifetime and 12-month alcohol dependence was 12.5% and 3.8%. Alcohol dependence was significantly more prevalent among men, whites, Native Americans, younger and unmarried adults, and those with lower incomes. Current alcohol abuse was more prevalent among men, whites, and younger and unmarried individuals while lifetime rates were highest among middle-aged Americans." They summarized their pertinent findings on comorbidity: "Comorbidity of alcohol dependence with other substance disorders appears due in part to unique factors underlying etiology for each pair of disorders studied while comorbidity of alcohol dependence with mood, anxiety, and personality disorders appears more attributable to factors shared among these other disorders. Persistent low treatment rates given the availability of effective treatments indicate the need for vigorous education efforts for the public and professionals" (Hasin et al., 2007). The picture is not much different for the substance use and abuse disorders in general. There is a high rate of personality disorders with those seeking treatment for the substance abuse disorders, and there is a strong association of antisocial, borderline, histrionic, and dependent personality disorders. Many of the individuals also had more than one personality disorder (Brady, Verduin, & Tolliver, 2007). However, with all of these comorbid patients, there are significant and increased complications for treatment.

Brady and colleagues concluded their review of the substance use disorder and comorbidity with psychiatric disorders: "Based on what we know, substance use disorders should always be specifically addressed in the treatment of all psychiatric disorders, preferably by the same treatment team. Expecting the patient to attend both a psychiatric clinic and a substance abuse clinic is not likely to be effective. This means that all psychiatrists should be trained in the treatment of substance use disorders, because they so commonly occur in the practice of psychiatry" (2007).

Therefore, comorbidities are indeed the more common condition. Unless we learn new ways of treating and preventing these ever increasing and self-perpetuating problems, the more our health care system and society will face an even greater peril than the one we face today. There is one additional age-old aggravating factor that we need to seriously consider here, and that is the role that trauma plays in the development of comorbidities. "Previous research has shown that traumatic life events are associated with a diagnosis of psychosis" (Shevlin, Houston, Dorahy, & Adamson, 2008). There is a high rate of multiple trauma experiences in people with severe mental illness, particularly with regard to interpersonal violence (Mueser et al., 1998). Brady and colleagues (2007) summarized: "The case for a trauma-psychosis link is however consistently supported by research that reports high rates of sexual abuse in childhood, in addition to other traumatic experiences, within psychotic populations (Masters, 1995; Mueser et al., 1998; Ross & Joshi, 1992). Indeed, in 1 study, over half of patients admitted as a result of first-episode psychosis reported incidents of childhood sexual abuse (Greenfield, Strakowski, Tohen, Batson, & Kolbrener, 1994)." It may be that trauma in one form or another, whether it is a singular event or a cascade of events, direct, or by omission, is the primary causal factor in the development of most if not all psychiatric disorders. To clarify this in respect to the personality disorder patient, I believe that the lack of or defective character that exhibits with the personality disorder patient results from the omission of the adequate and proper nurturing that is required in the early stages of development. The end result is that the child and adolescent will suffer from a form of psychological malnutrition during the critical stages of development, which in turn leads to an inadequacy in adulthood where the individual does not fit into society in a healthy and productive way. The latter in itself can be traumatic and then lead to anxiety, depression, poor relationships, and self-destructive behavior.

When using Kundalini yoga meditation protocols and exercise sets to help treat comorbid problems, there is one very basic and important principle: Treat the most severe, painful, and dangerous condition first. I first identify patients' immediate concerns, and this is usually why they have come to see me. They usually tell me what hurts most. In addition to the various disorder-specific protocols presented in this book, the complement to this book (Shannahoff-Khalsa, 2006) includes eight multipart disorder-specific protocols. These multipart protocols include: the 11-part protocol for obsessive-compulsive disorder (OCD); the 6-part protocol for acute stress disorder; the 6-part protocol for major depressive disorders (MDD); a 5-part protocol for bipolar disorders; a 7-part protocol for the addictive, impulse control, and eating disorders; a 9-part protocol for chronic fatigue syndrome (CFS); an 11-part protocol for attention-deficit/hyperactivity disorder (ADHD) and comorbid oppositional-defiant disorder and conduct disorder; and an 8-part protocol for post-traumatic stress disorder (PTSD) (Shannahoff-Khalsa, 2006). These eight protocols plus the five multipart protocols (one for the psychoses, three for the personality disorders, and a multipart protocol for PDD) and meditation substitution options in this book present a wide variety of options for treating patients. However, while there is a well-defined approach and protocol for treating the PDD, there is no further discussion of that population in this chapter. The reason is that the approach for treating autism and the autism spectrum disorders is singular and the initial challenge is simply to connect with the patient and get the patient to first implement the most elementary techniques; later the more advanced techniques can be taught that are also described in that chapter. So comorbidities with PDD are less of a concern at this point. Treating the PDD patient is more about bringing the patient into this world. When that is successful, and the patient continues to progress, comorbidities are less of a concern and are less likely to develop when there is early treatment. In addition, the dance of the heart protocol is also likely to help eliminate and reduce any comorbid conditions. It is also worth noting that there is a seven-part protocol for psycho-oncology patients (Shannahoff-Khalsa, 2005). This protocol is similar to the eight-part PTSD protocol; however, the psycho-oncology-specific protocol adds to the options for treating comorbid patients, especially for cancer patients.

I rarely have patients present who have had extensive therapy and a full diagnostic workup and inform me at the first visit of their multiple morbidities. Instead, they request help for a specific need, for example, OCD or a body dysmorphic disorder, bipolar disorder, CFS, PTSD, schizophrenia, depression, panic attacks, insomnia, or an addictive or substance abuse disorder. So by default, the approach to treatment is to implement therapy for their presenting concern. To them, that is what hurts most. Clearly, none of my patients ever say, "I also have a personality disorder, dependent personality disorder," or "I have borderline personality disorder," and so on. Also, these patients have almost never been diagnosed with personality disorders. So it may be some time before the picture becomes clear enough to start to work directly with them on their personality disorder. However, as an example of priorities, let's take the case of a woman who presents with CFS and also on the first encounter mentions that she was sexually abused by her father between the ages of 3 and 8. Here the primary complaint is the CFS. She is unemployed and does not have the energy to work. The obvious choice is to first focus on treating the CFS. Without fuel in the tank, an attempt at additional therapy is going to have little consequence since she is unlikely to be able to comply effectively with the PTSD protocol. In addition, the abuse issues are more latent and of less immediate concern, unless the patient is suicidal.

However, I had a patient present with OCD and then also mention that he had CFS (see case history 7, Shannahoff-Khalsa, 2006, pp. 86–87). But the reason that this fellow sought treatment was because of his severe OCD. OCD and CFS are a fairly dreadful combination. Here the mental anguish of the OCD in a severe case is nearly completely debilitating, but compliance with the OCD protocol is complicated by the patient's lack of energy. So this patient was taught two protocols in the beginning and both disorders began to improve. In time the patient was free from all comorbidities, except for "neurally mediated hypotension." This 46-year-old male presented not only with OCD and CFS but also social anxiety disorder, seasonal affective depression, and a learning disorder. When a patient first presents, my first question is essentially, "Where do you hurt?" If the patient says, "I am depressed," this is a symptom, but in a way it is really more of a referred pain. Often there is a good reason for the depression that is not always apparent or something that the patient wants to share. Perhaps there was an extensive history of childhood sexual abuse or spousal abuse. However, this may not be a history that the patient is willing to share early in treatment, and the PTSD symptoms are not immediately apparent. This may be because the patient does not recognize the symptoms as PTSD specific, and perhaps because he does not want to tell you about his tendency to dissociate and relive the incidents of trauma. But he does want help for depression. So in this case, the first attempt at treatment is the six-part protocol for MDD. After I work with the patient for some weeks, and he becomes more mentally clear, trusting, and relaxed, he is likely to reveal the relevant history about why he is depressed. At this point, the eight-part protocol for PTSD becomes the more appropriate therapy. It will help alleviate the anxiety, depression, and finally the other core symptoms of the trauma over time.

There is a second principle in therapy here. Help patients achieve substantial symptomatic relief on the first visit for the issue that is their primary concern. It is more important that patients achieve a temporary symptomatic relief on day one for what hurts most than to take a full history and explore more deeply. The patients that present to me have usually had extensive psychotherapy. In time, if patients achieve symptomatic relief for their primary complaints, they are more willing and able to share more deeply if this is relevant. The third principle is to take the most direct and simple approach to therapy at each respective stage of treatment.

It is also worth noting that the treatment of the primary pain or concern will usually lead to substantial relief with a range of other problems. For example, if the patient can work successfully to achieve a much-reduced severity of OCD symptoms, his general anxiety and depression will also be immediately relieved. There is the potential for every Kundalini yoga meditation protocol in my books to lead to quick and substantial relief for many symptoms. The reason is these protocols lead to a greater clarity and stability of mind. This brings about an inner peace and serenity that gives the patient new hope and a reason to continue therapy. Progress here is only based on the patient's direct and immediate experience. So the fourth principle in treatment is to set the "hooks" of experience deeper with each session. This means to take the patient into a state of greater remission with each treatment session. The fifth basic principle is not to expect too much from the patient and not to push the patient too hard. Inspire the patient.

Therefore, we now have a hierarchy and five principles for therapy: (1) treat the most severe, painful, and dangerous condition first; (2) help the patient achieve substantial symptomatic relief on the first visit; (3) take the most direct and simple approach to therapy at each respective stage of treatment; (4) set the hooks of experience more deeply with each new treatment session; and (5) do not push the patient too hard. Now let's consider a few representative and common cases for comorbidity.

Structuring Individual Treatment Plans

First, the case of Ms. E under Complex Case Histories of Treatment is worth reading as an example of a difficult and complex multimorbid disorder patient. Ms. E wrote her own case history, titled "A Complex Case With Severe Hallucinations and Delusions, Bipolar Disorder, and Narcissistic and Borderline Personality Disorders." She has been my most complex and difficult patient to date. Overall, while complex and difficult, she is not a one-of-a-kind patient. There are many Ms. Es in this world. Her treatment evolved over time, and initially her full diagnosis was not provided, in part because she was never correctly diagnosed at baseline. Her comorbidity with narcissistic personality disorder was missing and her psychiatrist later refined his diagnosis from bipolar disorder with psychotic features to bipolar disorder and schizophrenia. While Ms. E was initially hiding much about her condition from me, it would not have been possible from day 1 to prescribe for her a protocol that would eliminate all of her symptoms even if a full and accurate diagnosis was provided. The reason for this is that any single prescription would ultimately involve multiple protocols, and there is no way that she would have complied with what would be an overwhelming treatment plan after only one or two treatment sessions. So prescriptions evolve over time too, especially as the patient makes progress. However, let's consider two hypothetical but common and classic examples of multimorbid patients where the full diagnosis is known at baseline.

Case 1 is a female who suffers from moderate to severe OCD and also has depression, ADHD, bulimia nervosa, PTSD, dependent personality disorder, and self-mutilation. In this case, the bulimia and self-mutilation are secondary conditions that often result from extended trauma that evolves into PTSD. The ADHD is also a likely consequence of the unruly environmental circumstances and traumatic events. The three primary and independent disorders here are OCD, PTSD, and dependent personality disorder. So the initial focus on treatment would be to start with either the OCD-specific protocol (Shannahoff-Khalsa, 2006) or the PTSD-specific protocol (Shannahoff-Khalsa, 2006). The decision is mostly determined by which is the most severe at the time of presentation. If the patient is highly dissociative and the OCD is at only a moderate level, the multipart protocol for PTSD would be a good start. However, if the OCD is severe, then that is the first disorder to treat. While the OCD protocol would also eventually lead to remission for the PTSD, the reverse would not be true. The PTSD protocol will lead to the relief of some OCD symptoms, but it will not cure OCD. Once substantial progress is made with the OCD and PTSD, the attending problems with the personality disorder will also lessen. However, it is possible that the "clawlike" mentality of the dependent personality disorder will complicate the patient's adherence to therapy. These patients do best initially with a regular treatment schedule. The most critical factor here for progress is almost always determined by how much the patient is suffering. With substantial cases of OCD and PTSD, and the secondary symptoms, such patients can often be inspired to go forward with treatment if they receive immediate although only temporary relief in a treatment session. Much is also determined by how much is at stake for these patients. Complications in treatment are often created by cases of polypharmacy, which add additional and often substantial side effects to patients' primary suffering. Their basic health and financial condition also add to the potential of difficulties for a successful outcome. If one is unsure about which protocol to start with, the best choice is the OCD protocol since it also has multiple meditation techniques that help with anxiety and depression. If the self-destructive behavior is severe, then add the Meditation to Balance the Jupiter and Saturn Energies: A Technique Useful for Treating Depression, Focusing the Mind, and Eliminating Self-Destructive Behavior that is in both the MDD and PTSD protocols (Shannahoff-Khalsa, 2006). While there is an OCD-specific breath control meditation technique in the OCD protocol that is difficult to master, in my 17 years of experience, this technique is the only effective meditation technique that can lead to a complete remission of OCD. However, all of the other techniques in that protocol will also give substantial and immediate relief for PTSD patients and probably lead to a complete remission over time. However, the OCD protocol is more difficult to master than the PTSD protocol. But it should also be noted that even a temporary relief for OCD patients will be achieved with less than a complete mastery of the OCD protocol.

The rate of progress here is dependent on many factors. First, how severe are the various conditions? Second, what is the extent of the polypharmacy and drug-related side effects, and ultimately the inherent difficulties in reducing the medications regardless of the severity of the psychiatric disorders. Frequently, these patients are on at least one benzodiazepine, if not more. I have had a patient on as many as three different benzodiazepines, two antidepressants, and one atypical antipsychotic. This is the nightmare patient. The difficulty in treating this kind of patient may be increased by the attending psychiatrist being resistant to the patient lowering or eliminating medications over time, even if he is making progress. The improvement that this patient may make can be interpreted by the psychiatrist as meaning that the medications are working. However, the psychiatrist may forget that either he or the patient sought additional therapy because of the overall suffering that was not being reduced by the medications. Ultimately, the patient is faced with many decisions that are not easy to make.

Case 2 is a male diagnosed with schizophrenia and a schizoid personality disorder. He is disabled, unemployed, and a chronic cannabis abuser. He has managed his life independently for decades because of his family support system, but he has independent living quarters on the family property. He has Veteran Affairs disability support due to his condition, which originated with a mental breakdown in the military. His only reason for seeking treatment is that he is now increasingly haunted by auditory hallucinations. In the past, the voices only occurred intermittently and for much shorter periods of time, and only during his use of cannabis. He is unmedicated, does not use nicotine, and eats responsibly. However, he is a loner in his community. The pressures in his life are minimal and only consist of food shopping. His other basic needs are met, and he has no dreams of a future. His cannabis use is only considered to be at an abusive stage and he does not have a daily habit, but he uses on most days and has for 45 years. However, he has recently observed that its use is now leading to a worsening of the haunting voices. The formula here is simple. Get him started on the multipart protocol in Chapter 2, called A Protocol for Treating the Variants of Schizophrenia, and teach him A Four-Part Miniprotocol for Helping to Terminate Hallucinations that is also described in Chapter 2. This patient will likely only comply with therapy until the disturbing voices in his head come to an end. He may even be willing to permanently end his cannabis use once he realizes that his auditory hallucinations are worsened and probably caused by his extensive drug use. Given the grouping of his multimorbidities, it is not likely he will continue treatment beyond a reduction or elimination of his auditory hallucinations. Many patients are not motivated to go beyond a certain point in therapy. This gentleman is only interested in reducing his immediate suffering, and the voices are his only recognized source of suffering. He has been a loner and independent for decades and has no motivation or impetus to change his lifestyle. He has no responsibilities to others, nor any reason to become more involved in the world. He leads a lonely life of leisure, and he is perfectly adapted to this situation. While he begrudges others their material possessions and family-based lifestyles, he sees no chance of improving his condition or any reason to attempt to change his current living situation. His primary needs are met. He only wants relief from the disturbing voices. The one limitation with Kundalini yoga is that the patient must have a reason and motive to employ it. In my 35 years of experience with this therapeutic modality, I find that about 40% of patients who make an effort to employ it are only interested in titrating their misery to a tolerable level. Maybe 25% to 45% of people want to become completely cured of their condition and are willing to do whatever is necessary to achieve this end. The remainder choose to drop out of groups or individual treatment regardless of their suffering, frequently due to youth, anger, and immaturity.

When patients' motivation is lacking, or they want to progress more rapidly regardless of their diagnosis, there is one formula that can be employed to help expedite their growth and improvement if they are willing to add to the basics of their treatment protocol. This formula is a simple Kundalini yoga exercise set called Nabhi Kriya (see below). This exercise set was first taught by Yogi Bhajan in June 1971 (Bhajan & Khalsa, 1975). Nabhi Kriya works by empowering the third chakra, the personal power center that reflects our basic willpower, drive, stability, and sense of personal happiness. This power center in the martial arts is called the hara center. Without power here everything is difficult, even the ability to get a good night's sleep. Digestion of food is related to the power of this center, and so is the ability to digest and endure the psychological traumas of life. This center gives the positive sense of self: "I can do it all. I can conquer the mountaintops." When the navel point center, or third chakra, is weak, a patient will always have a problem engaging therapy and maintaining any sense of personal happiness or well-being. Nabhi Kriya is good for everyone as an adjunctive and supportive protocol. Ms. E employed it along with the True Glue protocol. This set on a minimal basis helps make life more bearable. Patients who feel empowered will never give in and give up. In the basic practice of yoga, it is probably the most neglected center because the exercises are not always so easy. But without power at the third chakra, there is very little power at any other chakra. The navel point is now our primary umbilical cord to the cosmos. Nabhi Kriya can be used to supplement any of the protocols in this book or *Kundalini Yoga Meditation* (Shannahoff-Khalsa, 2006). Even if it is practiced two or three times a week, a patient will make a much more rapid improvement regardless of the constellation of comorbidities, especially if willpower is an issue, for example, as it is vital to progress in overcoming the substance abuse disorders. To begin a practice with Nabhi Kriya, the patient can start with 3 to 5 minutes on the longer exercises (1, 2, and 4). Exercises 3, 5, and 6 are easy enough to do full times. Once patients achieve the full times on all of the exercises, there is really nothing that will stand in the way of their progress. Those patients will achieve the personal miracles that are sometimes required to achieve remission.

The individual claimed benefits for the different exercises in this set are the following (Bhajan & Khalsa, 1975): (1) is for lower digestive area; (2) is for upper digestion and solar plexus; (3) eliminates gas and relaxes the heart; (4) charges the magnetic field and opens the navel center; (5) sets the hips and lower spine; and (6) is for the entire spine, unleashing spinal fluid and expanding the aura. With some practice, the full times are not that difficult to achieve. This set will help heal many of the lower chakra problems that can manifest as fears (chakra 1), sexual dysfunction (chakra 2), and poor self-esteem, personal weakness, and depression (chakra 3).

Nabhi Kriya: A Basic and Elementary Exercise Set

Technique to Induce a Meditative State: Tuning In

Tuning in is employed here even if Nabhi Kriya is practiced alone and without including any additional meditations or exercise sets. Sit with a straight spine and with the feet flat on the floor if sitting in a chair (see Figure 2.1). Put the hands together at the center of the chest in prayer pose—the palms are pressed together with 10–15 pounds of pressure between the hands (a mild to medium pressure, nothing too intense). The area where the sides of the thumbs touch rests on the sternum with the thumbs pointing up (along the sternum), and the fingers are together and point up and out with a 60-degree angle to the ground. The eyes are closed and focused at the third eye. A mantra is chanted out loud in a 1½ breath cycle. Inhale first through the nose and chant "Ong Namo" with an equal emphasis on each word. Then immediately follow with a half-breath inhalation through the mouth and chant "Guru Dev Namo" with approximately equal emphasis on each word. (The *o* in Ong and Namo are each a long *o* sound; Dev sounds like *Dave*, with a long *a* sound. The practitioner should focus on the experience of the vibrations these sounds create on the upper palate and throughout the cranium while letting the mind be carried by the sounds into a new and pleasant mental space. This should be repeated a minimum of three times. This technique helps to create a protected meditative state of mind and is always used as a precursor to the other techniques.

1. Alternate Leg Lifts

Lie flat on your back and place your arms by your sides with the palms facing down. Inhale as you lift your left leg up to 90 degrees and perpendicular to the ground. Exhale as you lower it. Inhale and raise your right leg up perpendicular to the ground. Exhale and lower the right leg to the ground. Make every effort to keep the leg straight and the knees locked. Continue lifting alternate legs with deep, powerful breathing only through the nose. The maximum time is for 10 minutes. However, it is also possible to start with shorter times, and 3 to 5 minutes is an excellent time for beginners. Then slowly work up to 10 minutes.

2. Lifting Both Legs Together

Without pause after exercise 1, now lift both legs up to 90 degrees while inhaling through the nose and then lower both legs to the floor on the exhale through the nose. Either the arms are stretched straight up from the shoulders perpendicular to the ground with the palms facing each other or, if the patient has a lower back problem, then the preferred and safer method is to place the hands under the buttocks with palms facing the ground to reduce the pressure on the lower spine. Make an effort to keep the small of the back touching the ground during this exercise. The maximum time for this exercise is 5 minutes; however, even 1 to 3 minutes is excellent in the beginning.

3. Resting With the Knees Touching and Pulled Against the Chest

Bend your knees and clasp them to your chest with the arms wrapped around the legs just below the knees. Press the small of your back to the ground. Allow your head to relax flat on the ground with the eyes closed and breathe only through your nose. This rest position is held for a maximum time of 5 minutes. Two to three minutes is also a good time if the patient wants to expedite the practice.

4. Pavan Sodan Kriya

Start by holding the same position as in exercise 3 (see Figure 5.1). Then inhale through the nose and simultaneously open your arms straight out to your sides with the back of the hands touching the floor on the ground perpendicular to the direction of the body (see Figure 5.2) and at the same time extending your legs straight out and up to a 60-degree angle above the ground while keeping the heels together and locking the knees out to help keep the legs straight when they are extended. Remember to move the legs up and out at the same time that the arms are extended out to the sides. Exhale through the nose and return to the original position (see Figure 5.1). Repeat and continue for 3 to 5 minutes. The maximum time for Pavan Sodan Kriya is 15 minutes. Slowly build the time up to 15 minutes.

5. Raising and Lowering the Legs

While remaining flat on your back, bring your right knee to your chest, hold it there with both hands, and rapidly raise the left leg up to 90 degrees and then lower it to the ground. The breath is inhaled only through the nose when the leg is raised. Then the breath is exhaled only through the nose when the leg is lowered to the ground. Make every effort to keep the left leg straight with the knee locked out. Continue with only raising and lowering the left leg for 1 minute. Then reverse the legs and continue the same exercise for 1 minute but while raising and lowering only the right leg while the left leg is held against the chest. Then switch to raising and lowering only the left leg again for 1 minute. Finally, raise the right leg up and down for the final minute.

6. Standing Arm Stretch

After completing exercise 5, slowly stand up straight. Be careful to allow your blood pressure to equalize as you slowly and cautiously stand up. Once you are standing up, raise the arms straight up along

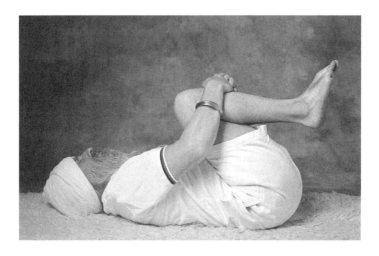

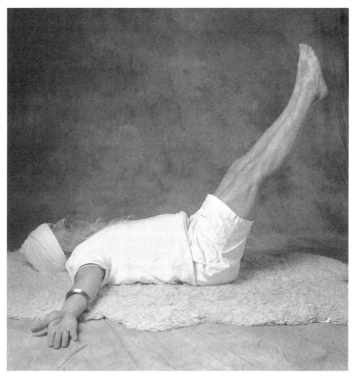

Figures 5.1 and 5.2
Parts A and B of Exercise 4 in Nabhi Kriya

the sides of the head with the upper arms touching the ears if possible. While in this erect position, press your fingers back so that your palms face up to the sky. This is the inhale posture and where the exercise begins. Exhale slowly through the nose as you bend forward at the waist to touch the ground with both hands flat if possible. As you exhale while slowly bending forward, and especially when you are fully forward, apply mulbhand (also called root lock), where the navel point is pulled back toward the spine. This is the down position. While keeping the arms straight and hugging the ears with the upper arms, inhale up slowly with a long deep breath through the nose until you again reach the standing posture. Continue at a slow pace for 2 minutes, then move more rapidly for 1 more minute.

7. Resting Pose

Completely relax flat on your back for 10 to 15 minutes while keeping the arms alongside the body with the palms facing up and the eyes closed. This posture is called corpse pose or shavasana. It is also possible to sit up and to begin a meditation technique without relaxing if desired.

Additional Health Concerns, Complications, and Modes of Alternative Treatment

One of the most serious health concerns for the psychotic, personality, and pervasive developmental disorder patients is the health hazards of the antipsychotic medications that are frequently prescribed, which can and often do induce what is called metabolic syndrome. This syndrome is defined as a cluster of clinical and laboratory abnormalities including abdominal obesity, insulin resistance, hypertension, low levels of high-density lipoprotein cholesterol, and high levels of triglycerides. Patients with metabolic syndrome have a two- to threefold increase in cardiovascular mortality and a twofold increase in all-cause mortality (Lakka et al., 2002). The atypical or second-generation antipsychotic medications are associated with an elevated risk of metabolic syndrome. There is overwhelming evidence linking them to weight gain, hyperglycemia, and lipid abnormalities (Newcomer, 2005). The antipsychotic drug considered most effective for treatment-resistant schizophrenia, called clozapine (Chakos, Lieberman, Hoffman, Bradford, & Sheitman, 2001), also has perhaps the most serious side effects. A meta-analysis of over 81 studies examining weight gain in several typical (first-generation) and atypical (second-generation) antipsychotics showed that clozapine treatment was associated with an average gain of 9.8 pounds over 10 weeks—the most of any antipsychotic drug (Allison et al., 1999). In the same analysis, a placebo over 10 weeks was associated with a mean weight reduction of 0.74 kilograms. "Among conventional agents, mean weight change ranged from a reduction of 0.39 kg with molindone to an increase of 3.19 kg with thioridazine. Among newer antipsychotic agents, mean increases were as follows: clozapine, 4.45 kg; olanzapine, 4.15 kg; sertindole, 2.92 kg; risperidone, 2.10 kg; and ziprasidone, 0.04 kg" (Allison et al., 1999). In addition, more case reports of clozapine-associated glucose abnormalities have been submitted to the Food and Drug Administration (Citrome & Jaffe, 2003) as well as published case reports compared to any other antipsychotic drug (Lamberti et al., 2005). Clozapine is also associated with high triglycerides (Meyer & Koro, 2004), increased levels of total cholesterol (Casey, 2004), and hypertension (Henderson et al., 2004). Another study showed that clozapine was linked to metabolic syndrome in 53.8% of patients compared to an epidemiologically normal comparison group, which had a rate of 20.7% (Lamberti et al., 2006). While clozapine is considered by many to be the most reliable antipsychotic medication, it also apparently has the worst record for metabolic parameters and metabolic syndrome. Other antipsychotics also show considerable and comparable problems, including the dreaded problem of tardive dyskinesia, which often leaves permanent effects. To quote Reynolds (2007) on one aspect of these problems, "Clearly there is much at stake; in 2005, Lilly made a settlement of over US$ 690 million in respect of claims for damages from users of olanzapine who developed diabetes-related conditions, and it is conceivable that there may be further claims against this or other pharmaceutical companies in respect of the metabolic consequences of antipsychotic drug treatment. . . . We must conclude that antipsychotic drug treatment, via effects on weight gain, raises the risk of developing type II diabetes."

The most expensive drug trial ever funded by the National Institute of Mental Health, the Clinical Antipsychotic Trials of Intervention Effectiveness (CATIE) Schizophrenia Trial initially included 1,460 subjects. In this trial the prevalence of metabolic syndrome was 40.9% and 42.7%, depending on two different criteria (McEvoy et al., 2005). Using these two criteria, metabolic syndrome in females occurred at a prevalence rate of 51.6% to 54.2%, compared with 36.0% and 36.6% for males, and 73.4% of all females met the waist circumference criterion compared to 36.6% of males. CATIE males were 138% more likely to have metabolic syndrome than the healthy matched sample, and CATIE females were 251% more likely than controls (McEvoy et al., 2005).

One of the great virtues of the CATIE trial was that it used patients that are typical of the U.S. schizophrenic population. This trial did not use exclusion criteria that would eliminate many patients who are otherwise eliminated in some trials because of comorbidities that are more likely to minimize the best possible results, which is standard practice for a pharmaceutical industry-based trial. However, one of the most disconcerting results of this expensive and well-designed multilevel trial was the relatively high discontinuation rate of patients on these antipsychotic drugs. The patients that quit did so either because of the intolerable side effects or because there was no positive response to treatment. To quote the discontinuation results:

> Overall, 74 percent of patients discontinued the study medication before 18 months (1061 of the 1432 patients who received at least one dose): 64 percent of those assigned to olanzapine, 75 percent

of those assigned to perphenazine, 82 percent of those assigned to quetiapine, 74 percent of those assigned to risperidone, and 79 percent of those assigned to ziprasidone. The time to the discontinuation of treatment for any cause was significantly longer in the olanzapine group than in the quetiapine $(P < 0.001)$ or risperidone $(P = 0.002)$ group, but not in the perphenazine $(P = 0.021)$ or ziprasidone $(P = 0.028)$ group. The times to discontinuation because of intolerable side effects were similar among the groups, but the rates differed $(P = 0.04)$; olanzapine was associated with more discontinuation for weight gain or metabolic effects, and perphenazine was associated with more discontinuation for extrapyramidal effects. (Lieberman et al., 2005)

The authors concluded, "The majority of patients in each group discontinued their assigned treatment owing to inefficacy or intolerable side effects or for other reasons. Olanzapine was the most effective in terms of the rates of discontinuation, and the efficacy of the conventional antipsychotic agent perphenazine appeared similar to that of quetiapine, risperidone, and ziprasidone. Olanzapine was associated with greater weight gain and increases in measures of glucose and lipid metabolism." Given the serious burden of the antipsychotic medications, whether they are first or second generation, and the much increased prevalence for metabolic syndrome, diabetes, and hypertension, there is one very important consideration here. The "consensus panel and other groups underscore the fact that monitoring for the components of metabolic syndrome should be considered the standard of care in the treatment of patients with schizophrenia" (McEvoy et al., 2005). Since a high percentage of psychotic patients are taking these drugs, it becomes imperative to attend to their medical needs in addition to their psychiatric problems. In time, we may find that Kundalini yoga is an important therapeutic modality for helping to reduce the dosages or the need for some patients with less severe conditions, with the schizophrenic, personality, and autistic patient populations.

In addition, there are threats to the general health in these three patient populations that result from the practice of polypharmacy, defined here as two or more psychiatric medications in the same patient. All too often, polypharmacy is a serious problem and one that has been given serious attention (NASMHPD, 2001). Polypharmacy has also been divided into the five following categories that describe the impact and appropriateness of polypharmacy in greater detail (NASMHPD, 2001):

1. Same-class polypharmacy: The use of more than one medication from the same medication class (e.g., two selective serotonin reuptake inhibitors, such as fluoxetine plus paroxetine).
2. Multiclass polypharmacy: The use of full therapeutic doses of more than one medication from different medication classes for the same symptom cluster (e.g., the use of lithium along with an atypical antipsychotic, such as fluoxetine plus olanzapine for treatment of mania).
3. Adjunctive polypharmacy: The use of one medication to treat the side effects or secondary symptoms of another medication from a different medication class (e.g., the use of trazodone along with buproprion for insomnia).
4. Augmentation: The use of one medication at a lower than normal dose along with another medication from a different medication class at its full therapeutic dose, for the same symptom cluster (e.g., the addition of a low dose of haloperidol in a patient with a partial response to risperidone) or the addition of a medication that would not be used alone for the same symptom cluster (e.g., the addition of lithium in a person with major depression who is currently taking an antidepressant).
5. Total polypharmacy: The total count of medications used in a patient, or total drug load. Consideration of total polypharmacy should include prescription medications, over-the-counter medications, alternative medical therapies, and illicit pharmacological agents.

This report also gives five very clear guidelines for treatment that are often violated (NASMHPD, 2001):

1. In general, same-class polypharmacy should not be used to treat the same symptoms in a patient. More than one medication from any of the following medication classes should not be used in a single patient:
   - Typical antipsychotics (e.g., haloperidol, fluphenazine)
   - Selective serotonin reuptake inhibitors (e.g., paroxetine, fluoxetine)
   - Tricyclic antidepressants (e.g., amitryptiline, imipramine)
   - Monoamine oxidase inhibitors (phenelzine, tranylcypromine)
   - Stimulants (methylphenidate, amphetamine)
   - Benzodiazepines (e.g., diazepam, alprazolam)
2. More than two antipsychotic medications, typical or atypical, should not be used simultaneously.
3. The dose of a medication should not be adjusted until the medication serum level has reached steady state and sufficient time to achieve therapeutic effect has passed.
4. Patients should not be discharged from an inpatient facility without allowing adequate time for the effects of the medication to be assessed. Patients on polypharmacy at the time of discharge from a facility are at a higher risk of subsequent medication problems. An increased level of monitoring and support should be considered when the patient is discharged with a complicated medication regimen. This statement should not be construed as support for outpatient commitment.

When patients are comorbid for psychiatric disorders, and a single medication is not adequate to provide symptomatic relief, many physicians resort to polypharmacy in an attempt to minimize the patient's suffering. However, for the most part, this is frequently a roll of the dice, and there can be severe consequences. A recent comment in a book review, "Polypharmacy in Psychiatry" (Ghaemi, 2002), deserves attention: "We are all aware that polypharmacy is a common practice—eminently rational when we engage in it but blatantly irrational in the hands of others" (Jefferson, 2003).

In addition, there are two very special populations that require great caution when multiple drugs are prescribed—children and the elderly. Pharmacological treatment of children with psychiatric disorders is increasing, despite the limited availability of supporting evidence for its effectiveness. A recent policy statement from the American Academy of Child and Adolescent Psychiatry briefly addressed polypharmacy, stating "little data exist to support advantageous efficacy for drug combinations," and "current clinical 'state-of-the-art' supports judicious use of combined medications, keeping such use to clearly justifiable clinical circumstances" (NASMHPD, 2001). This report noted that only five psychiatric drugs (methylphenidate, dextroamphetamine, imipramine, sertraline, and fluvoxamine) are currently approved by the U.S. Food and Drug Administration for use in children. The use of any other psychiatric medication with children is then considered off-label. However, they also noted, "The costs of and obstacles to medication trials in children are great, and continue to limit research in this area" (NASMHPD, 2001). We really do not know the long-term effects of many of these medications and what may result from the practice of polypharmacy.

The elderly patient also faces an increased and serious health risk due to polypharmacy.

> Multiple medical comorbidities in the elderly often lead to the use of multiple medications and treatment by multiple medical providers. . . . Medical comorbidity is common in elderly persons. The symptoms of disease and aging confound and complicate medication treatment. Health care providers are less able to distinguish the actual source of a patient's health problems. Medical comorbidities may render a patient more sensitive to the effects of medications and increase the likelihood of polypharmacy. The treatment of multiple medical conditions often requires multiple medications. In elderly patients, the use of polypharmacy is the rule rather than the exception. Elderly persons currently include 13% of the population and consume 33% of the medications in the United States. Elderly patients in the community take an average of six medica-

tions, and elderly patients in nursing homes take an average of nine. (NASMHPD, 2001)

It goes without saying that clinical trials have not been conducted to test the possible side effects of polypharmacy in the elderly. The risks and complications of polypharmacy are far too many to discuss here. However, the widespread practice deserves serious attention from both treating clinicians and those family members or others who play a role in the patient's welfare.

Clinical psychiatry and clinical medicine in general are in their infancy when it comes to clinical trials that compare multiple drugs or multiple modalities of treatment in a well-defined patient population. Little can be said definitively. However, a review of the literature with respect to complementary medical modalities gives us some insight to the potential for harm from these approaches to care. The authors reviewed the side effects of psychotherapy, body-work (without high-energy manipulations), mind-body medicine, body psychotherapy, sexology, clinical holistic medicine, and complementary and alternative medicine (Ventegodt & Merrick, 2009). They looked at reports in the literature from 1950 to 2009 and studies that included data on side effects and negative events. They found that "non-drug medicine did not have significant side effects (NNH [number needed to harm] > 18,000) and the only severe side effect was rare, brief reactive psychosis, a temporary illness with full recovery (NNH > 65,000). Non-drug therapy did not significantly cause re-traumatization, implanted memories, or induction of suicide (NNH > 100,000). The most intensive psychotherapy enhanced with psychotropic (hallucinogenic) drugs had serious, but rare side effects and only for the mentally ill, psychiatric patients: brief reactive psychosis (NNH = 556), suicide attempts (NNH = 833), and suicide (NNH = 2,500)." They concluded, "Non-drug (non-pharmaceutical) medicine seems to be safe even for seriously physically and mentally ill patients and, whenever efficient, therefore recommended as treatment of choice." However, it must be noted that this review only looked at the number of events of side effects, and it does not say anything definitive about the efficacy of these treatment modalities. The discussion of the potential benefits of therapeutic modalities other than Kundalini yoga are beyond the scope of this book. However, the use of Ayurvedic medicine and traditional Chinese medicine as well as other forms of meditation and mind-body therapies merit serious study in the treatment of the psychoses, personality, pervasive developmental, and multimorbid psychiatric disorders. In addition, it would be most valuable to do head-to-head trials comparing meditation techniques from various yogic and meditation lineages and to compare a variety of mind-body therapies with these patients.

A Complex Case History of Treatment

Case History 1: A Complex Case With Severe Hallucinations and Delusions, Bipolar Disorder, and Narcissistic and Borderline Personality Disorders

Ms. E has been my most problematic and complex case. Her condition with both bipolar disorder and schizophrenia were vastly complicated by her initial comorbid narcissistic and borderline personality disorders. She found me in my research office at UCSD and wanted to know about my work on the mind and body relationship. The sign on the door reads, The Research Group for Mind-Body Dynamics. When she entered my office, I initially thought she was a student on campus inquiring about my work. She did not state that she was looking for treatment or a solution to her psychiatric problems. Nor did she mention that she had any mental health problems or concerns. However, it quickly became apparent to me through Ms. E's language and behavior that she was not a balanced personality, and that she was severely troubled. She was the quintessential space cadet, making every effort to engage me in conversation. I distinctly remember telling her at the end of her second uninvited visit in March 2004, "Do not lie to people and do not try to manipulate people." After two visits, it was clear to me that she had talents with both deceit and manipulation. I realized that Ms. E needed help and I suggested that she attend my Kundalini yoga class at UCSD and that this class might also satisfy her inquisitiveness about my work. She took my suggestion and started to attend my yoga classes in the recreation department at UCSD in April 2004. However, I had no idea that she was being treated for schizophrenia and bipolar disorder. After several quarters in my yoga classes, her behavior in class became so erratic, along with intermittent obnoxious visits to my office, that I had to have her banned from the class and the administration was informed not to allow her to enter the building. After several occasions of being picked up by the police on campus and taken to a number of mental health services, she eventually began to see me on a professional basis for her bipolar condition. However, she did not reveal that she was hallucinating, nor did she realize that she had personality disorders. The following is her story in her own words.

I was born in 1977 in a small village in Peru. My mother, father, brother, and I lived in a single-room apartment with a stove as our only heating source, with a communal bathroom. My brother was 8 years older than me. From the beginning I showed signs of a troubled life. I cried often and did not want to play with the other kids, and frequently I would hurt myself by accident. My parents worked on the farms processing coca leaves. In time, our family's income improved due to my father's increased work status. My parents paid an older neighbor lady to look after me, despite the fact that I was clingy and threw temper tantrums when they left for work. When I was 3 or 4 years old my father became abusive to me and my mother. His brutal temperament even today brings me tears. I hated him, but at the same time I idolized him. He and mother fought often, and to me, for no apparent reason.

The first time that I went to school, I barricaded myself in the closet and I cried for hours. After I finished elementary school my parents were separated even though my father's income had improved a great deal. My father's connection with my brother was much closer than mine. My father would give me presents, but he was emotionally distant and rarely spent time with me. My brother had excelled in school, applied to college, and eventually got accepted by a university in the United States. My father gave us financial support to help us move to the United States and my mother found new work. However, once again I found myself in an impoverished setting. But this time, being in a predominantly materialistic culture, I reacted to my underprivileged status with an inner anger. While I loved my mother in Peru, I hated her in Houston, arguing all of the time and striking her on occasion. I became extremely self-conscious, wanting to fit in and wanting to hide the fact that we were poor. I had only a few friends. At times I felt inferior because of my background, and at other times, I thought it was a privilege for others to be my friend.

In 1992, my mother and I moved to San Diego, where my brother was finishing his master's degree at UCSD. My brother and I had been close when we were growing up, and I immediately made myself dependent on him when I saw him again. For my sake, and for my mother's, he did not go on to a PhD program but found work, and he moved in with us. He replaced the hole left by my father, and I enlisted him on my side against my mother as an unwanted tyrant. We often made fun of her because of her broken English. Except for dinner, the three of us seldom spent time together. As the years passed I became more and more eccentric. My preference for the iconoclastic echoed my antagonism as a child, and like a child I continued to throw temper tantrums well into my adolescence. With my parents' eventual divorce, and the awareness that we would never be a family again, I began to fantasize about a life that I would rather be living. I imagined that my father was an intellectual and a university professor in literature. So I studied literature in college.

When I went to the University of California in Los Angeles in 1996, I had no idea how to direct myself in a healthy pursuit of life. Once on my own, I was beginning to find even more manifestations of fantasies to enrich my emotionally deprived life. I made and broke friendships at will. Some peers called me a "user," others commented that I "waste people." Soon, I found myself in the psychedelic rave culture of the Hollywood scene, where we shared nothing but our stories of drug experiences, delusions, and thrills. I had all but lost myself and moved to the periphery of society. It seemed like it was all that I had ever wanted. My brother had "let go" of me after I wrote him a series of postcards about my romantic escapades, saying that I now had my own life. My mother did not know a thing about my drug history until much later, when my illness was made obvious.

With sex I was promiscuous to the extreme, juggling boyfriends with one-night stands. In my junior year I decided to study abroad and pushed my first serious boyfriend away. I had an epiphany of "free love." In my senior year at UCLA, I was swinging back and forth from being an agent of free love to that of asexuality. Eventually, with my last serious boyfriend, my out-of-control sexuality made it impossible to maintain a meaningful relationship. In addition to my lack of social understanding, my academic career also ended at graduation after 2000. While my degree in the humanities did not qualify me for any job besides that at an entry level, I was trying to cheat my way into the IT industry. At the advice of my brother I was fanatically trying to fabricate a résumé using people I knew as references. I used crystal methamphetamine to cram through computer books that I could not understand. In the end, I overcharged several credit cards, and filed for bankruptcy.

I came home to my mother in San Diego and I began to see a psychiatrist together with my mother. I was first diagnosed with depression, and I was prescribed the antidepressant Prozac. As it so happened, after 2 weeks, the Prozac triggered a manic episode after my mother and I made a trip back to Peru to see family. Something had happened to me, and in an instant, everything was changed. I was no longer the self that I knew, but a raging, wild force. I was hospitalized twice in Peru. The doctors were against releasing me because I could not be trusted to manage my life without outbursts. Finally, after some months of not reacting positively to medications, they performed electroconvulsive shock treatments over a 2-month period. I was stabilized and came back to America. My prescription was then 50 mg Topamax, 10 mg Zyprexa, and 600 mg lithium per day. This amount I continued to take after I moved back by myself to Los Angeles. I worked at temporary jobs until 2003, when my mania reemerged. I had been using drugs again and stopped my meds. My mother once again rescued me, bringing me back to San Diego, and she let me stay with her in her boyfriend's trailer.

Soon, I got into an argument with her boyfriend and started to act in bizarre ways. The neighbors in the trailer park petitioned the manager to drive me out. I was forced to sleep in my mother's car, and I had nowhere to go. My mother was taking me across San Diego to UCSD everyday, where I met David Shannahoff-Khalsa. I immediately recognized that Kundalini yoga could potentially heal me, and I began taking classes with him at the university. In the beginning I never told David about my problems or psychiatric history. In April 2004 I had my first Kundalini yoga class. Feeling almost high from rejuvenation, I had an outdoor picnic on campus. When a passerby sat on the bench next to me, I spat on him. The campus police were notified, and they tracked me down at a women's locker room about to take a shower. I was sent to the City Mental Health's emergency observation unit. From then on, I was picked up by the police repeatedly, because intermittently I would stop all of my medications because I was beginning to experience a clearer mental state from practicing Kundalini yoga. Unlike the jarring state of a hallucinogen-affected mind, Kundalini yoga connected my mind to a finite reality but with an expanded state of awareness. After my first class with David, I had an experience of peace and contentment that I had never experienced before. I reflected inward and saw my mind in a dormant and static state, trapped in my physical body. I had been too deeply enmeshed in drug-induced states, and, with mania, my mind had been further distorted.

Refusing adamantly to take any medications, I was tripping all the time. At times I felt that I was from a mythical world; at times, I was the cosmic body. A part of my mind was roaming breathlessly from one nonreality to the next, making connections between my distorted senses and a mental fantasy. I saw bodies arise out of energy which I alone could sense. I imagined that I was working for the heavenly spirits by wandering on the earth and healing everything, while other times destruction is called for. I believed that my thoughts controlled the environment. After a few ins and outs from the mental hospital, my mother found an apartment for me to start my life over. I began to practice the yoga sets from David's class on my own. But my wildness soon got me into trouble on the UCSD campus, and the campus police picked me up again. I was committed and then released from County Mental Health. My social worker made me bind to the condition that, in order to be sent back to my apartment, I would live in a board-and-care facility for at least 3 months and be medication compliant. There I made progress for the first time toward stability. I finally saw David in a private consultation where he first learned about my bipolar diagnosis. However, I did not tell him about my hallucinations. So he taught me the Kundalini yoga protocol for treating bipolar disorders, and I started practicing it several times a week. My medications at the time were 900 mg lithium, 20 mg Zyprexa, and 1,000 mg Depakote. I was compliant during the 3 months at the board-and-care facility. However, when I went back to my apartment, I stopped all of my medications again and I started drinking excessively. The neighbors called the police after I broke their window, and I was sent to a long-term, locked facility in the mountains in east San Diego County, called Alpine Special Treatment Center. I lost my apartment in March 2005.

I was still practicing Kundalini yoga daily on my own and I was making progress. After a few months, the doctor agreed that I was recovering and lowered my meds to 600 mg lithium and 10 mg Zyprexa. I got involved in the art therapy groups and found an outlet for my energy through painting. I felt that I was above the other patients, because of my yoga and my art. I daydreamed as if I was in a cocoon of my blossoming genius. With the Kundalini yoga and the medications, I stabilized around a light state of mania, with occasional delusions and hallucinations. After 8 months I was released and sent to a group home. I continued to paint and do Kundalini yoga, and was also attending David's UCSD yoga class. Five months later I began to throw away my medications, a little at a time, because the pills looked funny. In the ensuing orgiastic manic episode, I began to harass David and everyone around me, to the point of persecuting them. The group home owners called the police several times, but I acted normally and outwitted them. At last David took measures to block off contact. I got into a fight with one of my housemates, and finally, the police took me back to the Alpine facility. This time it was July 2006. I was to remain at Alpine for 11 months.

The second time in the same long-term facility without David's support brought out the worst in me. My grandiose behavior, swearing, and sarcasm soon brought about several assaults on me. Being a bitter victim, I further instigated more hostility, which soon snowballed. My medications were increased, but my mania worsened. I paced the corridor singing in a made-up language and began to experience olfactory hallucinations at mealtimes and in the shower. My delusions built up, never giving me a break. I got into more fights and was stripped of my privileges, which made me even more impossible. In September 2006 I had delusions of being pregnant. I felt something move in my abdomen area and pleaded with the doctor to stop my medications. When that failed, I refused the medications myself and, to everyone's surprise, my mania subsided. Apparently the high dosage of lithium induced intoxication. The doctor then discontinued all meds and ordered a biweekly injection of Risperdal Consta at a dosage of 25 mg. Although the psychiatrist told me that I could be discharged shortly, the administration insisted that I complete the program. It was November 2006. With the effect of Risperdal, I stabilized around a state of normalcy. By then I had been practicing intermittently the Kundalini yoga protocol for bipolar illness for close to 2 years. I then decided on my own to stop the daily practice, leaving it only for times when I felt the more severe symptoms, which were about twice a week. I began to experiment practicing a variety of Kundalini yoga meditation techniques that I found in manuals, and I started doing different techniques every day.

Unfortunately, my symptoms took a new manifestation unexpectedly. At a monthly day trip to the local park, I was observing the other patients as the day went on. I thought that they looked insane outside of the locked environment. A fear gnawed at me, and I felt an uncanny feeling that others were controlling me. I saw signs and symbols form around me out of the leaves on the ground, the paint on the walls, and the rocks on the hills. Back at the facility, I immediately practiced the Kundalini yoga meditation to "Prevent Freaking Out" for about an hour. The hallucination and the feelings of horror subsided, but the altered mental space, like that of an LSD flashback, came back persistently and without warning in the weeks to follow. When the hallucinations began, I would do the meditation to "Prevent Freaking Out" and the "Meditation for Insanity." After a few months of heightening stress from the population pressure in the facility, the attacks began to come daily at around 3:30 P.M. I then decided to do the two meditations every day for 40 days. After that, I did other meditations to strengthen my nerves and ease my mind, all lasting 40 days. The flashbacks were reduced to twice a week. When they came, I would meditate on a special prayer. My thoughts would jump out as words around me; my only consolation was seeing this particular prayer mentally appearing on the surfaces around me, again and again. Thus I chose to feed the hallucinatory state for lack of a better solution.

I took turns interacting with one or two people at a time, either patients or staff. Then, in a short time, I would become very emotionally involved, then I would turn against them, feeling that they were beginning to control me, or that they were too easily controlled by me. Then, I would isolate myself again, chanting loudly on the patio and singing songs while waiting for a meal. I was repeatedly reprimanded, was told that I should go to my room to chant and sing. But I ignored all corrections. I was alone in my mind, and every contact that I had with other patients and the staff encroached upon me. I lashed out left and right and tolerated no one. Then in a few days I would get close to someone again. The doctor wanted to increase my meds, but I refused. In the end the Risperdal Consta was upped to 50 mg biweekly. I continued to think that I was special. Roommates, one after another, were driven out by me yelling at them and by showing threatening behavior. I could only relate to my environment in a destructive way. Every-one around me was at the mercy of my distorted perception. Mo-ments of good behavior did not last. In the final months at Alpine, I became fixated on the delusion of the end of the world. I saw earthquakes and floods, and souls in torment. I was the only one that was saved.

In May 2007 I was in one of these delusions, and I was disrupt-ing a recreation group, and I was dragged out while yelling, "You are all damned!" I fought and bit the nurse who grabbed me on the arm. I was again sent to County Mental Health for observation for 3 days. The doctor in this facility additionally prescribed Prolixin to help with the delusions and paranoia. The change and quiet of environment there helped me to reflect on what I had done. I was affected at the core by catching a glimpse of my violent nature; I had finally gained some insight into my illness. When I went back to Alpine, there had been talk of sending me to the state hospital in Sacramento. My mother had intervened, and the administration decided to release me without having completed the program in June 2007. I was cooperative for the time being. The board-and-care home where I was sent was a small house in a residential neighborhood. My room, which was set up for two people, was empty when I got there. So I had the luxury of having my own room for a few weeks. The room was extremely small. When my roommate came, I alternated from being friendly to being hostile, and she became very upset. In the same week, when I was sup-posed to receive my injection of Risperdal Consta, my new clini-cian was 2 days late. I went into a state of shock when my mother came to visit me. Filled to the brim with feelings, I asked her about my life. We talked for hours, and for the first time in my life, my mother told me the details about her divorce with my father. I realized that it had been a fantasy of mine that he was a great person, and that he was even in my life. This new understanding changed my relationship with my mother dramatically. I then knew that she had stood by me through the most difficult times, and that she was committed to help me recover. I felt for the first time that I could trust her; I opened my shell and let her in. After that day, whenever she spoke concernedly about anything, I listened to find out what I could do, and not blame her for being too negative or thinking that she was trying to ruin my life. And if I saw that she was doing something she did not want to do, I would make compromises to ease her burden. For the first time in my life, I acted from gratitude.

The roommate situation did not improve. So my social worker arranged for me to move to a bigger facility, Fancor Guest Home. It happened to be near where my mother lives with her boyfriend. She came to visit often, and on weekends I went to stay with her (with her boyfriend's permission), so I could cook vegetarian meals for myself for the whole week. I had certain worries about the new place. It seemed like I had all but failed at so many opportunities at life. But I often had dreams that all turned out alright.

The onsite psychiatrist at Fancor changed my meds from Risperdal Consta to Clozaril at a dosage of 250 mg per day, keeping the Prolixin (10 mg/day). He said that all of his functioning patients use Clozaril, a drug for difficult-to-treat cases. I began to feel very well on the new medications, and this was just in time to enroll in a psychology class at the local community college. It was my mother's suggestion that I give psychology a try. My original ambition was in Oriental medicine. But my mother was strongly against it and would not fund me. She said that psychology is relevant to my own life experience, and so this will not turn into a dead end. Sure enough, since the start of my illness, I had entertained interests in fashion design, architecture, visual art, international relations, and massage therapy, all of which came to naught. As soon as I took a class in introductory psychology, I fell in love with the subject. It was intellectually engaging and helped to put my life into perspective. I took another class the next semester, and two more in fall 2008. At the time of the writing of this case history, I am enrolled in three classes including statistics.

A year and a half passed without crises. My mother's boyfriend was surprised at my enduring stability, considering my outrageous behavior 3 years ago. I was getting used to my hallucinations, which came on average two times a week, each time lasting anywhere from 6 to 10 hours. I was always looking for new meditation techniques to help me improve. I practiced different meditations for 40, 90, or 120 days at a time. Since I came to Fancor my hallucinations were images of my father and brother suspended in front of me accompanied by their voices, and on many occasions my thoughts appeared as visions of words all around me in both Spanish and English. In addition, I began to experience a memory trace, seeing the same person or car pass by me again and again after they had gone. After some time, the hallucinations changed again to images of blood, corpses, fires, genitals, and words. My mother was beginning to be able to detect when I was hallucinating, because I would have a certain look in my eyes. Almost every weekend when we saw each other there would be a hallucination episode. My mother began to worry, and I had no solutions. My mother then contacted David and requested that he see me again. This was 2 years after he stopped communicating with me due to my unwillingness to respect the appropriate boundaries of behavior. I was practicing a Kundalini yoga meditation at the time, but it had nothing to do with my healing. My mother pleaded with David to reconsider taking me as a patient. Since he had heard that my progress and behavior had improved, he decided to help me again on the condition that I would not violate any boundaries. I did not see him in person, but he sent me a new Kundalini yoga protocol that included an exercise set for my schizophrenia and other techniques for my personality disorder, and he then suggested a strict and arduous routine for me to practice. I immediately noticed that the new protocols that David recommended did not disassociate me from my normal consciousness, like some of the other meditations that I had been practicing. My hallucinations were soon reduced to once a week. After about a month the Prolixin was discontinued. The side effects had become unpleasant and I felt like they were interfering with my functioning. My symptoms improved even more, and my memory trace was also brought to a minimum. My "monkey mind" was coming under control.

Gradually and in stages, I came to experience my psychotic state as a state of light and vibration. The Kundalini yoga protocols that David recommended allowed me to go in and out of this state. At first, it was tremendously difficult to overcome the psychotic state, but with time I could go through it and reach stability. I also built a habit of mentally intoning the mantra Sat Nam with my breath during waking hours to help stabilize my mind. Sometimes feeling unreal or uncertain, the mantra greatly aided me in maintaining clarity and stability. David insisted that one of my major problems was not only my hallucinations and delusions, but that my behavior problems were also the result of having a personality disorder. He taught me nonreaction and restraint both normally and during hallucinations. My attacks became a blessing in disguise. Every time when an attack struck, I learned more about restraint and neutrality. And every time that I recovered from the hallucinatory state, my mind became a little more clear, and my spirit more strong. With the consistent practice of the Brain-Balancing Technique for Reducing Silliness, Focusing the Mind, and Controlling the Ego, my ego that was so previously enmeshed in my delusions began to lose its dominating effects. At David's suggestion, I was working on being a normal person instead of thinking that I was superior to others.

After 3 months of complying with the protocol, I had achieved a clearer state of mind. My medications were further reduced to 225 mg Clozaril per day. The hallucinations were much shorter, half an hour to 2 hours at the most. I learned to respect those around me with tolerance and peacefulness, and I felt like I had come in touch with my higher self during meditation. Whereas my lower self was filled with pain and suffering, my higher self had no pain but was filled with joy and acceptance. Kundalini yoga gave me the choice of having this relationship to my higher self. It gave me a sense of relief from the dependent and entangled relationships that I had with others, where in the past I would have wanted to cling to them. I became less judgmental of others and myself. Daily in life and in my Kundalini yoga practice, I go through the thickness of my suffering to healing. The hope that I had always had for improvement while practicing yoga on my own was now becoming a reality because of David's guidance that was leading to a real healing. My sense of being still wavers, and when I wake in the morning it takes some time to reorient myself. But I dive into my Kundalini yoga practice and emerge with a clear state of mind and emotions. Sometimes I still feel attached to isolation, but I am amazed at every person I see around me. Instead of being fixated on surface factors, I have trained my mind to be unattached and neutral. More recently I have been exploring my sense of identity. Previously, I had experienced only emptiness on an emotional level. Now, I not only have an accessible sense of joy, but I am beginning to experience a wider spectrum of emotions, naturally, and I feel less isolated. My dreams have become less "busy" and more lucid in some ways. I realize I still have a long way to go, but I have made a significant start.

Ms. E completed her case history in early February 2009 at the age of 31. In early November 2008, I had another consultation with Ms. E. This was the first contact that I had with her after some years. Her mother requested that I attempt to help her again. At that time I gave her the choice to see me in person or to communicate by e-mail. She chose e-mail. I knew she had enough experience with the Kundalini yoga meditation techniques that all she needed on that level was to read them, and then if necessary to ask questions to clarify any of the specifics for each technique. I also gave her instructions about what she needed to change in terms of her behavior and that she had to become very practical in her life. I have always been very direct with her, but only during the more recent times has she learned to really value my input. I then sent her a completely new routine since it was clear to me that she had more than the bipolar disorder to deal with. The bipolar condition is what she initially claimed was her diagnosis and condition when she first came to me professionally. After getting feedback from her, I realized she was also schizophrenic and that all of this was complicated by the additional problems of having both narcissistic and borderline personality disorders. During the interim of not seeing or communicating with her, her mother had kept me posted on the major events and changes in her life. Upon reconnecting, I told Ms. E that she also had schizophrenia. She initially denied having the condition and said that she only had bipolar disorder with psychotic features and borderline personality disorder. She resented my diagnosis, but several weeks later her psychiatrist also told her that she had schizophrenia and it was not just bipolar disorder with psychotic features. At this point, she was more willing to accept my diagnosis. Apparently she had been initially diagnosed with bipolar disorder with psychotic features, but she never shared the latter part about psychotic features. These disorders are frequently difficult to tease apart, and much has to do with what symptoms came first. They also tend to evolve over time, and therefore the diagnosis can frequently change. Those who make the diagnosis may also not have full insight and information on the patient's condition, especially if the patient is not willing to admit or recognize specific symptoms.

My new prescription for Ms. E, starting November 2008, included two very difficult Kundalini yoga routines that she was instructed to use on alternating days. Day 1 included the True Glue exercise set to be finished with 31 minutes of Sat Kriya instead of the normal 2 minutes that is standard for this set. She then rested on her back for at least 11 minutes and practiced the 5-minute Brain-Balancing Technique for Controlling the Ego. This was followed with 31 minutes of Gan Puttee Kriya, and finally followed immediately with 31 minutes of the Technique to Resolve the Bipolar Condition (Shannahoff-Khalsa, 2006). She was also told to do the Jupiter-Saturn meditation technique for 11 minutes at some point during the day (Shannahoff-Khalsa, 2006). On alternate days, she was instructed to practice the True Glue exercise set, again with Sat Kriya for 31 minutes, followed by the 5-minute Brain-Balancing Technique for Controlling the Ego. Then she was to follow this with Nabhi Kriya (Bhajan & Khalsa, 1975) for half times on the longer exercises, then practice the Meditation to Release Pressure From the Subconscious Mind, and finally end with the Jupiter-Saturn meditation technique for 11 minutes. From January 25, 2009, through October 2009 (this writing), she practiced the True Glue exercise set ending with 31 minutes of Sat Kriya every other day. All of the other meditations remained the same. Ms. E not only felt the benefits of what she had achieved, but she needed to have more time to devote to her psychology classes. As of October 20, 2009, Ms. E has had hallucinations lasting for only about 10 minutes to one hour with events occurring only every 15 to 18 days for the previous three months.

Ms. E had become somewhat disciplined with her previous Kundalini yoga practices. She also had an intense interest in the techniques, and she finally decided that she wanted to overcome her torturous condition. She had become fully aware of her condition and aware that if she was ever to have a normal life again, without the need to live in a special facility, she was going to have to commit to change both in her protocols for practice and with her behavior. If she did not have these complicating factors in her life, it is very unlikely that she would have complied with what is no doubt the most arduous Kundalini yoga practice that I have ever prescribed for a client. This long and difficult routine would challenge an advanced Kundalini yoga student or teacher. She also had youth on her side. She did not start with full times on Sat Kriya or the meditation to balance the ego, but soon developed the ability to comply with these routines with full times. Previously to this last intervention she had the ability to do the full times on Gan Puttee Kriya and the Technique to Resolve the Bipolar Condition. However, a few years earlier, when I had taught the Jupiter-Saturn meditation technique in my UCSD yoga classes, it was absolutely clear that this 11-minute technique was a torture for her and that she did not have the ability to do it full time or even correctly for a few minutes. Her fingers almost froze in motion and any additional movement of her fingers was simply painful after a minute or two. When I taught it to her again, I knew that this technique would help put her psyche through the changes that she required to learn both patience with herself and with others, and not to act out. This technique is very helpful for those with self-harming behavior and also for those who lose their patience with others. The Jupiter-Saturn meditation technique, the Meditation to Release Pressure From the Subconscious Mind, and the 5-minute technique for controlling the ego and reducing silly behavior were all included to help her overcome her personality disorders. I also knew that Gan Puttee Kriya would have a significant effect on her narcissistic and borderline personality disorders. She faced a near impossible challenge with this combination of disorders. Fortunately, when institutionalized she did not have access to drugs or alcohol. She soon realized that once she started to practice Kundalini yoga that her substance abuse problems and extraordinary sexual exploits had to be curbed entirely. I also knew that when I suspended contact with her that she had to realize through her hardship that she could not disrespect everyone in her life. She valued her initial contact with me and soon realized that she alone had ruined her opportunities for further study and treatment. Prior to the final break, I had warned her about crossing boundaries on several occasions. After the split, she attempted to seek guidance from other Kundalini yoga teachers, but these efforts did not lead to productive changes. In part, it was clear to others that her personality would be a major impediment in therapy, and indeed, the more one got to know her, the more apparent it became just how complex her case was in reality. At this time, I can say that many different factors have played a role in her progress. One of the most important factors was that she had to go through her self-created suffering to understand that it was indeed her responsibility to change her own behavior. After numerous events of being picked up by the police and the many months of institutionalization, her ego finally began to weaken and her delusions and fantasies were no longer effective support systems to explain her own situation in life. She indeed learned that she was not special or superior to others. I believe that the "torture" she had to endure in the various confined facilities was essential to this self-realization.

Due to Ms. E's intense interest and practice of Kundalini yoga techniques, and based on her own keen awareness of her condition and hallucinations, I decided to ask her to start to pay attention to which nostril was dominant during her hallucinations, thinking that there might be a clue on how to at least help her treat her acute state when experiencing her hallucinations. While I had a hunch that they might only occur during left nostril dominance, on January 20, 2009, she reported, "During the hallucinations my breath was left nostril dominant, and as soon as it was over my breath switched to right nostril dominant." I then asked her to continue to pay attention to her nasal dominance during the hallucinations. As of April 20, 2009, she has only had hallucinations during her left nostril dominant state, and only on a few occasions during the very brief transition period that leads into the left nostril dominant state. She has had approximately 15 different episodes of hallucination during this time, and they have only occurred during the left nostril dominant state, again with only a few occurring in the immediate transition state that occurs after the right nostril dominant state. But they have never occurred during the right nostril dominant state in her case.

I then asked her to start to practice slow deep right nostril breathing for up to 11 minutes during the hallucinations in an effort to help minimize the time and severity of the auditory and visual hallucinations, which routinely would last in her case for 6 to 10 hours. After her first report, she said, "Yesterday I had another hallucination episode. It was the 10th day since the last, and it lasted only 1 hour after 11 minutes of right-nostril breathing."

I then decided to construct a miniprotocol for her use during these acute episodes to see if it would help her to reduce and eliminate the hallucinations. The miniprotocol was to be used as soon as possible once she started to hallucinate. The techniques included four parts. First, she tuned in to Ong Namo Guru Dev Namo. Second was the Victory Breath technique for 3–5 minutes, or even longer if it seemed to help. Third was to do right nostril breathing while plugging the left nostril with the left thumb, breaking the breath into four equal parts on the inhalation and four equal parts on the exhalation. The four parts of the inhalation and exhalation were to be paired with the four respective syllables Sa Ta Na, and Ma for 5–11 minutes. So it is one cycle of the mantra Sa Ta Na Ma during the inhalation phase and one cycle of the mantra during the exhalation phase, where each syllable is paired with the respective four parts of the inhalation phase and each of the four parts of the exhalation phase. Finally, part 4 of the miniprotocol includes sitting straight while breathing only through the nose with Sa Ta Na Ma with the L-form vision unpaired with the breath cycle for up to 11 minutes. The latter is practiced with the eyes closed while mentally envisioning light and energy coming in through the top of the head, down to the middle of the head, and then out through the third eye. With each vision, the first sound of the Sa Ta Na Ma mantra first enters the top of the head such that the S sound of Sa starts at the top, moves down to the middle of the head, and then goes out the third eye as "ah," and then this is sequentially repeated for the other sounds. The first sound of each syllable starts as the light and energy are envisioned entering the head and moving to the middle of the head, and then exiting with the "ah" sound through the third eye. Ms. E was then instructed to lie down and relax if the hallucinations had not yet ended, but only lying on her left side to help engage and maintain the right nostril dominant state. She found that the use of this miniprotocol would frequently lead to a full remission of the hallucinations if she employed the full times for each technique, especially if she could sit down and practice the protocol quickly after the hallucinations started. Overall, when using the miniprotocol, even with shortened times for the four parts of the protocol, she found that her hallucinations would last for no more than 30 minutes to an hour. This was a major improvement on the 6–10 hours of hallucinations that she was having prior to the start of its use.

SIX

Epilogue

On the Future of the Prevention and Treatment
of Psychiatric Disorders

Meditation is the creative control of self where the Infinite
can talk to you.

> Yogi Bhajan, date unknown

Idiots think that saints do.

> Yogi Bhajan, date unknown

A new scientific truth does not triumph by convincing its
opponents and making them see the light, but rather because
its opponents eventually die, and a new generation grows up
that is familiar with it.

> Max Planck (1858–1947), *A Scientific Autobiography* (1949)

When contemplating the future of psychiatry and mental
health, let's first consider the present status of youth in
the United States and United Kingdom. While much has
already been presented on the prevalence and multimorbidities of
mental disorders and the poor efficacy of treatment, a striking and
illuminating commentary helps to encapsulate the present in "Edi-

torial: A Global Perspective on Child and Adolescent Mental Health" (Leckman & Leventhal, 2008). This editorial gives us the clearest possible picture in the shortest possible terms. The authors extracted information from a report by the United Nations Children's Fund Innocenti Research Center on the appraisal of child well-being in rich countries (UNICEF, 2007).

> This Report Card provides a comprehensive assessment of the lives and wellbeing of children and young people in 21 nations of the industrialized world. Its stated purpose is "to encourage monitoring, to permit comparison, and to stimulate the discussion and development of policies to improve children's lives." Although this first multidimensional overview can best be regarded as a work in progress, it is striking that the two countries at the very bottom of the rankings of child well-being were the two wealthiest English-speaking countries in the world, the United Kingdom and the United States. It is not just the developing countries of the world that need efficacious programs in child and adolescent mental health promotion. According to this report card, children growing up in the United Kingdom suffer greater deprivation, worse relationships with their parents and are exposed to more risks from alcohol, drugs, and unsafe sex than those in any other wealthy country in the world. The United States has the highest rate of children growing up in poverty (21.7%) and the highest rate of children living in single-parent homes (20.8%) in rich countries. Both countries have the highest percentage of young people rating their overall health as "fair or poor." In the United States our health care system is fragmented and too often biased toward serving the well-to-do and not serving individuals with mental disorders. (Leckman & Leventhal, 2008)

These authors also noted, "The future of our children and grandchildren in our global community is in jeopardy. We ignore this reality at our peril—and theirs."

The health care industry and insurance companies are primarily driven by market forces with an intention to first maximize profits. The academic medical community is not immune to these forces. At this writing, this nation faces the most serious challenge in its history on how to handle the current health care crisis. Ultimately, there is really only one solution to the health care crisis, and that is to invest in prevention. "Prevention also may be an easier concept for the public—the politics are less volatile, the logic more intuitive: it is better to prevent diseases than to concentrate resources on treating diseases after they become clinically apparent, when treatment may be too late to be effective" (Woolf, 2008). It is the view of this author that Kundalini yoga can be a very powerful therapy both for the prevention of psychiatric disorders and for treating the full syndrome and the multimorbid disorders, especially where conventional medicine has proven to show meager results.

On January 26, 1976, Yogi Bhajan gave the weekly lecture at the Salk Institute for Biological Studies. The title of his talk was "The Science of Meditation." He called meditation an "ancient technology of the mind" and he described Kundalini yoga as a "monstrous science." For the past 33 years I have been trying to bring attention and credibility to this ancient technology and monstrous science, and much of this work has now been published in books (Shannahoff-Khalsa, 2006, 2008). This work presents new insights for understanding psychophysiological states and the ultradian dynamics of mind-body interactions. This work also shows how to noninvasively augment these mind-body states, and all of the work is based on concepts that come from the teachings of Kundalini yoga as taught by Yogi Bhajan. These novel neuroscience studies demonstrate that our two cerebral hemispheres alternate in dominance during both waking and sleep, and these studies also help identify an important evolutionary step in the development of the nervous system that has otherwise been missed, ignored, or not understood (Shannahoff-Khalsa, 2008). The earliest studies here were conducted and published while the author was at the Salk Institute (Werntz, Bickford, Bloom, & Shannahoff-Khalsa, 1983; Werntz, Bickford, & Shannahoff-Khalsa, 1987). Early on, I had hoped that these novel discoveries would do more to help inspire interest in Kundalini yoga as a potential therapy for treating a variety of psychiatric disorders. The first clinical trial was an open uncontrolled trial (Shannahoff-Khalsa & Beckett, 1996) for treating OCD using the OCD-specific Kundalini yoga meditation protocol that is published in my first book. The second OCD study was funded by the National Institutes of Health, and it was a randomized controlled trial comparing the same OCD-specific Kundalini yoga meditation protocol against a comparison group that included two more common meditation techniques (Relaxation Response and Mindfulness Meditation) (Shannahoff-Khalsa, 1997; Shannahoff-Khalsa et al., 1999). The open trial showed efficacy that was at least equal to or better than conventional therapies, yielding a 55% improvement rate according to the Yale-Brown Obsessive Compulsive Scale (Y-BOCS). The second trial showed results that surpassed conventional modalities, with a 71% improvement rate using the Y-BOCS. At 3 months the two groups were merged since the control group showed no efficacy with any of the six psychological scales (Shannahoff-Khalsa et al., 1999).

The problem at this stage is understandable. The vastness of Kundalini yoga as a science is beyond what people can either imagine or believe, unless they have direct personal experience of the techniques. Otherwise, it is too difficult for most people to accept that humans were once far more advanced in their consciousness than they are today. It is estimated that Yogi Bhajan taught about 5,000 different Kundalini yoga meditation techniques over 35 years (Shannahoff-Khalsa, 2004, 2006), not including the many hundreds of different sequence-specific exercise sets that all have different properties and claimed benefits. In *Kundalini Yoga Meditation*, there are 64 different meditation techniques and eight disorder-specific multipart Kundalini yoga meditation protocols for treating Axis I disorders (Shannahoff-Khalsa, 2006). These eight protocols include an 11-part protocol for obsessive-compulsive disorder; a 6-part protocol for acute stress disorder; a 6-part protocol for major depressive disorders; a 5-part protocol for bipolar disorders; a 7-part protocol for the addictive, impulse control, and eating disorders; a 9-part protocol for chronic fatigue syndrome (CFS); an 11-part protocol for attention-deficit/hyperactivity disorder and comorbid disorders (oppositional defiant disorder and conduct disorder); and an 8-part protocol for post-traumatic stress disorder (PTSD) (Shannahoff-Khalsa, 2006). A list of meditation techniques in that book that are not also included in this book are categorized as the following: 14 techniques for couples therapy, 10 techniques for the abused and battered psyche, 6 meditation techniques specific for generalized anxiety, 2 for depression, 1 for fear, and 1 each for OCD, panic attacks, phobias, grief, resolving bipolar disorders, treating the manic phase of bipolar disorder, treating the depressed phase of bipolar disorder, addictions, impulsive behaviors, insomnia, nightmares, inducing deep super-efficient sleep, CFS, learning disabilities, dyslexia, patience and temperament, a normal or supernormal state of consciousness, and for commanding your own consciousness to a higher state of consciousness. The seven-part psycho-oncology protocol also adds to the diversity of these techniques and their condition-specific benefits (Shannahoff-Khalsa, 2005).

Four meditation techniques are included in this book that also appear in *Kundalini Yoga Meditation*: Gan Puttee Kriya, A Meditation to Balance and Synchronize the Cerebral Hemispheres, the mantra technique for anger, and the Victory Breath.

These meditation techniques are not taught in other yogic or meditation lineages. They are unique to Kundalini yoga as taught by Yogi Bhajan and belong to the teachings of the House of Guru Ram Das. While these 15 different multipart protocols (8 in *Kundalini Yoga Meditation*, 6 in this book, and the psycho-oncology protocol) are specific for their respective psychiatric disorders, they would also be beneficial for any individual that wants to help improve his or her own mental health or for preventing the onset of a psychiatric disorder. For example, while PTSD results from either a single traumatic event (e.g., rape), or a series of traumatic events (e.g., extended combat missions), immediate or continued use of these techniques will do a great deal to either prevent or minimize the severity of the disorder. In general, these techniques can play an important role in helping solve the current mental health care crisis. In addition, these techniques can be a powerful means for helping to awaken the dormant mental and spiritual potential of the practitioner. Another very important use for these techniques is in helping to prevent interest in the use and abuse of drugs or alcohol. These techniques are very potent, and they can quickly help the practitioner experience a natural high and state of intoxication, but one that has incredible clarity, stability, and much greater awareness. There is clearly a great need to help children and adolescents find a healthy substitute for illicit drugs, prescription drugs, and alcohol. Kundalini yoga can become a powerful deterrent for substance abuse. In addition, these techniques are likely to give young people another reason not to smoke. They will quickly learn how valuable their breath is for higher purposes.

The ancient yogis learned techniques for treating the variants of the psychiatric disorders as we know them today, and these same disorders have all existed since the origins of the human race. However, one of the most exciting possibilities here is to exploit these techniques to help enhance normal neurodevelopmental growth, or what the yogis call awakening the mystical or spiritual potential, the path toward enlightenment. Yogis view consciousness as having eight different and distinct levels. Each level of consciousness is represented by a chakra, a center or vortex of energy within the body that also extends into the spiritual bodies. Today, the biggest problem that we face is that the majority of individuals are limited by having their consciousness confined to one of their three lower chakras: (1) a survival mentality consciousness, as the first chakra dominates when an individual is in a state of fear or acting out of perversion; (2) the consciousness that relates solely to sexual activity and reproduction; and (3) the consciousness of "me" versus "we"—the state of mind where the individual wants to dominate, conquer, and control others. It is only the fourth chakra that begins to support the more humane qualities of the human. This is the chakra that is active in the state of compassion and heartfelt love, where the individual knows the greater virtues of living in a "we" state of consciousness at the expense of the "me" state of consciousness. The individual living with an active heart chakra has learned the virtues of being a giver. These four chakras and chakras 5 through 8 are each discussed in greater depth elsewhere, along with how yogis view the concept of the five "elements" (ether, air, fire, water, and earth) and how they relate to the fabric of consciousness (Shannahoff-Khalsa, 2006).

In sum, as a nation we are not exploiting the higher states of consciousness that give life the richness and reward that can help cure the otherwise excessive and neurotic needs that lead to the maladies of our present world condition. Nor are we finding effective solutions to treat the maladies that occur when the lower three chakras are damaged and out of balance. Medications at best are useful for treating symptoms, and frequently psychotherapy alone will also not suffice. The ancients believed that there are only five true diseases—lust, anger, greed, pride, and attachment—and when any one of these five factors is excessive or inappropriately expressed, there is a consequence in the mind. This consequence is also eventually expressed in the body in the form of what we call disease. Therefore, the diseases that we commonly acknowledge today are all actually symptomatic of an imbalance in a previous or current state of consciousness, which can include the karmas of a previous lifetime. On a spiritual plane, there is purpose and a fate or a destiny for each individual soul. These symptomatic diseases are learning experiences for that host individual.

Yogic therapy was meant to be a system for healing and renewal, and a highly technical aid to help augment the natural stages of development to ultimately awaken the higher states of consciousness that give us the fullest experience of the self. Without this self-realization, we are plagued by preconceived notions of reality and the true nature of our identity. This book covers three topics of abnormal neurodevelopment: the variants of psychoses, the personality, and the pervasive developmental disorders. Each disorder results from either direct or indirect traumatic events that

326

impair the development of a natural and healthy state of being. These disorders can be corrected, and it is unlikely that we will ever discover drugs that can heal the residuals of trauma as effectively as the ancient yogic techniques. These techniques are the heritage of humanity, and they will again help to heal and elevate humanity for a better future.

References

Alegria, M., Nakash, O., Lapatin, S., Oddo, V., Gao, S., Lin, J., et al. (2008). How missing information in diagnosis can lead to disparities in the clinical encounter. *Journal of Public Health Management and Practice, 14*(Suppl.), S26–S35.

Allison, D. B., Mentore, J. L., Heo, M., Chandler, L. P., Cappelleri, J. C., Infante, M. C., et al. (1999). Antipsychotic-induced weight gain: A comprehensive research synthesis. *American Journal of Psychiatry, 156,* 1686–1696.

Alwin, N., Blackburn, R., Davidson, K., Hilton, M., Logan, C., & Shine, J. (2006). *Understanding personality disorder: A professional practice board report by the British Psychological Society.* Leicester, UK: British Psychological Society, St. Andrews House.

Anahata, C. (2001). *Healing sounds of the ancients*, Vol. 3 (Ardas Bhaee and Har Har Gobinde Mukande).

Angst, J., Sellaro, R., & Ries Merikangas, K. (2002). Multimorbidity of psychiatric disorders as an indicator of clinical severity. *European Archives of Psychiatry and Clinical Neuroscience, 252*(4), 147–154.

APA. (1987). *Diagnostic and statistical manual of mental disorders* (3rd ed. rev.). Washington, DC: American Psychiatric Association.

APA. (1994). *Diagnostic and statistical manual of mental disorders* (4th ed.). Washington, DC: American Psychiatric Association.

APA. (2000). *Diagnostic and statistical manual of mental disorders* (4th ed., text rev). Arlington, VA: American Psychiatric Association.

APA. (2001). Practice guidelines for the treatment of patients with borderline personality disorder. *American Journal of Psychiatry, 158* (Suppl.), 1–52.

Appelbaum, P. S., Robbins, P. C., & Roth, L. H. (1999). Dimensional approach to delusions: Comparison across types and diagnoses. *American Journal of Psychiatry, 156,* 1938–1943.

Arnevik, E., Wilberg, T., Urnes, O., Johansen, M., Monsen, J. T., & Karterud, S. (2008). Psychotherapy for personality disorders: Short-term day hospital psychotherapy versus outpatient individual therapy—a randomized controlled study. *European Psychiatry.* Epub December 19.

Augstein, H. F. (1996). J C Prichard's concept of moral insanity—a medical theory of the corruption of human nature. *Medical History, 40*(3), 311–343.

Bailey, A., Le Couteur, A., Gottesman, I., Bolton, P., Simonoff, E., Yuzda, E., et al. (1995). Autism as a strongly genetic disorder: Evidence from a British twin study. *Psychological Medicine, 25*(1), 63–77.

Bartels, S. J., & Drake, R. E. (1988). Depressive symptoms in schizophrenia: Comprehensive differential diagnosis. *Comprehensive Psychiatry, 29,* 467–483.

Bateman, A., & Fonagy, P. (1999). Effectiveness of partial hospitalization in the treatment of borderline personality disorder: A randomized controlled trial. *American Journal of Psychiatry, 156,* 1563–1569.

Bateman, A., & Fonagy, P. (2001). Treatment of borderline personality disorder with psychoanalytically oriented partial hospitalization: An 18-month follow-up. *American Journal of Psychiatry, 158,* 36–42.

Bates, M. E., Bowden, S. C., & Barry, D. (2002). Neurocognitive impairment associated with alcohol use disorders: Implications for treatment. *Experimental and Clinical Psychopharmacology, 10*(3), 193–212.

Bazargan-Hejazi, S., Bazargan, M., Hardin, E., & Bing, E. G. (2005). Alcohol use and adherence to prescribed therapy among under-served Latino and African-American patients using emergency department services. *Ethnicity and Disease, 15*(2), 267–275.

Beer, M. D. (1995). Psychosis: From mental disorder to disease concept. *History of Psychiatry, 6*(22 Pt. 2), 177–200.

Beer, M. D. (1996). Psychosis: A history of the concept. *Comprehensive Psychiatry, 37*(4), 273–291.

Benjet, C., Borges, G., & Medina-Mora, M. E. (2008). DSM-IV personality disorders in Mexico: Results from a general population survey. *Revista Brasileira de Psiquiatria, 30*(3), 227–234.

Bentall, R. (2006). Madness explained: Why we must reject the Kraepelinian paradigm and replace it with a "complaint-orientated" approach to understanding mental illness. *Medical Hypotheses, 66*(2), 220–233.

Bhajan, Y. (2000). *Self-experience: Kundalini yoga as taught by Yogi Bhajan.* Espanola, NM: Kundalini Research Institute.

Bhajan, Y. (2002). *Reaching me in me*. Espanola, NM: Kundalini Research Institute.

Bhajan, Y., & Khalsa, G. (1975). *Kundalini meditation manual for intermediate students*. Espanola, NM: Kundalini Research Institute.

Bhajan, Y., & Khalsa, G. (1998). *The mind: Its projections and multiple facets* (1st ed.). Espanola, NM: Kundalini Research Institute.

Binks, C. A., Fenton, M., McCarthy, L., Lee, T., Adams, C. E., & Duggan, C. (2006). Psychological therapies for people with borderline personality disorder. *Cochrane Database of Systematic Reviews* (1), CD005652.

Bird, H. R., Gould, M. S., & Staghezza, B. M. (1993). Patterns of diagnostic comorbidity in a community sample of children aged 9 through 16 years. *Journal of the American Academy of Child and Adolescent Psychiatry, 32,* 361–368.

Bleuler, P. (1908). Who named it? Retrieved January 23, 2008, from http://www.whonamedit.com/doctor.cfm/1294.html

Blumer, J. L. (1999). Off-label uses of drugs in children. *Pediatrics, 104*(3 Pt. 2), 598–602.

Boddaert, N., Belin, P., Chabane, N., Poline, J. B., Barthelemy, C., Mouren-Simeoni, M. C., et al. (2003). Perception of complex sounds: Abnormal pattern of cortical activation in autism. *American Journal of Psychiatry, 160,* 2057–2060.

Bohus, M., Haaf, B., Simms, T., Limberger, M. F., Schmahl, C., Unckel, C., et al. (2004). Effectiveness of inpatient dialectical behavioral therapy for borderline personality disorder: A controlled trial. *Behaviour Research and Therapy, 42,* 487–499.

Bohus, M., Haaf, B., Stiglmayr, C., Pohl, U., Bohme, R., & Linehan, M. (2000). Evaluation of inpatient dialectical-behavioral therapy for borderline personality disorder—a prospective study. *Behaviour Research and Therapy, 38,* 875–887.

Boyd, J. H. (1986). Use of mental health services for the treatment of panic disorder. *American Journal of Psychiatry, 143,* 1569–1574.

Boyd, J. H., Burke, J. D., Jr., Gruenberg, E., Holzer, C. E., 3rd, Rae, D. S., George, L. K., et al. (1984). Exclusion criteria of DSM-III. A study of co-occurrence of hierarchy-free syndromes. *Archives of General Psychiatry, 41,* 983–989.

Brady, K. T., Verduin, M. L., & Tolliver, B. K. (2007). Treatment of patients comorbid for addiction and other psychiatric disorders. *Current Psychiatry Reports, 9*, 374–380.

Brawman-Mintzer, O., Lydiard, R. B., Emmanuel, N., Payeur, R., Johnson, M., Roberts, J., et al. (1993). Psychiatric comorbidity in patients with generalized anxiety disorder. *American Journal of Psychiatry, 150*, 1216–1218.

Breier, A., & Berg, P. H. (1999). The psychosis of schizophrenia: Prevalence, response to atypical antipsychotics, and prediction of outcome. *Biological Psychiatry, 46*, 361–364.

Breier, A., Schreiber, J. L., Dyer, J., & Pickar, D. (1991). National Institute of Mental Health longitudinal study of chronic schizophrenia. Prognosis and predictors of outcome. *Archives of General Psychiatry, 48*, 239–246.

Brink, T. L. (1980). Idiot savant with unusual mechanical ability: An organic explanation. *American Journal of Psychiatry, 137*, 250–251.

Brown, T. A., & Barlow, D. H. (1992). Comorbidity among anxiety disorders: Implications for treatment and DSM-IV. *Journal of Consulting and Clinical Psychology, 60*, 835–844.

Buckley, P. F., Miller, B. J., Lehrer, D. S., & Castle, D. J. (2009). Psychiatric comorbidities and schizophrenia. *Schizophrenia Bulletin, 35*, 383–402.

Burgmair, W., Engstrom, E., & Weber, M. (2000–2006). *Emil Kraepelin* (Vols. 1–6). Munich: Belleville.

Byrne, M., Agerbo, E., Eaton, W. W., & Mortensen, P. B. (2004). Parental socio-economic status and risk of first admission with schizophrenia—a Danish national register based study. *Social Psychiatry and Psychiatric Epidemiology, 39*(2), 87–96.

Caetano, R., Nelson, S., & Cunradi, C. (2001). Intimate partner violence, dependence symptoms and social consequences from drinking among white, black and Hispanic couples in the United States. *American Journal of Addiction, 10* (Suppl.), 60–69.

Casey, D. E. (2004). Dyslipidemia and atypical antipsychotic drugs. *Journal of Clinical Psychiatry, 65*(Suppl. 18), 27–35.

Chakos, M., Lieberman, J., Hoffman, E., Bradford, D., & Sheitman, B. (2001). Effectiveness of second-generation antipsychotics in patients with treatment-resistant schizophrenia: A review and meta-analysis of randomized trials. *American Journal of Psychiatry, 158*, 518–526.

Chen, E. Y., Matthews, L., Allen, C., Kuo, J. R., & Linehan, M. M. (2008). Dialectical behavior therapy for clients with binge-eating disorder or bulimia nervosa and borderline personality disorder. *International Journal of Eating Disorders, 41*, 505–512.

Chou, S. P., Dawson, D. A., Stinson, F. S., Huang, B., Pickering, R. P., Zhou, Y., et al. (2006). The prevalence of drinking and driving in the United States, 2001–2002: Results from the national epidemiological survey on alcohol and related conditions. *Drug and Alcohol Dependence, 83,* 137–146.

Ciompi, L. (1980a). Catamnestic long-term study on the course of life and aging of schizophrenics. *Schizophrenia Bulletin, 6,* 606–618.

Ciompi, L. (1980b). The natural history of schizophrenia in the long term. *British Journal of Psychiatry, 136,* 413–420.

Citrome, L. L., & Jaffe, A. B. (2003). Relationship of atypical antipsychotics with development of diabetes mellitus. *Annals of Pharmacotherapy, 37,* 1849–1857.

Clarkin, J. F., Levy, K. N., Lenzenweger, M. F., & Kernberg, O. F. (2007). Evaluating three treatments for borderline personality disorder: A multiwave study. *American Journal of Psychiatry, 164,* 922–928.

Coid, J., Yang, M., Tyrer, P., Roberts, A., & Ullrich, S. (2006). Prevalence and correlates of personality disorder in Great Britain. *British Journal of Psychiatry, 188,* 423–431.

Copeland, W. E., Miller-Johnson, S., Keeler, G., Angold, A., & Costello, E. J. (2007). Childhood psychiatric disorders and young adult crime: A prospective, population-based study. *American Journal of Psychiatry, 164,* 1668–1675.

Cougnard, A., Marcelis, M., Myin-Germeys, I., De Graaf, R., Vollebergh, W., Krabbendam, L., et al. (2007). Does normal developmental expression of psychosis combine with environmental risk to cause persistence of psychosis? A psychosis proneness-persistence model. *Psychological Medicine, 37,* 513–527.

Crawford, T. N., Cohen, P., First, M. B., Skodol, A. E., Johnson, J. G., & Kasen, S. (2008). Comorbid axis I and axis II disorders in early adolescence: Outcomes 20 years later. *Archives of General Psychiatry, 65,* 641–648.

Dane, S., & Balci, N. (2007). Handedness, eyedness and nasal cycle in children with autism. *International Journal of Developmental Neuroscience, 25,* 223–226.

Daschner, F., & Mutter, J. (2007). [Special vote on "Amalgam: Statement on its environmental medical impact," report of the commission "Methods and Quality Assurance in Environmental Medicine" of the Robert Koch Institute, Berlin]. *Bundesgesundheitsblatt Gesundheitsforschung Gesundheitsschutz, 50,* 1432–1433.

de Groot, E. R., Verheul, R., & Trijsburg, R. W. (2008). An integrative perspective on psychotherapeutic treatments for borderline personality disorder. *Journal of Personality Disorders, 22,* 332–352.

Deister, A., & Marneros, A. (1993). Long-term stability of subtypes in schizophrenic disorders: A comparison of four diagnostic systems. *European Archives of Psychiatry and Clinical Neuroscience, 242*, 184–190.

DeLong, R. (1999). Autism: New data suggest a new hypothesis. *Neurology*, 52, 911–916.

Dolan-Sewell, R., Krueger, R., & Shea, M. (2001). Co-occurrence with syndrome disorders. In W. Livesley (Ed.), *Handbook of personality disorders: Theory, research and treatment* (pp. 84–104). New York: Guilford.

Dominick, K. C., Davis, N. O., Lainhart, J., Tager-Flusberg, H., & Folstein, S. (2007). Atypical behaviors in children with autism and children with a history of language impairment. *Research in Devopmental Disabilities, 28*, 145–162.

Douglas, C. J. (2008). Teaching supportive psychotherapy to psychiatric residents. *American Journal of Psychiatry, 165*, 445–452.

Duraiswamy, G., Thirthalli, J., Nagendra, H. R., & Gangadhar, B. N. (2007). Yoga therapy as an add-on treatment in the management of patients with schizophrenia—a randomized controlled trial. *Acta Psychiatrica Scandinavica, 116*, 226–232.

Dyck, I. R., Phillips, K. A., Warshaw, M. G., Dolan, R. T., Shea, M. T., Stout, R. L., et al. (2001). Patterns of personality pathology in patients with generalized anxiety disorder, panic disorder with and without agoraphobia, and social phobia. *Journal of Personality Disorders, 15*(1), 60–71.

Engstrom, E. J., Weber, M. M., & Burgmair, W. (2006). Emil Wilhelm Magnus Georg Kraepelin (1856–1926). *American Journal of Psychiatry, 163*, 1710.

Escalante-Mead, P. R., Minshew, N. J., & Sweeney, J. A. (2003). Abnormal brain lateralization in high-functioning autism. *Journal of Autism and Developmental Disorders, 33*, 539-543.

Fan, X., Henderson, D. C., Nguyen, D. D., Cather, C., Freudenreich, O., Evins, A. E., et al. (2008). Posttraumatic stress disorder, cognitive function and quality of life in patients with schizophrenia. *Psychiatry Research, 159*(1–2), 140–146.

Farrell, J. M., Shaw, I. A., & Webber, M. A. (2009). A schema-focused approach to group psychotherapy for outpatients with borderline personality disorder: A randomized controlled trial. *Journal of Behavior Therapy and Experimental Psychiatry, 40*, 317:328.

Fazel, S., Gulati, G., Linsell, L., Geddes, J. R., & Grann, M. (2009). Schizophrenia and violence: Systematic review and meta-analysis. *PLoS Medicine*, 6(8), e1000120.

Fazel, S., Langstrom, N., Hjern, A., Grann, M., & Lichtenstein, P. (2009). Schizophrenia, substance abuse, and violent crime. *JAMA, 301*, 2016–2023.

Feuchtersleben, E. v. (1845). *Lehrbuch der arzlichen seelenkunde.* Vienna, Austria: Gerold.

Filipek, P. A., Steinberg-Epstein, R., & Book, T. M. (2006). Intervention for autistic spectrum disorders. *NeuroRx, 3*(2), 207–216.

Fombonne, E. (2005). Epidemiology of autistic disorder and other pervasive developmental disorders. *Journal of Clinical Psychiatry, 66*(Suppl. 10), 3–8.

Fonagy, P. (1998). An attachment theory approach to treatment of the difficult patient. *Bulletin of the Menninger Clinic, 62*(2), 147–169.

Fonagy, P., Kächele, R., Krause, E., Jones, R., & Perron, R. (2002). An open door review of outcome studies in psychoanalysis. *Pszichoterápia, 11*(4), 245–248.

Gabbard, G. O. (2001). Psychoanalysis and psychoanalytic psychotherapy. In W. Livesley (Ed.), *Handbook of personality disorders: Theory, research, and treatment* (pp. 359–376). New York: Guilford.

Gabbard, G. O. (2005a). From the guest editor. *Focus, 3*(3), 361.

Gabbard, G. O. (2005b). Psychoanalysis. In J. M. Oldham, A. E. Skodol, & D. S. Bender (Eds.), *The American Psychiatric Publishing textbook of personality disorders* (pp. 257–273). Washington, DC: American Psychiatric Publishing.

Geier, D. A., Kern, J. K., & Geier, M. R. (2009). A prospective study of prenatal mercury exposure from maternal dental amalgams and autism severity. *Acta Neurobiologiae Experimentalis (Warsaw), 69*(2), 189–197.

Geschwind, N., & Galaburda, A. M. (1987). *Cerebral lateralization: Biological mechanisms, associations, and pathology.* Cambridge, MA: MIT Press.

Ghaemi, S. N. (Ed.). (2002). *Polypharmacy in psychiatry.* New York: Marcel Dekker.

Giesen-Bloo, J., van Dyck, R., Spinhoven, P., van Tilburg, W., Dirksen, C., van Asselt, T., et al. (2006). Outpatient psychotherapy for borderline personality disorder: Randomized trial of schema-focused therapy vs transference-focused psychotherapy. *Archives of General Psychiatry, 63*, 649–658.

Goisman, R. M., Goldenberg, I., Vasile, R. G., & Keller, M. B. (1995). Comorbidity of anxiety disorders in a multicenter anxiety study. *Comprehensive Psychiatry, 36*, 303–311.

Goldner, E. M., Hsu, L., Waraich, P., & Somers, J. M. (2002). Prevalence and incidence studies of schizophrenic disorders: A systematic review of the literature. *Canadian Journal of Psychiatry, 47*, 833–843.

Goldsmith, R. J., & Garlapati, V. (2004). Behavioral interventions for dual-diagnosis patients. *Psychiatric Clinics of North America, 27*, 709–725.

Goodman, C., Finkel, B., Naser, M., Andreyev, P., Segev, Y., Kurs, R., et al. (2007). Neurocognitive deterioration in elderly chronic schizophrenia patients with and without PTSD. *Journal of Nervous and Mental Disease, 195*, 415–420.

Goodwin, R., Lyons, J. S., & McNally, R. J. (2002). Panic attacks in schizophrenia. *Schizophrenia Research, 58*(2–3), 213–220.

Gordon, C. T., State, R. C., Nelson, J. E., Hamburger, S. D., & Rapoport, J. L. (1993). A double-blind comparison of clomipramine, desipramine, and placebo in the treatment of autistic disorder. *Archives of General Psychiatry, 50*, 441–447.

Gould, R., Mueser, K., Bolton, E., Mays, V., & Goff, D. (2004). Cognitive therapy for psychosis in schizophrenia: An effect size analysis. *Focus, 2*(1), 95–101.

Grant, B. F., Chou, S. P., Goldstein, R. B., Huang, B., Stinson, F. S., Saha, T. D., et al. (2008). Prevalence, correlates, disability, and comorbidity of DSM-IV borderline personality disorder: Results from the wave 2 national epidemiologic survey on alcohol and related conditions. *Journal of Clinical Psychiatry, 69*, 533–545.

Grant, B. F., Hasin, D. S., Stinson, F. S., Dawson, D. A., Goldstein, R. B., Smith, S., et al. (2006). The epidemiology of DSM-IV panic disorder and agoraphobia in the United States: Results from the national epidemiologic survey on alcohol and related conditions. *Journal of Clinical Psychiatry, 67*, 363–374.

Great Britain, Department of Health. (2003). *Personality disorder: No longer a diagnosis of exclusion.* London: Department of Health, National Institute for Mental Health in England.

Green, J., Gilchrist, A., Burton, D., & Cox, A. (2000). Social and psychiatric functioning in adolescents with Asperger syndrome compared with conduct disorder. *Journal of Autism and Developmental Disorders, 30*, 279–293.

Greenfield, S. F., Strakowski, S. M., Tohen, M., Batson, S. C., & Kolbrener, M. L. (1994). Childhood abuse in first-episode psychosis. *British Journal of Psychiatry, 164*, 831–834.

Gunderson, J. G. (2001). *Borderline personality disorder: A clinical guide.* Washington, DC: American Psychiatric Press.

Gunderson, J. G., Frank, A. F., Ronningstam, E. F., Wachter, S., Lynch, V. J., & Wolf, P. J. (1989). Early discontinuance of borderline patients from psychotherapy. *Journal of Nervous and Mental Disease, 177*(1), 38–42.

Gunderson, J. G., Gratz, K. L., Neuhaus, E. C., & Smith, G. W. (2005). Levels of care in treatment. In J. M. Oldham, A. E. Skodol, & D. S. Bender (Eds.), *Textbook of personality disorders* (pp. 239-255). Washington, DC: American Psychiatric Publishing.

Hafner, H., Maurer, K., & Loffler, W. (1999). Onset and prodromal phase as determinants of the course. In W. Gattaz & H. Hafner (Eds.), *Search for the causes of schizophrenia, vol. IV: Balance of the century* (pp. 35–58). Darmstadt, Germany: Steinkopf Springer.

Harwood, R., Fountain, D., & Livermore, G. (1998). *The economic costs of alcohol and drug abuse in the United States, 1992.* Bethesda, MD: National Institute on Alcohol Abuse and Alcoholism and National Institute on Drug Abuse.

Hasin, D. S., Stinson, F. S., Ogburn, E., & Grant, B. F. (2007). Prevalence, correlates, disability, and comorbidity of DSM-IV alcohol abuse and dependence in the United States: Results from the national epidemiologic survey on alcohol and related conditions. *Archives of General Psychiatry, 64,* 830–842.

Hauser, S., DeLong, G., & Rosman, N. (1975). Pneumographic findings in the infantile autism syndrome. *Brain, 98,* 667–688.

Hellerstein, D. J., & Markowitz, J. C. (2008). Developing supportive psychotherapy as evidence-based treatment. *American Journal of Psychiatry, 165,* 1355–1356; author reply 1356.

Henderson, D. C., Daley, T. B., Kunkel, L., Rodrigues-Scott, M., Koul, P., & Hayden, D. (2004). Clozapine and hypertension: A chart review of 82 patients. *Journal of Clinical Psychiatry, 65,* 686–689.

Herbert, M. R. (2008). Treatment guided research: Helping people now with humility, respect and boldness. *Autism Advocate, 1,* 8–14.

Hertz-Picciotto, I., & Delwiche, L. (2009). The rise in autism and the role of age at diagnosis. *Epidemiology, 20*(1), 84–90.

Herve, H., & Yuille, J. C. (2007). *The psychopath: Theory, research, and practice.* Mahwah, NJ: Erlbaum.

Hill, A. L. (1977). Idiot savants: Rate of incidence. *Perceptual and Motor Skills, 44*(1), 161–162.

Hoffman, P. D., & Fruzzetti, A. E. (2005). Psychoeducation. In J. M. Oldham, A. E. Skodol, & D. S. Bender (Eds.), *Textbook of personality disorders* (pp. 375–385). Washington, DC: American Psychiatric Publishing.

Hofvander, B., Delorme, R., Chaste, P., Nyden, A., Wentz, E., Stahlberg, O., et al. (2009). Psychiatric and psychosocial problems in adults with normal-intelligence autism spectrum disorders. *BMC Psychiatry, 9,* 35.

Hollander, E., Phillips, A., Chaplin, W., Zagursky, K., Novotny, S., Wasserman, S., et al. (2005). A placebo controlled crossover trial of liquid fluoxetine on repetitive behaviors in childhood and adolescent autism. *Neuropsychopharmacology, 30,* 582–589.

Huang, Y., Kotov, R., de Girolamo, G., Preti, A., Angermeyer, M., Benjet, C., et al. (2009). DSM-IV personality disorders in the WHO World Mental Health Surveys. *British Journal of Psychiatry, 195*, 46–53.

Isohanni, M., Murray, G. K., Jokelainen, J., Croudace, T., & Jones, P. B. (2004). The persistence of developmental markers in childhood and adolescence and risk for schizophrenic psychoses in adult life. A 34-year follow-up of the northern Finland 1966 birth cohort. *Schizophrenia Research, 71*(2–3), 213–225.

James, D. J., & Glaze, L. E. (2006). Mental health problems of prison and jail inmates. Washington, DC: U.S. Department of Justice, Office of Justice Programs. Retrieved November 11, 2009, from http://www.ojp.usdoj.gov/bjs/pub/pdf/mhppji.pdf

Jefferson, J. W. (2003). Book forum: Psychopharmacology. *American Journal of Psychiatry, 160*, 1198–1199.

Jibson, M., Glick, I., & Tandon, R. (2004). Schizophrenia and other psychotic disorders. *Focus, 2*(1), 17–30.

Johnson, C. P., & Myers, S. M. (2007). Identification and evaluation of children with autism spectrum disorders. *Pediatrics, 120*, 1183–1215.

Johnson, J. G., Smailes, E. M., Cohen, P., Brown, J., & Bernstein, D. P. (2000). Associations between four types of childhood neglect and personality disorder symptoms during adolescence and early adulthood: Findings of a community-based longitudinal study. *Journal of Personality Disorders, 14*, 171–187.

Kahn, R. S., Fleischhacker, W. W., Boter, H., Davidson, M., Vergouwe, Y., Keet, I. P., et al. (2008). Effectiveness of antipsychotic drugs in first-episode schizophrenia and schizophreniform disorder: An open randomized clinical trial. *Lancet, 371*, 1085–1097.

Katerndahl, D. A., & Realini, J. P. (1993). Lifetime prevalence of panic states. *American Journal of Psychiatry, 150*(2), 246–249.

Kaur, N. *Humee hum and peace and tranquility* (audio recording). Available at http://www.spiritvoyage.com/

Keefe, R. S., Mohs, R. C., Bilder, R. M., Harvey, P. D., Green, M. F., Meltzer, H. Y., et al. (2003). Neurocognitive assessment in the Clinical Antipsychotic Trials of Intervention Effectiveness (CATIE) project schizophrenia trial: Development, methodology, and rationale. *Schizophrenia Bulletin, 29*(1), 45–55.

Kelly, T., Soloff, P., Cornelius, J., George, A., Lis, J., & Ulrich, R. (1992). Can we study (treat) borderline patients? Attrition from research and open treatment. *Journal of Personality Disorders, 6*, 417–433.

Kessler, R. C., Crum, R. M., Warner, L. A., Nelson, C. B., Schulenberg, J., & Anthony, J. C. (1997). Lifetime co-occurrence of DSM-III-R alcohol abuse and dependence with other psychiatric disorders in the national comorbidity survey. *Archives of General Psychiatry, 54,* 313–321.

Kessler, R. C., McGonagle, K. A., Zhao, S., Nelson, C. B., Hughes, M., Eshleman, S., et al. (1994). Lifetime and 12-month prevalence of DSM-III-R psychiatric disorders in the United States. Results from the national comorbidity survey. *Archives of General Psychiatry, 51,* 8–19.

Kessler, R. C., Nelson, C. B., McGonagle, K. A., Liu, J., Swartz, M., & Blazer, D. G. (1996). Comorbidity of DSM-III-R major depressive disorder in the general population: Results from the US national comorbidity survey. *British Journal of Psychiatry Supplement,* (30), 17–30.

Kessler, R. C., Stein, M. B., & Berglund, P. (1998). Social phobia subtypes in the national comorbidity survey. *American Journal of Psychiatry, 155,* 613–619.

Kessler, R. C., & Wang, P. S. (2008). The descriptive epidemiology of commonly occurring mental disorders in the United States. *Annual Review of Public Health, 29,* 115–129.

Khalsa, H. K. (2006). *Infinity and me—Kundalini yoga as taught by Yogi Bhajan.* Espanola, NM: Kundalini Research Institute.

Khalsa, S. K. (2000). *Tantric har and har haray haree wahe guru* (Audio recording). Available at http://www.spiritvoyage.com

Kilcommons, A. M., & Morrison, A. P. (2005). Relationships between trauma and psychosis: An exploration of cognitive and dissociative factors. *Acta Psychiatrica Scandinavica, 112,* 351–359.

Kim-Cohen, J., Caspi, A., Moffitt, T. E., Harrington, H., Milne, B. J., & Poulton, R. (2003). Prior juvenile diagnoses in adults with mental disorder: Developmental follow-back of a prospective-longitudinal cohort. *Archives of General Psychiatry, 60,* 709–717.

King, B. H., & Bostic, J. Q. (2006). An update on pharmacologic treatments for autism spectrum disorders. *Child and Adolescent Psychiatric Clinics of North America, 15*(1), 161–175.

King, B. H., Hollander, E., Sikich, L., McCracken, J. T., Scahill, L., Bregman, J. D., et al. (2009). Lack of efficacy of citalopram in children with autism spectrum disorders and high levels of repetitive behavior: Citalopram ineffective in children with autism. *Archives of General Psychiatry, 66,* 583–590.

Kitamura, T., Okazaki, Y., Fujinawa, A., Takayanagi, I., & Kasahara, Y. (1998). Dimensions of schizophrenic positive symptoms: An exploratory factor analysis investigation. *European Archives of Psychiatry and Clinical Neuroscience, 248*(3), 130–135.

Kleindienst, N., Limberger, M. F., Schmahl, C., Steil, R., Ebner-Priemer,

U. W., & Bohus, M. (2008). Do improvements after inpatient dialectical behavioral therapy persist in the long term? A naturalistic follow-up in patients with borderline personality disorder. *Journal of Nervous and Mental Disease, 196*, 847–851.

Klin, A., Pauls, D., Schultz, R., & Volkmar, F. (2005). Three diagnostic approaches to Asperger syndrome: Implications for research. *Journal of Autism and Developmental Disorders, 35*, 221–234.

Koch, J. L. (1891). *Die Psychopatischen Minderwertigkeiter*. Ravensburg, Germany: Meier.

Kool, S., Dekker, J., Duijsens, I. J., de Jonghe, F., & Puite, B. (2003). Changes in personality pathology after pharmacotherapy and combined therapy for depressed patients. *Journal of Personality Disorders, 17*(1), 60–72.

Koons, C. R., Robins, C. J., JL, T., Lynch, T., Gonzalez, A., Morse, J., et al. (2001). Efficacy of dialectical behavior therapy in women veterans with borderline personality disorder: A randomized controlled trial. *Behavior Therapy, 32*, 371–390.

Kotsaftis, A., & Neale, J. M. (1993). Schizotypal personality disorder 1: The clinical syndrome. *Clinical Psychology Review, 13*, 451–472.

Kovacs, M. (1990). Comorbid anxiety disorders in childhood-onset depression. In J. Maser & R. Cloninger (Eds.), *Comorbidity of mood and anxiety disorders* (pp. 271–282). Washington, DC: American Psychiatric Press.

Kraepelin, E. (1913). *Psychiatrie: Ein Lehrbuch* (8th ed., vol. 3). Leipzig, Germany: Barth.

Kroll, J. L. (2007). New directions in the conceptualization of psychotic disorders. *Current Opinion in Psychiatry, 20*, 573–577.

Krueger, R. F., Skodol, A. E., Livesley, W. J., Shrout, P. E., & Huang, Y. (2007). Synthesizing dimensional and categorical approaches to personality disorders: Refining the research agenda for DSM-IV axis II. *International Journal of Methods in Psychiatry Research, 16* (Suppl. 1), S65–S73.

Kuban, K. C., O'Shea, T. M., Allred, E. N., Tager-Flusberg, H., Goldstein, D. J., & Leviton, A. (2009). Positive screening on the modified checklist for autism in toddlers (M-CHAT) in extremely low gestational age newborns. *Journal of Pediatrics, 154*, 535–540, e531.

Kuehn, B. M. (2007). CDC: Autism spectrum disorders common. *JAMA, 297*, 940.

Lakka, H. M., Laaksonen, D. E., Lakka, T. A., Niskanen, L. K., Kumpusalo, E., Tuomilehto, J., et al. (2002). The metabolic syndrome and total and cardiovascular disease mortality in middle-aged men. *JAMA, 288*, 2709–2716.

Lamberti, J. S., Costea, G. O., Olson, D., Crilly, J. F., Maharaj, K., Tu, X., et al.

(2005). Diabetes mellitus among outpatients receiving clozapine: Prevalence and clinical-demographic correlates. *Journal of Clinical Psychiatry, 66,* 900–906.

Lamberti, J. S., Olson, D., Crilly, J. F., Olivares, T., Williams, G. C., Tu, X., et al. (2006). Prevalence of the metabolic syndrome among patients receiving clozapine. *American Journal of Psychiatry, 163,* 1273–1276.

Lauriello, J. (2004). Schizophrenia (editorial). *Focus, 2*(1), 5.

Laursen, T. M., Agerbo, E., & Pedersen, C. B. (2009). Bipolar disorder, schizoaffective disorder, and schizophrenia overlap: A new comorbidity index. *Journal of Clinical Psychiatry,* Epub, June 16.

Leckman, J. F., & Leventhal, B. L. (2008). Editorial: A global perspective on child and adolescent mental health. *Journal of Child Psychology and Psychiatry, 49,* 221–225.

Leff, J., Sartorius, N., Jablensky, A., Korten, A., & Ernberg, G. (1992). The international pilot study of schizophrenia: Five-year follow-up findings. *Psychological Medicine, 22*(1), 131–145.

Leichsenring, F., & Leibing, E. (2003). The effectiveness of psychodynamic therapy and cognitive behavior therapy in the treatment of personality disorders: A meta-analysis. *American Journal of Psychiatry, 160,* 1223–1232.

Lemoine, P., Harousseau, H., Borteyru, J. P., & Menuet, J. C. (2003). Children of alcoholic parents—observed anomalies: Discussion of 127 cases. *Therapeutic Drug Monitoring, 25*(2), 132–136.

Lenzenweger, M. F. (2008). Epidemiology of personality disorders. *Psychiatric Clinics of North America, 31,* 395–403, vi.

Lenzenweger, M. F., Lane, M. C., Loranger, A. W., & Kessler, R. C. (2007). DSM-IV personality disorders in the national comorbidity survey replication. *Biological Psychiatry, 62,* 553–564.

Leonard, K. (1999). *Classification of endogenous psychoses and their differentiated etiology* (2nd ed.). Vienna: Springer.

Lewinsohn, P. M., Rohde, P., & Seeley, J. R. (1995). Adolescent psychopathology: III. The clinical consequences of comorbidity. *Journal of the American Academy of Child and Adolescent Psychiatry, 34,* 510–519.

Lieberman, J. A., Stroup, T. S., McEvoy, J. P., Swartz, M. S., Rosenheck, R. A., Perkins, D. O., et al. (2005). Effectiveness of antipsychotic drugs in patients with chronic schizophrenia. *New England Journal of Medicine, 353,* 1209–1223.

Linehan, M. M. (1987). Dialectical behavior therapy for borderline personality disorder. Theory and method. *Bulletin of the Menninger Clinic, 51*(3), 261–276.

Linehan, M. M. (1993). *Cognitive-behavioral treatment of borderline personality disorder*. New York: Guilford.

Linehan, M. M., Armstrong, H. E., Suarez, A., Allmon, D., & Heard, H. L. (1991). Cognitive-behavioral treatment of chronically parasuicidal borderline patients. *Archives of General Psychiatry, 48*, 1060–1064.

Linehan, M. M., Heard, H. L., & Armstrong, H. E. (1993). Naturalistic follow-up of a behavioral treatment for chronically parasuicidal borderline patients. *Archives of General Psychiatry, 50*, 971–974.

Linehan, M. M., McDavid, J. D., Brown, M. Z., Sayrs, J. H., & Gallop, R. J. (2008). Olanzapine plus dialectical behavior therapy for women with high irritability who meet criteria for borderline personality disorder: A double-blind, placebo-controlled pilot study. *Journal of Clinical Psychiatry, 69*, 999–1005.

Liu, X. Q., Paterson, A. D., & Szatmari, P. (2008). Genome-wide linkage analyses of quantitative and categorical autism subphenotypes. *Biological Psychiatry, 64*, 561–570.

Lord, C., Bristol-Power, M., Cafiero, J. M., Filipek, P. A., Gallagher, J. J., Harris, S. L., et al. (2002). NAS workshop papers. *Journal of Autism and Developmental Disorders, 32*, 349–350.

Maki, P., Veijola, J., Jones, P. B., Murray, G. K., Koponen, H., Tienari, P., et al. (2005). Predictors of schizophrenia—a review. *British Medical Bulletin, 73/74*, 1–15.

Mandell, D. S., Morales, K. H., Marcus, S. C., Stahmer, A. C., Doshi, J., & Polsky, D. E. (2008). Psychotropic medication use among Medicaid-enrolled children with autism spectrum disorders. *Pediatrics, 121*, 441–448.

Markowitz, J. C. (2005). Interpersonal therapy. In J. M. Oldham, A. E. Skodol, & D. S. Bender (Eds.), *Textbook of personality disorders* (pp. 321–334). Washington, DC: American Psychiatric Publishing.

Markowitz, J. C., Skodol, A. E., & Bleiberg, K. (2006). Interpersonal psychotherapy for borderline personality disorder: Possible mechanisms of change. *Journal of Clinical Psychology, 62*, 431–444.

Martin, R. L., Cloninger, C. R., Guze, S. B., & Clayton, P. J. (1985). Frequency and differential diagnosis of depressive syndromes in schizophrenia. *Journal of Clinical Psychiatry, 46*(11 Pt. 2), 9–13.

Massion, A. O., Warshaw, M. G., & Keller, M. B. (1993). Quality of life and psychiatric morbidity in panic disorder and generalized anxiety disorder. *American Journal of Psychiatry, 150*, 600–607.

Masters, K. J. (1995). Environmental trauma and psychosis. *Journal of the American Academy of Child and Adolescent Psychiatry, 34*, 12581259.

Maudsley, H. (1874). *Responsibility in mental disease*. London: King.

McCracken, J. T., McGough, J., Shah, B., Cronin, P., Hong, D., Aman, M. G., et al. (2002). Risperidone in children with autism and serious behavioral problems. *New England Journal of Medicine, 347,* 314–321.

McDougle, C. J., Naylor, S. T., Cohen, D. J., Volkmar, F. R., Heninger, G. R., & Price, L. H. (1996). A double-blind, placebo-controlled study of fluvoxamine in adults with autistic disorder. *Archives of General Psychiatry, 53,* 1001–1008.

McEvoy, J. P., Lieberman, J. A., Stroup, T. S., Davis, S. M., Meltzer, H. Y., Rosenheck, R. A., et al. (2006). Effectiveness of clozapine versus olanzapine, quetiapine, and risperidone in patients with chronic schizophrenia who did not respond to prior atypical antipsychotic treatment. *American Journal of Psychiatry, 163,* 600–610.

McEvoy, J. P., Meyer, J. M., Goff, D. C., Nasrallah, H. A., Davis, S. M., Sullivan, L., et al. (2005). Prevalence of the metabolic syndrome in patients with schizophrenia: Baseline results from the Clinical Antipsychotic Trials of Intervention Effectiveness (CATIE) schizophrenia trial and comparison with national estimates from NHANES III. *Schizophrenia Research, 80*(1), 19–32.

McGlashan, T. H., Grilo, C. M., Skodol, A. E., Gunderson, J. G., Shea, M. T., Morey, L. C., et al. (2000). The collaborative longitudinal personality disorders study: Baseline axis I/II and II/II diagnostic co-occurrence. *Acta Psychiatrica Scandinavica, 102,* 256–264.

McGrath, J., Saha, S., Welham, J., El Saadi, O., MacCauley, C., & Chant, D. (2004). A systematic review of the incidence of schizophrenia: The distribution of rates and the influence of sex, urbanicity, migrant status and methodology. *BMC Medicine, 2,* 13.

McGrath, J. J. (2005). Myths and plain truths about schizophrenia epidemiology—the Nape lecture 2004. *Acta Psychiatrica Scandinavica, 111,* 4–11.

Messias, E. L., Chen, C. Y., & Eaton, W. W. (2007). Epidemiology of schizophrenia: Review of findings and myths. *Psychiatric Clinics of North America, 30,* 323–338.

Meyer, J. M., & Koro, C. E. (2004). The effects of antipsychotic therapy on serum lipids: A comprehensive review. *Schizophrenia Research, 70*(1), 1–17.

Miller, B. L., Cummings, J., Mishkin, F., Boone, K., Prince, F., Ponton, M., et al. (1998). Emergence of artistic talent in frontotemporal dementia. *Neurology, 51,* 978–982.

Millon, T., & Davis, R. (2000). *Personality disorders in modern life.* New York: Wiley.

Mirenda, P. (2001). Autism, augmentative communication, and assistive technology: What do we really know? *Focus on Autism and Other Developmental Disabilities, 16*, 141–151.

Moran, P. (1999). The epidemiology of antisocial personality disorder. *Social Psychiatry and Psychiatric Epidemiology, 34*, 231–242.

Morgan, C., & Fisher, H. (2007). Environment and schizophrenia: Environmental factors in schizophrenia: Childhood trauma—a critical review. *Schizophrenia Bulletin, 33*(1), 3–10.

Morrison, J. R. (1974). Changes in subtype diagnosis of schizophrenia: 1920–1966. *American Journal of Psychiatry, 131*, 674–677.

Mueser, K. T., Goodman, L. B., Trumbetta, S. L., Rosenberg, S. D., Osher, C., Vidaver, R., et al. (1998). Trauma and posttraumatic stress disorder in severe mental illness. *Journal of Consulting and Clinical Psychology, 66*, 493–499.

Murray, R. M., & Lewis, S. W. (1987). Is schizophrenia a neurodevelopmental disorder? *British Medical Journal (Clinical Research Edition), 295*, 681–682.

Mutter, J., Naumann, J., & Guethlin, C. (2007). Comments on the article "The toxicology of mercury and its chemical compounds" by Clarkson and Magos (2006). *Critical Reviews of Toxicology, 37*, 537–549; discussion 551–532.

NASMHPD. (2001). *Technical report on psychiatric polypharmacy*. Alexandria, VA: National Association of State Mental Health Program Directors.

Newcomer, J. W. (2005). Second-generation (atypical) antipsychotics and metabolic effects: A comprehensive literature review. *CNS Drugs, 19*(Suppl. 1), 1–93.

Newschaffer, C. J., Croen, L. A., Daniels, J., Giarelli, E., Grether, J. K., Levy, S. E., et al. (2007). The epidemiology of autism spectrum disorders. *Annual Review of Public Health, 28*, 235–258.

NRC. (2001). *Educating children with autism*. Washington, DC: National Academy Press Committee on Educational Interventions for Children with Autism. Division of Behavioral and Social Sciences and Education.

Oldham, J. M. (2005). Personality disorders. *FOCUS: The Journal of Lifelong Learning in Psychiatry, 3*, 372–382.

Oldham, J. M., Skodol, A. E., & Bender, D. S. (2005). *The American Psychiatric Publishing textbook of personality disorders*. Washington, DC: American Psychiatric Publishing.

Oldham, J. M., Skodol, A. E., Kellman, H. D., Hyler, S. E., Doidge, N., Rosnick, L., et al. (1995). Comorbidity of axis I and axis II disorders. *American Journal of Psychiatry, 152*, 571–578.

Oswald, D. P., & Sonenklar, N. A. (2007). Medication use among children with autism spectrum disorders. *Journal of Child and Adolescent Psycho-pharmacology, 17*, 348–355.

Parks, C. E. (2007). Psychoanalytic approaches to work with children with severe developmental and biological disorders. Panel report. *Journal of the American Psychoanalytic Association, 55*, 923–935.

Perry, J. C., Banon, E., & Ianni, F. (1999). Effectiveness of psychotherapy for personality disorders. *American Journal of Psychiatry, 156*, 1312–1321.

Petersen, B., Toft, J., Christensen, N. B., Foldager, L., Munk-Jorgensen, P., Lien, K., et al. (2008). Outcome of a psychotherapeutic programme for patients with severe personality disorders. *Nordic Journal of Psychiatry, 62*, 450–456.

Pinel, P. (1801). *Traite medico-philosophique sur l'alienation mentale.* Paris: Richard, Caille et Ravier.

Pinel, P., & Maudsley, H. (1977). *Treatise on insanity; Responsibility in mental disease: two works. series C medical psychology. Vol. 3.* Bethesda, MD: University Publications of America.

Piper, W. E., & Ogrodniczuk, J. S. (2004). Brief group therapy. In J. Delucia-Waack, D. A. Gerrity, C. Kalodner, et al. (Eds.), *Handbook of group counseling and psychotherapy* (pp. 641–650). Beverly Hills, CA: Sage.

Piper, W. E., & Ogrodniczuk, J. S. (2005). Group treatment. In J. M. Oldham, A. E. Skodol, & D. S. Bender (Eds.), *Textbook of personality disorders* (pp. 347–357). Washington, DC: American Psychiatric Publishing.

Pokos, V., & Castle, D. J. (2006). Prevalence of comorbid anxiety disorders in schizophrenia spectrum disorders: A literature review. *Current Psychiatry Reviews, 2*, 285–307.

Polimeni, M. A., Richdale, A. L., & Francis, A. J. (2005). A survey of sleep problems in autism, Asperger's disorder and typically developing children. *Journal of Intellectual Disability Research, 49*(Pt. 4), 260–268.

Posey, D. J., & McDougle, C. J. (2000). The pharmacotherapy of target symptoms associated with autistic disorder and other pervasive developmental disorders. *Harvard Review of Psychiatry, 8*(2), 45–63.

Prichard, J. C. (1835). *A treatise on insanity, and other disorders affecting the mind.* London: Sherwood, Gilbert and Piper.

Pulay, A. J., Dawson, D. A., Ruan, W. J., Pickering, R. P., Huang, B., Chou, S. P., et al. (2008). The relationship of impairment to personality disorder severity among individuals with specific axis I disorders: Results from the national epidemiologic survey on alcohol and related conditions. *Journal of Personality Disorders, 22*, 405–417.

Pulay, A. J., Stinson, F. S., Dawson, D. A., Goldstein, R. B., Chou, S. P., Huang, B., et al. (2009). Prevalence, correlates, disability, and comorbidity of DSM-

IV schizotypal personality disorder: Results from the wave 2 national epidemiologic survey on alcohol and related conditions. *Prim Care Companion to the Journal of Clinical Psychiatry, 11*(2), 53–67.

Raine, A. (2006). Schizotypal personality: Neurodevelopmental and psychosocial trajectories. *Annual Review of Clinical Psychology, 2*, 291–326.

Ram, R., Bromet, E. J., Eaton, W. W., Pato, C., & Schwartz, J. E. (1992). The
natural course of schizophrenia: A review of first-admission studies. *Schizophrenia Bulletin, 18*(2), 185–207.

Regier, D. A., Farmer, M. E., Rae, D. S., Locke, B. Z., Keith, S. J., Judd, L. L., et
al. (1990). Comorbidity of mental disorders with alcohol and other drug
abuse. Results from the epidemiologic catchment area (ECA) study.
JAMA, 264, 2511–2518.

Regier, D. A., Rae, D. S., Narrow, W. E., Kaelber, C. T., & Schatzberg, A. F.
(1998). Prevalence of anxiety disorders and their comorbidity with mood
and addictive disorders. *British Journal of Psychiatry Supplement*, (34), 24–
28.

Remington, G., Sloman, L., Konstantareas, M., Parker, K., & Gow, R. (2001).
Clomipramine versus haloperidol in the treatment of autistic disorder: A
double-blind, placebo-controlled, crossover study. *Journal of Clinical Psychopharmacology, 21*, 440–444.

Reynolds, G. P. (2007). Schizophrenia, antipsychotics and metabolic disease.
Journal of Psychopharmacology, 21, 355–356.

Richler, J., Bishop, S. L., Kleinke, J. R., & Lord, C. (2007). Restricted and repetitive behaviors in young children with autism spectrum disorders. *Journal of Autism and Developmental Disorders, 37*(1), 73–85.

Rimland, B. (1978a). *Infantile autism: The syndrome and its implications for a
neural theory of behavior*. New York: Appleton-Century-Crofts.

Rimland, B. (1978b). Savant capabilities of autistic children and their cognitive implications. In G. Serban (Ed.), *Cognitive defects in the development of
mental illness*. New York: Brunner/Mazel.

Robins, C., Ivanoff, A., & Linehan, M. M. (2001). Dialectical behavior therapy. In W. Livesley (Ed.), *Handbook of personality disorders: Theory, research, and treatment* (pp. 117–139). New York: Guilford.

Robins, L. N., & Regier, D. A. (Eds.). (1991). *Psychiatric disorders in America:
The Epidemiological Catchment Area Study*. New York: Free Press.

Ross, C. A., & Joshi, S. (1992). Schneiderian symptoms and childhood trauma
in the general population. *Comprehensive Psychiatry, 33*, 269–273.

Rusch, N., Schiel, S., Corrigan, P. W., Leihener, F., Jacob, G. A., Olschewski,
M., et al. (2008). Predictors of dropout from inpatient dialectical behavior

therapy among women with borderline personality disorder. *Journal of Behavior Therapy and Experimental Psychiatry, 39,* 497–503.

Rush, B. (1812). *Medical inquiries and observations upon the diseases of the mind.* Philadelphia, PA: Kimber and Richardson.

Rutter, M., Kim-Cohen, J., & Maughan, B. (2006). Continuities and discontinuities in psychopathology between childhood and adult life. *Journal of Child Psychology and Psychiatry, 47*(3–4), 276–295.

SAMSA. (2008). *Results from the 2007 national survey on drug use and health: National findings.* Washington, DC: Substance Abuse and Mental Health Services Administration Office of Applied Studies.

Sanders, A. R., Duan, J., Levinson, D. F., Shi, J., He, D., Hou, C., et al. (2008). No significant association of 14 candidate genes with schizophrenia in a large European ancestry sample: Implications for psychiatric genetics. *American Journal of Psychiatry, 165,* 497–506.

Sanderson, W. C., DiNardo, P. A., Rapee, R. M., & Barlow, D. H. (1990). Syndrome comorbidity in patients diagnosed with a DSM-III-R anxiety disorder. *Journal of Abnormal Psychology, 99,* 308–312.

Schechter, R., & Grether, J. K. (2008). Continuing increases in autism reported to California's developmental services system: Mercury in retrograde. *Archives of General Psychiatry, 65*(1), 19–24.

Scheller-Gilkey, G., Moynes, K., Cooper, I., Kant, C., & Miller, A. H. (2004). Early life stress and PTSD symptoms in patients with comorbid schizophrenia and substance abuse. *Schizophrenia Research, 69*(2–3), 167–174.

Schlesinger, A., & Silk, K. R. (2005). Collaborative treatment. In J. M. Oldham, A. E. Skodol, & D. S. Bender (Eds.), *Textbook of personality disorders* (pp. 431–446). Washington, DC: American Psychiatric Publishing.

Schneider, K. (1958). *Psychopathic personalities* (9th ed., M. Hamilton, trans.). London: Cassell.

Shannahoff-Khalsa, D. (2008). Psychophysiological states: The ultradian dynamics of mind-body interactions. San Diego, CA: Academic Press/Elsevier.

Shannahoff-Khalsa, D. (2009). A single case history of hallucinations, nostril dominance, and unilateral forced nostril breathing. Manuscript submitted for publication.

Shannahoff-Khalsa, D., & Bhajan, Y. (1988). Sound current therapy and self-healing: The ancient science of NAD and mantra yoga. *International Journal of Music, Dance and Art Therapy, 1*(4), 183–192.

Shannahoff-Khalsa, D., & Bhajan, Y. (1991). The healing power of sound:

Techniques from yogic medicine. In R. Droh & R. Spintge (Eds.), *Music-medicine* (pp. 179–193).,Gilsum, NH: Barcelona Publishers.

Shannahoff-Khalsa, D., Ray, L., Levine, S., Gallen, C., Schwartz, B., & Sidorowich, J. (1999). Randomized controlled trial of yogic meditation techniques for patients with obsessive compulsive disorders. *CNS Spectrums: The International Journal of Neuropsychiatric Medicine, 4*(12), 34–46.

Shannahoff-Khalsa, D. S. (1997). Yogic techniques are effective in the treatment of obsessive compulsive disorders. In E. Hollander & D. Stein (Eds.), *Obsessive-compulsive disorders: Diagnosis, etiology, and treatment* (pp. 283–329). New York: Marcel Dekker.

Shannahoff-Khalsa, D. S. (2003). Kundalini yoga meditation techniques in the treatment of obsessive compulsive and OC spectrum disorders. *Brief Treatment and Crisis Intervention, 3,* 369–382.

Shannahoff-Khalsa, D. S. (2004). An introduction to Kundalini yoga meditation techniques that are specific for the treatment of psychiatric disorders. *Journal of Alternative and Complementary Medicine, 10*(1), 91–101.

Shannahoff-Khalsa, D. S. (2005). Patient perspectives: Kundalini yoga meditation techniques for psycho-oncology and as potential therapies for cancer. *Integrated Cancer Therapies, 4*(1), 87–100.

Shannahoff-Khalsa, D. S. (2006). *Kundalini Yoga meditation: Techniques specific for psychiatric disorders, couples therapy, and personal growth.* New York: Norton.

Shannahoff-Khalsa, D. S. (2007). Selective unilateral autonomic activation: Implications for psychiatry. *CNS Spectrums: The International Journal of Neuropsychiatric Medicine, 12,* 625–634.

Shannahoff-Khalsa, D. S., & Beckett, L. R. (1996). Clinical case report: Efficacy of yogic techniques in the treatment of obsessive compulsive disorders. *International Journal of Neuroscience, 85*(1–2), 1–17.

Shevlin, M., Dorahy, M., Adamson, G., & Murphy, J. (2007). Subtypes of borderline personality disorder, associated clinical disorders and stressful life-events: A latent class analysis based on the British psychiatric morbidity survey. *British Journal of Clinical Psychology, 46*(Pt. 3), 273–281.

Shevlin, M., Houston, J. E., Dorahy, M. J., & Adamson, G. (2008). Cumulative traumas and psychosis: An analysis of the national comorbidity survey and the British psychiatric morbidity survey. *Schizophrenia Bulletin, 34*(1), 193–199.

Sholevar, G. P. (2005). Family therapy. In J. M. Oldham, A. E. Skodol, & D. S. Bender (Eds.), *Textbook of personality disorders* (pp. 359–373). Washington, DC: American Psychiatric Publishing.

Simpson, E. B., Yen, S., Costello, E., Rosen, K., Begin, A., Pistorello, J., et al.

(2004). Combined dialectical behavior therapy and fluoxetine in the treatment of borderline personality disorder. *Journal of Clinical Psychiatry, 65,* 379–385.

Singh, J. (1996). *Sat nam wahe guru # 2 tantric version.* Retrieved July 30, 2009, from http://ahw.stores.yahoo.net/16317.html

Skodol, A. E., Gunderson, J. G., McGlashan, T. H., Dyck, I. R., Stout, R. L., Bender, D. S., et al. (2002). Functional impairment in patients with schizotypal, borderline, avoidant, or obsessive-compulsive personality disorder. *American Journal of Psychiatry, 159,* 276–283.

Soeteman, D. I., Hakkaart-van Roijen, L., Verheul, R., & Busschbach, J. J. (2008). The economic burden of personality disorders in mental health care. *Journal of Clinical Psychiatry, 69,* 259–265.

Soler, J., Pascual, J. C., Campins, J., Barrachina, J., Puigdemont, D., Alvarez, E., et al. (2005). Double-blind, placebo-controlled study of dialectical behavior therapy plus olanzapine for borderline personality disorder. *American Journal of Psychiatry, 162,* 1221–1224.

Soloff, P. (2005). Somatic treatments. In J. M. Oldham, A. E. Skodol, & D. S. Bender (Eds.), *Textbook of personality disorders* (pp. 387–403). Washington, DC: American Psychiatric Publishing.

Stanley, B., & Brodsky, B. (2005). Dialectical behavior therapy. In J. M. Oldham, A. E. Skodol, & D. S. Bender (Eds.), *Textbook of personality disorders* (pp. 307–320). Washington, DC: American Psychiatric Publishing.

Stanley, B., Bundy, E., & Beberman, R. (2001). Skills training as an adjunctive treatment for personality disorders. *Journal of Psychiatric Practice, 7,* 324–335.

Starling, J., & Dossetor, D. (2009). Pervasive developmental disorders and psychosis. *Current Psychiatry Reports, 11*(3), 190–196.

Steinbrook, R. (2002). Testing medications in children. *New England Journal of Medicine, 347,* 1462–1470.

Stinson, F. S., Dawson, D. A., Goldstein, R. B., Chou, S. P., Huang, B., Smith, S. M., et al. (2008). Prevalence, correlates, disability, and comorbidity of DSM-IV narcissistic personality disorder: Results from the wave 2 national epidemiologic survey on alcohol and related conditions. *Journal of Clinical Psychiatry, 69,* 1033–1045.

Stoffers, J., Lieb, K., Vollm, B., et al., (in press). Pharmacotherapy of borderline personality disorder. *Cochrane Database of Systematic Reviews.*

Stompe, T., Ortwein-Swoboda, G., Ritter, K., Marquart, B., & Schanda, H. (2005). The impact of diagnostic criteria on the prevalence of schizophrenic subtypes. *Comprehensive Psychiatry, 46,* 433–439.

Strauss, J. L., Calhoun, P. S., Marx, C. E., Stechuchak, K. M., Oddone, E. Z.,

Swartz, M. S., et al. (2006). Comorbid posttraumatic stress disorder is associated with suicidality in male veterans with schizophrenia or schizoaffective disorder. *Schizophrenia Research, 84*(1), 165–169.

Stroup, T. S., Lieberman, J. A., McEvoy, J. P., Swartz, M. S., Davis, S. M., Rosenheck, R. A., et al. (2006). Effectiveness of olanzapine, quetiapine, risperidone, and ziprasidone in patients with chronic schizophrenia following discontinuation of a previous atypical antipsychotic. *American Journal of Psychiatry, 163,* 611–622.

Stroup, T. S., McEvoy, J. P., Swartz, M. S., Byerly, M. J., Glick, I. D., Canive, J. M., et al. (2003). The National Institute of Mental Health Clinical Antipsychotic Trials of Intervention Effectiveness (CATIE) project: Schizophrenia trial design and protocol development. *Schizophrenia Bulletin, 29*(1), 15–31.

Szatmari, P., Paterson, A. D., Zwaigenbaum, L., Roberts, W., Brian, J., Liu, X. Q., et al. (2007). Mapping autism risk loci using genetic linkage and chromosomal rearrangements. *Nature Genetics, 39,* 319–328.

Tamminga, C. A. (2006). Practical treatment information for schizophrenia. *American Journal of Psychiatry, 163,* 563–565.

Tanguay, P. (1973). *A tentative hypothesis regarding the role of hemispheric specialization in early infantile autism.* Unpublished manuscript, Los Angeles.

Tanielian, T. L., Marcus, S. C., Suarez, A. P., & Pincus, H. A. (2001). Datapoints: Trends in psychiatric practice, 1988–1998: II. Caseload and treatment characteristics. *Psychiatric Services, 52,* 880.

Teusch, L., Bohme, H., Finke, J., & Gastpar, M. (2001). Effects of client-centered psychotherapy for personality disorders alone and in combination with psychopharmacological treatment. *Psychotherapy and Psychosomatics, 70,* 328–336.

Toneatto, T., & Nguyen, L. (2007). Does mindfulness meditation improve anxiety and mood symptoms? A review of the controlled research. *Canadian Journal of Psychiatry, 52,* 260–266.

Torgersen, S. (2005). Epidemiology. In J. M. Oldham, A. E. Skodol, & D. S. Bender (Eds.), *Textbook of personality disorders* (pp. 129–141). Washington, DC: American Psychiatric Publishing.

Torgersen, S., Kringlen, E., & Cramer, V. (2001). The prevalence of personality disorders in a community sample. *Archives of General Psychiatry, 58,* 590–596.

Treffert, D. (1989). *Extraordinary people: Understanding savant syndrome.* New York: Harper & Row.

Treffert, D. A. (2006). *Savant syndrome: An extraordinary condition, a synopsis: Past, present, future.* Madison, WI: Wisconsin Medical Society.

Tsai, L. Y. (2007). Asperger syndrome and medication treatment. *Focus on Autism and Other Developmental Disabilities, 22*(3), 138–148.

UNICEF. (2007). *Innocenti report card 7: Child poverty in perspective: An overview of child well-being in rich countries.* New York: United Nations Children's Fund.

van Asselt, A. D., Dirksen, C. D., Arntz, A., Giesen-Bloo, J. H., van Dyck, R., Spinhoven, P., et al. (2008). Out-patient psychotherapy for borderline personality disorder: Cost-effectiveness of schema-focused therapy V. Transference-focused psychotherapy. *British Journal of Psychiatry, 192,* 450–457.

Ventegodt, S., & Merrick, J. (2009). A review of side effects and adverse events of non-drug medicine (nonpharmaceutical complementary and alternative medicine): Psychotherapy, mind-body medicine and clinical holistic medicine. *Journal of Complementary and Integrative Medicine, 6*(1), 1–28.

Verheul, R., & Herbrink, M. (2007). The efficacy of various modalities of psychotherapy for personality disorders: A systematic review of the evidence and clinical recommendations. *International Review of Psychiatry, 19*(1), 25–38.

Verheul, R., Van Den Bosch, L. M., Koeter, M. W., De Ridder, M. A., Stijnen, T., & Van Den Brink, W. (2003). Dialectical behavior therapy for women with borderline personality disorder: 12-month, randomized clinical trial in the Netherlands. *British Journal of Psychiatry, 182,* 135–140.

Verheul, R., & Widiger, T. A. (2004). A meta-analysis of the prevalence and usage of the personality disorder not otherwise specified (PDNOS) diagnosis. *Journal of Personality Disorders, 18,* 309–319.

Volkmar, F. R. (2009). Citalopram treatment in children with autism spectrum disorders and high levels of repetitive behavior. *Archives of General Psychiatry, 66,* 581–582.

Volkow, N. D. (2009). Substance use disorders in schizophrenia—clinical implications of comorbidity. *Schizophrenia Bulletin, 35,* 469–472.

Waldman, M., Nicholson, S., Adilov, N., & Williams, J. (2008). Autism prevalence and precipitation rates in California, Oregon, and Washington counties. *Archives of Pediatrics and Adolescent Medicine, 162,* 1026–1034.

Webber, M. A., & Farrell, J. M. (2008). Pharmacotherapy of borderline personality disorder. *Psychopharmacology Review, 42*(11), 83–90.

Weber, N. S., Cowan, D. N., Millikan, A. M., & Niebuhr, D. W. (2009). Psychiatric and general medical conditions comorbid with schizophrenia in the national hospital discharge survey. *Psychiatric Services, 60,* 1059–1067.

Weinberger, D. R. (1995). From neuropathology to neurodevelopment. *Lancet, 346,* 552–557.

Weiner, D. B. (1999). *Comprendre et soigner: Philippe Pinel (1745–1826): La médecine de l'esprit. Penser la médecine.* Paris: Fayard.

Weissman, M. M. (1993). The epidemiology of personality disorders—a 1990 update. *Journal of Personality Disorders, 7,* 44–62.

Weissman, M. M., Markowitz, J. C., & Klerman, G. L. (2000). *Comprehensive guide to interpersonal psychotherapy.* New York: Basic Books.

Werntz, D. A., Bickford, R. G., Bloom, F. E., & Shannahoff-Khalsa, D. S. (1983). Alternating cerebral hemispheric activity and the lateralization of autonomic nervous function. *Human Neurobiology, 2*(1), 39–43.

Werntz, D. A., Bickford, R. G., & Shannahoff-Khalsa, D. (1987). Selective hemispheric stimulation by unilateral forced nostril breathing. *Human Neurobiology, 6*(3), 165–171.

WHO. (1992). *Mental and behavioral disorders* (Chapter 5). Geneva: World Health Organization.

WHO. (2003). *F84. Pervasive developmental disorders.* Geneva: World Health Organization.

WHO. (2007). *International statistical classification of diseases and related health problems: 10th revision version for 2007.* Geneva: World Health Organization.

Wilberg, T., Hummelen, B., Pedersen, G., & Karterud, S. (2008). A study of patients with personality disorder not otherwise specified. *Comprehensive Psychiatry, 49,* 460–468.

Wilberg, T., Karterud, S., Urnes, O., Pedersen, G., & Friis, S. (1998). Outcomes of poorly functioning patients with personality disorders in a day treatment program. *Psychiatric Services, 49,* 1462–1467.

Woolf, S. H. (2008). The power of prevention and what it requires. *JAMA, 299,* 2437–2439.

Yeomans, F. E., Clarkin, J. F., & Levy, K. N. (2005). Psychodynamic psychotherapies. In J. M. Oldam, A. E. Skodol, & D. S. Bender (Eds.), *Textbook of personality disorders* (pp. 275–287). Washington, DC: American Psychiatric Publishing.

Young, J., & Klosko, J. (2005). Schema therapy. In J. M. Oldham, A. E. Skodol, & D. S. Bender (Eds.), *Textbook of personality disorders* (pp. 289–306). Washington, DC: American Psychiatric Publishing.

Young, J. E. (1999). *Cognitive therapy for personality disorder*. Sarasota, FL: Professional Resources Press.

Young, J. E., Klosko, J. S., & Weishaar, M. E. (2003). *Schema therapy: A practitioner's guide*. New York: Guilford.

Yrigollen, C. M., Han, S. S., Kochetkova, A., Babitz, T., Chang, J. T., Volkmar, F. R., et al. (2008). Genes controlling affiliative behavior as candidate genes for autism. *Biological Psychiatry, 63*, 911–916.

Index